# The Gut Microbiome

The influence of the gut microbiome on human health and disease has been established in recent years through advances in high-throughput DNA sequencing. *The Gut Microbiome: Bench to Table* presents a scientific introduction to this topic and analyzes the research on how the microbiome is affected by nutrients and how dietary modifications can alter the microbiome.

*The Gut Microbiome: Bench to Table* is divided into three sections. The first section details the current state of laboratory-scale analysis of gut microbiome samples and how we can identify the communities and their functional repertoire. Section II explains the next phase of translational research models such as preclinical animal studies, proof of concept safety, and efficacy human trials. The third section demonstrates the effectiveness of therapeutic treatments in larger populations. It addresses how diet influences the gut microbiome and presents an array of approaches that have been reported, including a discussion of issues of the safety of probiotics and selected supplements and micronutrients.

This book is essential for clinicians, dietitians, and food and nutrition professionals who wish to have the most up-to-date knowledge in understanding gut microbiome and diet.

# The Gut Microbiome
## Bench to Table

Edited by
## Vivian C.H. Wu

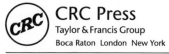

**CRC Press**
Taylor & Francis Group
Boca Raton London New York

CRC Press is an imprint of the
Taylor & Francis Group, an **informa** business

First edition published 2023
by CRC Press
6000 Broken Sound Parkway NW, Suite 300, Boca Raton, FL 33487-2742

and by CRC Press
4 Park Square, Milton Park, Abingdon, Oxon, OX14 4RN

*CRC Press is an imprint of Taylor & Francis Group, LLC*

© 2023 Taylor & Francis Group, LLC

*Library of Congress Cataloging-in-Publication Data*
Names: Wu, Vivian C. H., editor.
Title: The gut microbiome : bench to table / edited by Vivian C.H. Wu, Ph.D.
Description: First edition. | Boca Raton : CRC Press, 2023. |
Includes bibliographical references and index. |
Identifiers: LCCN 2022022597 (print) | LCCN 2022022598 (ebook) |
ISBN 9781032295442 (hardback) | ISBN 9781032295435 (paperback) |
ISBN 9781003302070 (ebook)
Subjects: LCSH: Gastrointestinal system–Microbiology. |
MESH: Gastrointestinal Microbiome | Gastrointestinal Tract–microbiology
Classification: LCC QR171.G29 G886 2023  (print) |
LCC QR171.G29 (ebook) | DDC 612.3/601579–dc23/eng/20220601
LC record available at https://lccn.loc.gov/2022022597
LC ebook record available at https://lccn.loc.gov/2022022598

ISBN: 9781032295442 (hbk)
ISBN: 9781032295435 (pbk)
ISBN: 9781003302070 (ebk)

DOI: 10.1201/b22970

Typeset in Times
by codeMantra

# Dedication

---

*This book is wholeheartedly dedicated to my parents and grandmother for their dear unsurpassed love and support.*

*To my husband and the greatest gift from God, my son for their love, patience, and understanding.*

*To my brother, sister-in-law, and nephews for their love and care.*

*To God for giving me strength and power of mind and for enabling me to live, learn, love, and inspire.*

# Contents

## SECTION I  T0 Benchwork, Including Techniques for Microbiome Studies

## SECTION II  T1 Preclinical Animal Studies, and Safety and Efficacy Trial in Humans

# SECTION III    T2–3 Effectiveness Trials in General Population and Regulatory Limitations

# Preface

The human fascination with diet and its impact on health is not new and quite ancient. The link between what goes into the body and what comes out is obvious and indisputable. The history of medicine in the West, the East, and the Americas focused on the amelioration of disease through the impact of foods, herbs, and elixirs on digestion. Stool testing was commonly used in medicine long before the understanding of microbes and their role in the digestive process. A common historical example was the madness of King George III. His intermittent bouts of mania were associated with abdominal pain, constipation, and discoloration of the urine. Twentieth-century scientists would later pore over meticulous documentation of stool samples and posthumously diagnose the king with porphyria. While dissecting stool samples for signs of melancholic dysphoria seems arcane, the medical profession at the time was ironically on the right track. Today medical science has reinforced the evidence suggesting that the gut microbiome is associated with conditions like major depression.

What has evolved from this fascination with the elimination product from digestion is the understanding of the individual components and key players in the digestive process. Today there are numerous tools to investigate the gut microbiome and the impact of diet. The influence of the gut microbiome on human health and disease has been established through numerous advances in high-throughput DNA sequencing. Genome-enabled biology provides an effective tool for investigating the members of a microbial community, their adaption to the environment, and downstream effects on their host. While we might seem quite advanced compared with the standard medical practices of the 18th century, we are still excavating just the tip of the iceberg. With every advance in genomics, metabolomics, proteomics, and other -omics, scientists are coming up with more questions than answers. This book will attempt to answer some of these questions and posit the question to be addressed in the future.

The subtitle *Bench to Table* depicts the journey of knowledge from small laboratory investigations to more extensive clinical trials. This book borrows from the National Institutes of Health guidelines for translational medicine. Translational research is the process of integrating laboratory, clinical, and population-based research with the long-term aim of improving public health. The translational approach uses a multidisciplinary team of experts to bring knowledge generated in small-scale laboratory experiments to a clinical setting in an attempt to bridge the gap between the bench and bedside. T0 research is conducted in laboratories with the aim of achieving tools and resources enabling microbiome studies. T1 research expedites the movement between laboratory research and clinical research by investigating the preclinical outcomes such as safety and efficacy. T2 research facilitates the movement of knowledge gained toward the general population with clinical trials investigating which factors contribute to better patient outcomes, implementation of best practices, and improved health status in communities. T3 research promotes the interaction between laboratory-based research and population-based research through larger-scale clinical trials to stimulate a robust scientific understanding of human health and disease. The book addresses the modulation of the gut microbiota through dietary modulation. Such knowledge in understanding gut microbiome and diet may offer innovative strategies for targeted product development.

# Acknowledgments

This book would not have been possible without the trust and effort of each of the chapter contributors. Special thanks go to Dr. Alison Lacombe for her countless hours assisting with the chapters. We began our world of the microbiome in Maine and accomplished the book of gut microbiome we promised in California.

I thank my publishers, CRC Press/Taylor & Francis Group, LLC, especially Randy Brehm and Tom Connelly, for their assistance in this book project. Thanks to Joseph Eckenrode for approaching me and encouraging me to develop this book. Thanks also to Susan Farmer for connecting the right place for this book.

Acknowledgment is also given to Wu's group from Maine to California and to all over the world. If I have ever made an impact on the science of microbiology, that is from the hard work of Wu's group.

My deep gratitude and heartfelt appreciation go to Dr. Daniel Y. C. Fung, my M.S. and Ph.D. advisor, for teaching and inspiring me with everything about food microbiology.

I am grateful, as always, to my beloved family.

# Editor

**Vivian C.H. Wu, Ph.D., Professor Research Leader Produce Safety and Microbiology Research Unit USDA-ARS Western Regional Research Center** Dr. Vivian C.H. Wu is the Research Leader of the Produce Safety and Microbiology Research Unit, one of the six Research Units at the U.S. Dept. of Agriculture (USDA)-Agriculture Research Service (ARS) Western Regional Research Center in Albany, California. Before joining USDA ARS, Dr. Wu served as a Full Professor at the University of Maine, where she led the Pathogenic Microbiology Laboratory. Dr. Wu and her team's cutting-edge science have immensely benefitted the food sector and have significantly impacted food supplies and public health. Dr. Wu received a multitude of awards, including the 2012 International Bimbo Pan-American Nutrition, Food Science and Technology Award for her achievement in the development of biosensors, the 2012 Distinguished Service Award from the Chinese American Food Society for her service contribution to society, and 2019 USDA Technology Transfer Innovation Fund Award for the commercialization of her biosensors. She received the Chinese American Food Society (CAFS) Professional Achievement Award in 2020. Dr. Wu received National Chung-Hsing University Distinguished Alumni Achievement Award in 2020 for her outstanding professional achievement. She received the 2022 Institute of Food Technologists (IFT) Achievement Award in Microbial Research for Food Safety in Honor of Gerhard J. Haas for her innovative research into the microbial aspects of food safety. Her research accomplishments have also been translated into successfully training undergraduate and graduate students and postdoctoral research scientists. Dr. Wu is the Editor-in-Chief of the *Journal of Food Safety.*

# Contributors

**Raphael D. Ayivi**
Department of Food and Nutritional
  Sciences
North Carolina A&T State University
University of North Carolina
Greensboro, North Carolina
Department of Nanoscience, Joint
  School of Nanoscience and
  Nanoengineering
University of North Carolina
Greensboro, North Carolina

**Reza V. Bakhshayesh**
Department of Food Biotechnology,
  Branch for Northwest &
  West Region, Agricultural
  Research, Education and
  Extension Organization (AREEO)
Agricultural Biotechnology Research
  Institute of Iran
Tabriz, Iran
Department of Food Science and
  Technology
University of Tabriz
Tabriz, Iran

**Claudia Caglioti**
Digestive Disease Center
Catholic University of Rome
Rome, Italy

**Yu-Chieh Cheng**
Agricultural Biotechnology Research
  Center
Academia Sinica
Taipei, Taiwan
Biotechnology Center in Southern
  Taiwan
Academia Sinica
Tainan, Taiwan

**Hafize Fidan**
Department of Nutrition and Tourism
University of Food Technology
Plovdiv, Bulgaria

**Rabin Gyawali**
Department of Food and Nutritional
  Sciences
North Carolina A&T State University
Greensboro, North Carolina

**Gianluca Ianiro**
Digestive Disease Center
Catholic University of Rome
Rome, Italy

**Salam A. Ibrahim**
Department of Food and Nutritional
  Sciences
North Carolina A&T State University
Greensboro, North Carolina

**Dorothy Klimis-Zacas**
School of Food and Agriculture
University of Maine
Orono, Maine

**Aleksandra S. Kristo**
Department of Food Science and Nutrition
California Polytechnic
  State University
San Luis Obispo, California

**Alison Lacombe**
Produce Safety and Microbiology
  Research Unit, Agricultural
  Research Service
United States Department of
  Agriculture
Albany, California

**Robert W. Li**
Agriculture Research Service, Animal
  Genomics and Improvement
  Laboratory
United States Department of Agriculture
Beltsville, Maryland

**Yen-te Liao**
Produce Safety and Microbiology
  Research Unit, Agricultural
  Research Service, Western Regional
  Research Center
United States Department of
  Agriculture
Albany, California

**Jianan Liu**
Agriculture Research Service, Animal
  Genomics and Improvement
  Laboratory
United States Department of Agriculture
Beltsville, Maryland

**Saeed Paidari**
Department of Food Science and
  Technology, Science and Research
  Branch
Islamic Azad University
Tehran, Iran

**Somanshu Sharma**
Produce Safety and Microbiology
  Research Unit, Agricultural
  Research Service, Western Regional
  Research Center
United States Department of
  Agriculture
Albany, California

**Angelos K. Sikalidis**
Department of Food Science and
  Nutrition
California Polytechnic State University
San Luis Obispo, California

**Logan Tom**
Produce Safety and Microbiology
  Research Unit, Agricultural
  Research Service, Western Regional
  Research Center
United States Department of
  Agriculture
Albany, California

**Marta Vernero**
Department of Medical Sciences
University of Pavia
Pavia, Italy

**Vivian C.H. Wu**
Produce Safety and Microbiology
  Research Unit, Agricultural
  Research Service, Western Regional
  Research Center
United States Department of
  Agriculture
Albany, California

**Yujie Zhang**
Produce Safety and Microbiology
  Research Unit, Agricultural
  Research Service, Western Regional
  Research Center
United States Department of
  Agriculture
Albany, California

# Introduction

Our planet is inhabited by millions of species that have coevolved to either share or compete for the same resources. The collective way multiple species interact is generically known as *symbiosis*. There are many forms of symbiotic relationships that are apparent to the naked eye, for example, the honeybee and flowering plants. With nature, what is seen at the macrocosmic level is often reflected in the microcosm. The result is an infinite "doll" of interconnected microorganisms forever adapting and evolving in an ever-changing environment. The gut microbiome is a perfect representation of the continuing dialogue that occurs with organisms in a constantly changing environment. Fed by the host's diet, the microorganisms that inhabit the gastrointestinal tract (GIT) compete for resources, and the resulting relationship is categorized as follows: mutualism, commensalism, predation, parasitism, and competition. The human large intestine is an intensively colonized area containing microorganisms that are health promoting as well as pathogenic. This has led to functional food developments that fortify the former at the expense of the latter.

Translational research is the process of integrating laboratory, clinical, and population-based research with the long-term aim of improving public health. The translational approach uses a multidisciplinary team of experts to bring knowledge generated in small-scale laboratory experiments to a clinical setting to bridge the gap between the bench and bedside and table. Basic research (T0) is conducted in laboratories with the aim of determining the efficacy of an intervention and its potential mechanism. In the next stage, T1 research expedites the movement between laboratory research and clinical research by investigating the preclinical outcomes such as safety and efficacy. T2 research facilitates the movement of knowledge gained toward the general population with clinical trials investigating which factors contribute to better patient outcomes, implementation of best practices, and improved health status in communities. Finally, T3 research promotes the interaction between laboratory-based research and population-based research through larger-scale clinical trials to stimulate a robust scientific understanding of human health and disease. To properly examine the interactions between human health and the gut microbiome, each step of the translational approach is needed. For example, a specific phytochemical may demonstrate promising anti-inflammatory properties *in vitro*, but have poor bioavailability when studied in animals or humans.

This book will discuss some of the challenges, such as complex relationships between human hosts, gut microbiome, and diet. The book will explore the population complexity and diversity between individuals when studying gut microbiota and how to improve the techniques available for microbiota research. To advance the knowledge in this area and understand how gut microbiota adapts to humans' changing lifestyle involves understanding the gut microbiomes' involvement in human development. In addition, we need detailed information about the specific aspects of host–microbe relationships and the mechanisms underlying them. There is a complex bidirectional symbiosis that exists between the gut microbiome and its host. The holistic composition of the human microbiome is governed by genetics, environment, and diet. In turn, the microbiome influences host metabolism, calorie absorption, immune reactions, and behavior. The gut microbiome modulates its host environment by releasing its own metabolites, modifying the metabolites of the host, and synthesizing vitamins and enzymes.

Consumers are aware of the potential healing properties of dietary regimens and foods and have fueled the demand for products that promote health. The desire for food that meets nutritional needs and can improve health has led food scientists to develop the concept of functional foods. Dietary supplements/nutrients offer new tools for improving host health by either preventing or ameliorating the symptoms of immune disorders, cancer, obesity, and other diseases. This book will discuss the microbes used as probiotics and the best industrial practices for optimal use. One future direction is optimizing the composition of infant formulas and other food products in maintaining gut health.

As the concept of gut health continues to evolve, researchers investigate the potential benefits of enhancing beneficial species through diet or other interventions. There are many possible sources of beneficial products for the gut, which can be found in the natural environment or synthesized based on research indicating certain functional groups with benefits. However, more work is needed to determine which prebiotic regimen is best for dietary recommendations, although recommendations cannot probably be applied ubiquitously across the population. This opens a fascinating field of inquiry into tailoring probiotic and prebiotic regimens for optimum health. Using a translation approach with different models, research can begin to elucidate the causal relationship between the diet, the host genetics, and the gut microbiome.

# Section I

TO Benchwork,
Including Techniques for
Microbiome Studies

# 1 Tools and Resources Enabling Marker Gene–Based Microbiome Studies

*Jianan Liu and Robert W. Li*
United States Department of Agriculture

## CONTENTS

DOI: 10.1201/b22970-2

## INTRODUCTION

The microbiome is referred to as "the entire habitat, including the microorganisms (bacteria, archaea, lower and higher eukaryotes, and viruses), their genomes (i.e., genes), and the surrounding environmental conditions" (Marchesi and Ravel, 2015). Trillions of microorganisms from archaea, bacteria, and eukarya and their viruses colonize the gastrointestinal tract of humans and animals from birth and play critical roles in their development and disease. It is still debatable whether the placenta is sterile. Most studies show that the detection of the placental microbiome is largely due to contamination (Kuperman et al., 2019; Theis et al., 2019). However, a recent study of a human fetus microbiome revealed the possibility of the exposure of the fetus to bacteria and their metabolites *in utero* (Stinson et al., 2019). Moreover, questions have been raised about the widely quoted notion that the total number of microbial cells outnumbers human cells by 10 to 1. The latest study suggests that the estimated number of bacteria in the human body is $3.8 \times 10^{13}$, approximately a 1:1 ratio with the number of human cells (Sender et al., 2016). Nevertheless, the microbiome plays vital functions in host physiology and nutrition, including modulating the host immunity, protecting the host against invading pathogens, and affecting the host organ development. It has long been known that microorganisms in the gastrointestinal tract act as a metabolic organ and are responsible for nutrient production and utilization. For ruminant species, the microorganisms in the rumen and hindgut convert carbohydrates (mainly plant fiber) into readily absorbable short-chain fatty acids, which provide up to 75% of their total metabolizable energy (Li et al., 2012). In monogastric species, such as humans and pigs, microbial fermentation in the hindgut allows the host to harvest extra energy from otherwise indigestible carbohydrates. Numerous gut bacteria, especially those from *Prevotella*, also participate in dietary protein degradation, including oligopeptide degradation and deamination. In addition, gut microorganisms produce vitamins for the host (LeBlanc et al., 2013). As a result, ruminants do not need a dietary supply of water-soluble vitamins, while a significant portion of our daily vitamin requirement, particularly water-soluble B vitamins and vitamin K, are synthesized by gut microbes. Gut microorganisms also affect host organ development. Evidence accumulated from studies of germ-free animals suggests the gut microbiome is essential for proper intestinal motility, morphology, function, and epithelial renewal (Sommer and Bäckhed, 2013). Most notably, the gut microbiome is instrumental in promoting the development of both innate and adapted immune systems (Duerkop et al., 2009; Sansonetti and Di Santo, 2007). Indeed, the strong induction of innate immunity followed by the stimulation of adaptive immune responses can be detected only four days after colonization of germ-free mice with the total fecal microbial community (El Aidy et al., 2012). Microbiome-derived metabolites, including short-chain fatty acids, directly regulate innate and adaptive immune cells (Rooks and Garrett, 2016). However, disruption of the homeostasis of the host microbiome can result in severe pathological consequences, such as chronic inflammation and metabolic dysfunction (Sommer and Bäckhed, 2013). The gut microbiome has been linked to the development of obesity and metabolic disorders, such as diabetes and insulin resistance (Ley, 2010). The intestinal microbiome affects the pathogenesis of inflammatory bowel diseases, such as Crohn's disease and ulcerative colitis (Baker et al., 2009; Joossens et al., 2011; Schwiertz et al., 2010). Inflammatory bowel disease patients tend to have an aberrant microbiome, characterized by the depletion of commensal bacteria, notably members of the phyla Firmicutes and Bacteroidetes. Furthermore, the altered microbiome has been suggested to affect the carcinogenesis of several tumors, including colorectal gastric tumors and cancerous liver tumors (Fox et al., 2010). Evidence also suggests the gut microbiome affects viral infection (Wilks and Golovkina, 2012) and plays a role in HIV progression (Ellis et al., 2011). As a result, the gut microbiome has been touted as a therapeutic target or as a drug target (Cani and Delzenne, 2011).

While the structure and functions of the gut microbiome have been extensively explored in the past few years, the complex interrelationships of the microbiome within a host still require higher-resolution studies using comprehensive toolsets to promote new discoveries (Heintz-Buschart and Wilmes, 2018). Because of the complexity and functional importance of the microbiome, numerous methods and bioinformatic tools have been developed in recent years to conduct comprehensive microbiome studies using culture-independent approaches. For example, enzymes that catalyze chemical reactions are encoded by genes present in microbial communities from a broad spectrum of environmental conditions. Therefore, functional screening has become an increasingly important tool to discover novel biomolecules for applications in biotechnology and medicine. This approach, also termed functional metagenomics, provides direct access to largely unexploited microbial genetic diversity in the environment. In the meantime, the rapid advancement of ultra-low cost and high-throughput or parallel sequencing technologies and the development of bioinformatics tools and various databases have stimulated sequencing-based microbiome studies, including whole genome shotgun–based computational metagenomics and marker gene–based microbiome studies. The former allows us to have a holistic assessment of the functional capacity and metabolic potential of the microbial community in its habitat.

Marker gene–based microbiome profiling is a rapid alternative to whole genome shotgun–based approaches in quantifying the structure and composition of microbial communities. Due to their functional constancy and highly conserved nature, small subunits (SSUs) of the rRNA gene, especially the 16S rRNA gene, have been used the most as phylogenetic markers for genus and species identification and taxonomic classification of bacteria and archaea. The 16S rRNA gene is large enough (~1,500 nucleotides) compared to 5S rRNA genes to carry adequate information for comparisons and is small enough compared to 23S rRNA genes (~2,900 nucleotides) to be conveniently analyzed. As a homologue of prokaryotic 16S rRNA genes, the eukaryotic 18S rRNA gene is also widely used as a phylogenetic marker for fungi and other eukaryotes. The presence of hypervariable (HV) regions in these genes reflects the evolutionary divergence of microorganisms and can be explored to differentiate even highly related species (Woese, 1987). The internal transcribed spacer (ITS), located between the 18S and 5.8S rRNA genes, is used as a marker specifically to identify a broad range of fungi. The ITS is more variable than the 18S rRNA genes and is therefore more appropriate as the genetic marker to study intraspecific genetic diversity (Schoch et al., 2012). Furthermore, many protein-coding single-copy genes, such as the RNA polymerase β subunit gene (rpoB), have also been explored as molecular markers for microbial ecology studies (Case et al., 2007).

Many molecular methods have been developed in the past to characterize SSUs of rRNA genes, such as polymerase chain reaction (PCR)–based cloning and traditional sequencing and culture-independent molecular approaches, including denaturing gradient gel electrophoresis/temperature gradient gel electrophoresis, PCR-restriction fragment length polymorphism (RFLP), and terminal restriction fragment length polymorphism (TRFLP). Additionally, 16S probe-based fluorescent *in situ* hybridization (FISH) is a powerful tool for the visualization and identification of microorganisms in their native habitats (Crocetti et al., 2000; Ginige et al., 2004). The recent renaissance of the microbial marker gene–based study to characterize the gut microbiome is largely driven by rapid advances in next-generation DNA sequencing technologies (Gloor et al., 2010; Tringe and Hugenholtz, 2008) and the development of related data analysis pipelines and databases (Balvočiūtė and Huson, 2017; Caporaso et al., 2010). Moreover, several new concepts and computational tools are in rapid development. In this chapter, we will focus on recent advances in marker gene–based approaches and bioinformatics tools essential for microbiome studies.

## HISTORICAL PERSPECTIVE OF MICROBIOME STUDIES

Traditional culturing methods, accompanied with morphological and biochemical studies of cultured strains, were developed gradually for the characterization of single microorganisms in the late 19th century (Schaechter, 2015). However, by the 1980s, it was recognized that the population of prokaryotes in the environment is vast and incredibly diverse (Whitman et al., 1998). Because of the complexity of microbial communities, only a limited portion of the bacteria in the environment can be successfully isolated and cultured. The discovery of viable but nonculturable microorganisms (Oliver, 2005) motivated scientists to develop alternative methods to study them in their habitat. SSU rRNA genes gradually attracted attention. These genes were later found to be an appropriate phylogenetic marker of microorganisms because of their highly conservative sequences and functional specificity (Woese, 1987; Woese and Fox, 1977; Woese et al., 1990).

Since the invention of Sanger sequencing and PCR techniques, scientists have developed culture-independent methods for sequencing cloned 16S rRNA genes from microbial populations (Pace et al., 1986). The clone library of 16S and/or 18S rRNA genes was sequenced, followed by phylogenetic analysis. This conventional clone-and-sequencing method targeting SSU rDNA was developed to study complex microorganism populations without prior microbial cultivation. The process involves the cloning of targeted genes by creating a population of host bacteria, such as *E. coli*, that carries plasmids containing the inserted DNA. With the development of available databases, taxonomy identification can be achieved for the obtained sequences, with similarity thresholds from 80% at the phylum level to 97% at the species level

(DeSantis et al., 2007). The advantage of this conventional cloning method is that the clean sequence of the entire 16S rRNA gene can be obtained and then sequenced, which provides a reliable and precise picture of prokaryotes in a microbial community. However, the heavy workload makes the method extremely time-consuming, laborious, and expensive (Green and Sambrook, 2012).

A variety of molecular methods were then developed to overcome the issues associated with conventional cloning. Most of these methods utilize DNA hybridization and DNA length and sequence polymorphisms to study microbial communities. In 1993, a method called denaturing gradient gel electrophoresis was applied to analyze the genetic diversity of complex prokaryotic communities (Muyzer et al., 1993). Shortly after, a similar method called temperature gradient gel electrophoresis was developed. Denaturing gradient gel electrophoresis examines microbial genetic patterns via a chemical gradient to denature the PCR-amplified 16S molecules as they move across an acrylamide gel, while temperature gradient gel electrophoresis is based on melting point differences in DNA molecules with a linear temperature gradient in the gel (Muyzer et al., 1993; Muyzer and Smalla, 1998). These two methods are more rapid and reproducible than the conventional cloning method.

Two other efficient methods, PCR-RFLP and TRFLP, are based on RFLP. These methods can be applied to 16S rRNA, ITS-5.8S rRNA-ITS2, or 23S rRNA genes to characterize microbial diversity (Guillamón et al., 1998; Leaw et al., 2006). For PCR-RFLP, PCR products amplified from SSU rRNA genes are digested with restriction enzymes to generate DNA fragments that are then separated by gel electrophoresis based on their size. In TRFLP, PCR products are generated with 5″-fluorescent-labeled primers before endonuclease digestion to generate the terminal restriction fragments (Marsh, 1999). The mixture of DNA fragments can then be analyzed in an automated DNA sequencer, but only the terminal fragments with labels can be detected and displayed. Several bioinformatics methods have been developed for peak identification and taxonomic assignment for TRFLP results, such as T-REX (**T-R** FLP analysis **EX** pedited) (Culman et al., 2009), web-based TRFMA (Nakano et al., 2006), and Excel-based tools (Fredriksson et al., 2014). TRFLP simplifies complex banding pattern analysis compared to PCR-RFLP and allows for the more rapid identification of microbial composition in a community.

Although RFLP-based methods are able to provide fingerprint patterns to detect community structure, problems exist, including the introduction of PCR bias and variation caused by the choice of restriction enzymes (Osborn et al., 2000; v. Wintzingerode et al., 1997). Phylogenetic oligonucleotide arrays, an amplification-independent method, were developed to overcome these pitfalls. PhyloChip, developed at Lawrence Berkeley National Laboratory, is the most comprehensive and high-density phylogenetic oligonucleotide array to detect the presence of bacteria and archaea from direct microbial DNA or PCR products with a broad dynamic range. The platform developed its own proprietary bioinformatics pipelines to identify variations in 16S rRNA gene sequences. The latest version of PhyloChip (PhyloChip G4), currently available from Second Genome, Inc., can identify and measure the relative abundance of more than 50,000 individual microbial taxa. PhyloChip has been used to characterize microbial communities in a variety of samples and environments. In one case, spatial patterns of microbial species in a rough environment, salt crusts of the hyper-arid Atacama Desert, were examined using PhyloChip G3. The results from this study identified two dominant species, Halobacteriales and Bacteroidetes, and the existence of a few algal and cyanobacterial species in low abundance levels (Finstad et al., 2017) in this extreme habitat.

FISH is another powerful method that evolved from non-FISH in 1980 (Bauman et al., 1980). FISH targeting microbial SSU rRNA genes can be used to determine the spatial distribution and genome structure of microbes. Typically, probes targeting the 16S rRNA gene are generally 18–30 nucleotides in length with fluorescence labels. These probes can penetrate through the cell membrane and eventually hybridize to the target 16S rRNA genes *in situ* (Hugenholtz et al., 2002). Hybridized target genes within the individual cells can then be visualized using a fluorescence or confocal microcopy, which allow exploring the spatial location of the targeted genes in addition to taxonomic identifications. With recent technical innovations, FISH has been combined with several other cutting-edge biological tools to visualize and elucidate genome structures of microorganisms. A powerful example is the integration of FISH with Hi-C to reveal the 3D structure of chromosomes (Abbas et al., 2019). This method was also used to define the chromosome structure of *Mycoplasma pneumoniae*. By using Hi-C with a 10kb resolution to generate 3D models of the stationary *M. pneumoniae* chromosome and then applying FISH to visualize and measure distances between genomic regions, Trussart et al. (2017) concluded that transcriptional regulation can be affected by chromosome organization.

## HIGH-THROUGHPUT SEQUENCING TECHNOLOGIES

In the past decade, rapid technological advances in next-generation sequencing (NGS) and the concomitant development of bioinformatics tools and database resources have revolutionized microbiome studies. Unlike traditional Sanger sequencing, NGS platforms can generate (hundreds of) millions of sequences during a single run. The development history of the traditional and NGS technologies, the basic features and performance comparisons and the application potential between various sequencing platforms have been extensively reviewed (Ambardar et al., 2016; Besser et al., 2018; Gužvić, 2013. Lam et al., 2012). In this chapter, we limit our discussion to the technologies more relevant to SSU marker gene–based studies.

### 454 PYROSEQUENCING AND SUPPORTED
### OLIGONUCLEOTIDE LIGATION AND DETECTION

The introduction of large-scale parallel pyrosequencing technology by 454 Life Sciences in 2005 initiated the NGS revolution. Roche then acquired this technology and released the 454 GS FLX Titanium system in 2008 with improved average read length (up to 700 bp) and accuracy (up to 99.997%). The GS FLX system can sequence ~400–600 Mb of DNA per 10-hour run (Voelkerding et al., 2009). The long read length facilitates *de novo* sequencing and microbiome studies. However, the labor-intensive nature of the sample preparation, the high reagent cost, and the high error rates in homopolymer regions are some of the obstacles that are difficult to overcome. Because Roche later decided to stop supplying the hardware and reagents, this platform is now defunct.

Supported Oligonucleotide Ligation and Detection was originally invented by Applied Biosystems Instruments and later acquired by Life Technologies (Thermo Fisher Scientific). The platform relies on a ligation-based sequencing technology that uses DNA ligase and fluorescently labeled oligonucleotide probes for sequencing in either the 3′ to 5′ direction or the 5′ to 3′ direction. While the current 5,500 W Series Genetic Analysis Systems offer a highly accurate and flexible sequencing solution with adequate output, the short read length they generate (up to 75 bp) and the long running time (days) make Supported Oligonucleotide Ligation and Detection suboptimal for SSU amplicon sequencing.

## ILLUMINA PLATFORM

The Illumina platform relies on the "sequencing by synthesis" technology invented by Solexa (Bentley et al., 2008). In contrast to various costly enzymes used by pyrosequencing in the 454 platform, sequencing by synthesis uses only DNA polymerase. Specifically, in the flow cell, DNA templates are amplified using isothermal bridging amplification, which relies on arching over and hybridizing to an adjacent oligonucleotide anchor by DNA strands. Numerous amplification cycles make the single-molecule DNA template into a clonally amplified arching cluster of approximately 1,000 clonal molecules. As each Deoxynucleotide triphosphates (dNTP) is inserted, a fluorescently marked reversible terminator is recorded and then cleaved to allow the next base to be integrated. The ultimate result is a base-by-base sequencing that allows a wide range of applications with accurate sequencing data (Bentley et al., 2008).

Illumina has since acquired this technology from Solexa and marketed several systems that differ in terms of sequencing capacities. HiSeq ($2 \times 150$ bp) and MiSeq ($2 \times 250 \sim 300$ bp) series have long been the dominant high-throughput sequencers. In recent years, Illumina has launched several new systems, such as NovaSeq 6000. The HiSeq X system is the world's first to break the $1,000 genome barrier for human whole genome sequencing. The system contains a set of 10 HiSeq X ultra-high-throughput instruments. Illumina will discontinue its support for HiSeq 2500 and X series after 2023 and 2024, respectively. NovaSeq 6000 is a relatively new comprehensive Illumina system that enables cost-effective sequencing. Notably, it is a scalable platform that allows the loading of individual flow cell lanes with different library types to suit a wide range of project sizes or needs with the NovaSeq Xp workflow. It also comes with single and dual flow cell modes with different flow cell types to generate several combinations of read length and coverage depth, with read lengths up to $2 \times 250$ bp (paired-end).

Illumina MiSeq is another powerful sequencer that enables the generation of approximately 25 million sequencing reads with up to $2 \times 300$ bp read lengths. In November 2013, the US Food and Drug Administration approved the marketing of the NGS system, Illumina's MiSeqDx, as a diagnostic device for human genome sequencing. The marketing approval of the first high-throughput genome sequencer represents a significant step forward in producing genomic data to aid diagnosis and eventually improve patient care. MiSeq is suitable for amplicon-based microbiome studies because of its longer read length. Merging its paired-end reads can result in up to 550 bp assembled reads while allowing for an overlap of 50 bp. As a result, it is advisable to use paired-end MiSeq sequencing to cover more than one HV region on SSU marker genes. The selection of target HV regions and primers is a critical factor for consideration for SSU marker gene sequencing using MiSeq. Various HV regions have discriminatory differences in terms of the groups of microbes (D'Amore et al., 2016). It is known that V1 works best in differentiating across *Staphylococcus aureus* and coagulase-negative *Staphylococcus* species, whereas V2 and V3 perform better in distinguishing bacterial species up to the genus level, except for the closely related species in *Enterobacteriaceae*. V6 differentiates across all select agents defined by the Centers for Disease Control and Prevention (Chakravorty et al., 2007). More recent studies demonstrate that V4 is generally more informative than other regions, and combining HV regions is highly recommended (D'Amore et al., 2016; Soergel et al., 2012). For example, the selection of 341F/785R (or 805R) across V3 to V4 regions is recommended over using V4 only, as longer amplicon length is reported to improve species-level assignment and provide higher phylogenetic diversity (Klindworth et al., 2012; Thijs et al., 2017). Besides universal primers, archaea- and bacteria-specific primers should also be selected depending on the objectives of a specific project. A study of the human archaeome found that the archaea-specific primer pair 349af/519ar outperforms universal primers in identifying archaeal operational taxonomic unit (OTU) and Amplicon Sequence Variant (ASV) (Koskinen et al., 2017).

One recent trend is full-length sequencing of the 16S rRNA gene using existing platforms with improved combinational chemistry and novel bioinformatic tools. For example, the recently developed LoopSeq technique is able to sequence DNA or mRNA molecules with synthetic long reads based on Illumina sequencers (Wu et al., 2019). Its core technology lies in a set of unique barcodes that attach to each individual DNA molecule. Every molecule is amplified with its unique barcode, and the copies get sequenced next to each randomly distributed barcode. Short reads with the same barcodes are assembled with linked-read *de novo* assembly. Full length in combination with high sequence accuracy from proved sequencing platforms makes species-level taxonomic specificity possible (Wu et al., 2019).

## ION TORRENT

While the Ion Torrent platform uses sequencing by synthesis and emulsion PCR somewhat similarly to Illumina chemistry and 454 pyrosequencing, respectively, its method of detection is unique. If a nucleotide is incorporated into a strand of DNA, an $H^+$ ion is released. The charge from $H^+$ ions alters the solution pH value, which can be detected by a proprietary ion sensor. An Ion Torrent sequencer is essentially a solid-state pH meter. Because the detection is direct and rapid without the need for scanners, cameras, or light (and without the need for fluorescence and chemiluminescence reagents), the cost of sequencers is low, and running time is short (<7 hours). While high error rates in sequencing homopolymer stretches and repeats (similar to the 454 platform) are undesirable, Ion Torrent generates a mean read length up to 400 bp, which is quite appealing for SSU amplicon sequencing.

Salipante et al. (2014) compared the performance of two common benchtop NGS sequencers, Illumina MiSeq and Ion Torrent Personal Genome Machine (PGM), for bacterial community profiling by 16S rRNA (V1–V2) amplicon sequencing using a mock microbial community consisting of 20 known species and human samples. Two issues with Ion Torrent PGM, comparatively higher error rates and premature sequence truncation, are documented in this study. The latter results in organism-specific biases in community profiles. While results are generally in good agreement between the two platforms with protocol optimization in Ion Torrent, organism-dependent differences in sequence error rates and premature sequence truncation pose a challenge for certain microorganisms when using Ion Torrent technology.

## Long Read Sequencing Platforms

Given limited read lengths, only one or two adjacent HV regions of the 16S rRNA gene can be sequenced using the second-generation sequencing technologies. Short reads may not be effective for species- or subspecies-level identification. New platforms with long read sequencing, also termed the third-generation sequencing technologies—such as those developed by Pacific Biosciences (PacBio) and Oxford Nanopore—have increasingly gained popularity.

PacBio Sequel Systems use a single-molecule, real-time sequencing technology to provide highly accurate long reads. Single-molecule, real-time cells contain millions of zero-mode waveguides (ZMWs). A single DNA molecule is immobilized in each ZMW and is repeat sequenced with real-time detection of base incorporation. Each of the four nucleotides A, C, G, and T are labeled with different fluorescent dyes on their terminal phosphates. Light is emitted during DNA synthesis through the template in the ZMW and recorded as nucleotide sequences. The sequencing reads can reach up to tens of Kb. However, one key issue with the technology in the past is a high sequencing error rate, sometimes up to 11%–15%. PacBio tries to reduce the error rate by utilizing a consensus accuracy function to reduce systematic errors. Specifically, both DNA strands in one ZMW can be sequenced multiple times to generate multiple reads (subreads); a consensus sequence of these subreads can yield higher accuracy (Rhoads and Au, 2015). The newest release is the Sequel II System, which produces exceptional results with faster running time, affordable expense, and highly accurate long reads. PacBio has recently been successfully used in SSU sequencing projects to cover the full length of 16S rRNA genes (Callahan et al., 2019; Earl et al., 2018).

Oxford Nanopore is another promising DNA sequencing technology designed to have essentially no reagent costs, little sample preparation, and ultra-long read length to reduce the need for complicated assembly algorithms and reveal the long-range structure of the genome at the same time (Branton et al., 2010). The principle of Nanopore is that when a strand of DNA passes through a nanopore, the current is changed as the bases T, C, G, and A pass through in different combinations. Several sequencers, such as MinION, GridION, and PromethION, that differ in device size, nanopore channels, and sample prep procedures are currently available. Nanopore technology has also been successfully applied to sequence full-length 16S rRNA genes. One study analyzed the mouse gut microbiome by full-length 16S rRNA amplicon sequencing using Nanopore and compared the results with short-read sequencing data (Shin et al., 2016). The study found no significant differences in major taxonomic assignment between the two methods. However, the difference becomes apparent at species-level identification. Empowered with long reads, Nanopore is able to identify more species than short-read platforms, which improves the classification accuracy of community bacterial composition (Shin et al., 2016). It is conceivable that this technology will play a critical role in field microbial ecology and microbiome studies with anticipated significant reduction of the sequencing error rate in the near future.

## SSU REFERENCE DATABASES

The accuracy and robustness of taxonomic classification and phylogenetic affiliation of sequence reads obtained in amplicon-based sequencing are dependent on the coverage and quality of SSU reference databases. Resulting from many years of community effort, these databases are vital resources in microbiome studies.

### GREENGENES

Greengenes is a database for full-length 16S rRNA genes of bacteria and archaea that aims to provide a curated taxonomy for users based on *de novo* tree inference (DeSantis et al., 2006; McDonald et al., 2012). The latest Greengenes version is gg_13_8, released in August 2013, and is a minor improvement over the previous version (the gg_13_5 released in May 2013). The improvement addressed the missing genus and species names. If a genus or species name is missing for a particular OTU, the National Center for Biotechnology Information (NCBI) taxonomy of cluster members was checked, and the most supported names were then selected to update the taxonomy of representative sequences. The taxonomic name was then transferred to all the lower similarity representative sequences. The number of sequences in Greengenes and other databases is listed in Table 1.1.

Although Greengenes has not been updated since 2013, this curated, chimera-checked database is still robust and is one of the most used databases in 16S gene sequencing analysis. Several analysis tools, such as the Quantitative Insights into Microbial Ecology (QIIME) analysis pipeline and the metagenome function prediction

---

**TABLE 1.1**

**Commonly Used Databases on Marker Gene–Based Microbiome Studies and Their Number of Sequences**

| Database | Latest Version | Release Date | Number of Sequences |
|---|---|---|---|
| Greengenes | gg_13_8 | Aug 2013 | 1262,986 (16S rRNA sequence) |
| SILVA | SILVA 132 | Dec 2017 | 2,090,668 (SSU Ref), 695,171 (SSU Ref NR) |
| RDP | Release 11.5 | Sep 2016 | 3,356,809 (16S rRNA sequences), 125,525 (28S rRNA sequences) |
| EzBioCloud | Version 20191112 | Nov 2019 | 65,050 (16S rRNA sequences), bacterial genomes |
| UNITE | Version 8.1 | Sep 2019 | 98,183 (fungal SH with DOIs at 1.5% threshold) |
| PR$^2$ | Version 4.12.0 | Aug 2019 | 183,949 (eukaryotic SSU) |

software package Phylogenetic Investigation of Communities by Reconstruction of Unobserved States (PICRUSt) (Langille et al., 2013), have chosen Greengenes as their default database or have been developed based on Greengenes.

## SILVA

SILVA (from Latin *silva*, forest) is a comprehensive rRNA gene web resource dedicated to providing the taxonomy information for bacteria, archaea, and eukarya (Pruesse et al., 2007; Quast et al., 2012). It contains the ribosomal RNA sequence datasets of aligned small (16S/18S, SSU) and large subunit (23S/28S, LSU) rRNA sequences, which are quality checked and regularly updated. The latest full release is the SILVA SSU/LSU version 132, released in December 2017. The preliminary release information of SILVA 138 is available on its website, and the version is expected to launch around the end of 2019. SILVA is highly recommended by the widely used analysis platform mothur as its default reference database. The SILVA database contains different sections of rRNA genes. "SSU Parc" includes all aligned sequences with an alignment identity value $\geq 50$, alignment quality value $\geq 40$, and base-pair score or sequence quality $\geq 30$. "SSU Ref" was created by excluding sequences shorter than 1,200 bases (for bacteria and eukarya) and below 900 bases (for archaea) or an alignment identity lower than 70 or an alignment quality value lower than 50 from the SSU Parc dataset. Additionally, SILVA offers a nonredundant (NR) version of the SSU Ref dataset, "SSU Ref NR," where highly identical sequences are removed by applying UCLUST with a 99% identity criterion, yet sequences from cultivated species have been kept in all cases. By adding all sequences to the SSU Ref tree of SILVA release 128, a guide tree was calculated. Similarly, for LSU rRNA databases, SILVA also contains "LSU Parc" and "LSU Ref" datasets based on different criteria of LSU gene sequences. "LSU Ref" also contains a calculated guide tree.

In addition, SILVA provides several online data processing and analysis functions, including probe and primer evaluation with "TestProbe" and "TestPrime," sequence alignment and classification, and an online data analysis service, SILVAngs, for rRNA NGS amplicon reads. SILVAngs uses the taxonomies and alignments of the SILVA rRNA gene database, supports reads classification, and offers many user-friendly output files in table, chart, and sequence formats.

### Ribosomal Database Project

The ribosome database project (RDP) offers quality-controlled bacterial and archaeal SSU rRNA sequence alignments and annotation, as well as data analysis tools. Besides the SSU rRNA genes of bacteria and archaea, the RDP also adds a collection of fungal LSU 28S rRNA sequences (Cole et al., 2009; Cole et al., 2013). The latest release is RDP 11.5, which was released in September 2016. The RDP implements improved alignments and also provides collections of tools for rRNA analysis. Newly obtained sequences are aligned and classified with the RDP Aligner and Classifier with its own phylogenetic assessment. Specifically, the RDP utilizes the infernal secondary structure-aware aligner to improve its alignment quality, speed, and consistency. The RDP Classifier is a powerful and widely used method in taxonomy classification for SSU rRNA data analysis. The RDP Classifier and RDP Hierarchy Browser Bacteria and Archaea hierarchy model has been updated to training set no. 16, to which over 300 new genera and 2000 new sequences have been added. Notably, the RDP provides its resource files for the NCBI LinkOut service, which enables users to switch from the sequence records in the Nucleotide and BioProject databases of the NCBI directly to the corresponding RDP sequence records. The RDP also provides an online RDPipeline for high-throughput amplicon analysis and offers multiple tools, such as primer-probe examination, approximate phylogenetic building of user-submitted sequences, chimera removal, and automated alignment (Cole et al., 2013).

## EzBioCloud

EzBioCloud is a curated and taxonomically united database of 16S rRNA gene sequences and whole genome assemblies for bacteria and archaea (Yoon et al., 2017). It filters the low-quality whole genome assemblies from the NCBI Assembly Database and contains a bioinformatics composite identification pipeline using gene-based searches followed by average nucleotide identity calculations to construct a database with 61,700 species/phylotypes. These include 13,132 validly published names and 62,362 whole genome assemblies. Using a combination of a gene-based search and Orthologous Average Nucleotide Identity (OrthoANI) (Lee et al., 2016) calculations, all genomes are taxonomically defined at the genus, species, or subspecies level. The hierarchy is based on the 16S maximum likelihood phylogenetic tree, taking into account the currently accepted classification. The website also provides a complete set of EzBioCloud 16S databases in formats compatible with QIIME or mothur pipelines. One of the unique features of EzBioCloud is that it enables identifying a bacterial isolate using either 16S rRNA or genome data. EzBioCloud also offers a cloud service called Microbiome Taxonomic Profiling with several bioinformatics tools. Users are able to compare their own data with the published microbiome data in this Microbiome Taxonomic Profiling service and perform comprehensive species-level profiling using closed-reference OTU picking.

## UNITE

The ITS region is the most widely used fungal marker to identify fungi and explore fungal diversity in the environment. The UNITE is a web-based database and sequence management environment dedicated to the molecular identification of fungi using ITS regions as markers (Nilsson et al., 2018). UNITE is arguably the most commonly used database for classifying and annotating fungi with ITS high-throughput sequencing. It includes ~1000,000 public fungal ITS sequences that are clustered into ~459,000 species hypotheses for reference and assigned DOIs to reduce ambiguity among studies. UNITE redesigned how it handles unclassifiable species hypotheses, integrated the Global Biodiversity Information Facility's taxonomic backbone, and supports parallel taxonomic classification systems (Nilsson et al., 2018). Users can also compare sequences to species hypotheses through Basic Local Alignment Search Tool (BLAST), probabilistic method for taxonomical classification (PROTAX) (Abarenkov et al., 2018) and other query tools through UNITE. In addition to taxonomic annotation, UNITE also adds relevant metadata, such as the host of collection and voucher specimens. Importantly, UNITE supports web-based third-party annotations to update taxonomy and nomenclature information and to correct suboptimal taxonomic annotation and other metadata across public DNA sequences (Nilsson et al., 2018). With these efforts, UNITE identifies fungi from ITS sequence data with assembling and disseminating taxonomic, ecological, and geographical metadata. UNITE acts as a data provider for a number of metabarcoding software tools and exchanges data with all major fungal sequence databases and other community resources on a regular basis.

## PR²

The Protist Ribosomal Reference (PR²) database offers exclusive access to the ribosomal RNA and DNA sequences of eukaryotic SSU 18S with curated taxonomy (Guillou et al., 2013). The majority of sequences in this database are nuclear-encoded protistan sequences. Yet PR² also contains sequences from metazoans, land plants, macrosporic fungi, and eukaryotic organelles (mitochondrion, plastid, and others), which is useful for high-throughput sequencing data analysis. PR² also carefully checks introns and putative chimeric sequences. Additionally, there are web tools one can use to search the database by sequence similarity (Guillou et al., 2013).

## MARKER GENE SEQUENCE ANALYSIS PIPELINES

## QIIME 1 AND QIIME 2

To facilitate marker gene–based microbiome studies, several data analysis pipelines have been developed (Figure 1.1). QIIME (Caporaso et al., 2010) is a widely used pipeline for analyzing SSU rRNA amplicon sequencing data of microbial community studies, including 16S, 18S, and ITS sequence data. QIIME incorporates many third-party tools and algorithms that make it a robust pipeline to achieve a wide range of analyses and visualizations. It can handle SSU data generated from various sequencing platforms.

The QIIME pipeline starts with preprocessing raw sequences with a mapping file (sample metadata) and performs primer removal, demultiplexing, and quality filtering. For paired-end data, two methods, fastq-join (default) and SeqPrep, are available to merge forward and reverse reads. Barcode and primer sequences from the mapping file are used to demultiplex and clean raw sequences. Low-quality sequence reads can be removed based on Phred-score and user-defined parameters. After preprocessing, three types of OTU-picking strategies, *de novo*, closed-reference, and open-reference, are available. QIIME provides multiple OTU clustering tools, such as cd-hit, mothur, BLAST, Trie, uclust, usearch, sumaclust, sortmerna, and swarm. The default OTU-picking tool is uclust with a similarity threshold of 97% and several flexible parameter options. The QIIME team recommends open-reference OTU picking because it offers a trade-off between running time and the possibility of new diversity discovery. During OTU clustering, a representative sequence is selected for

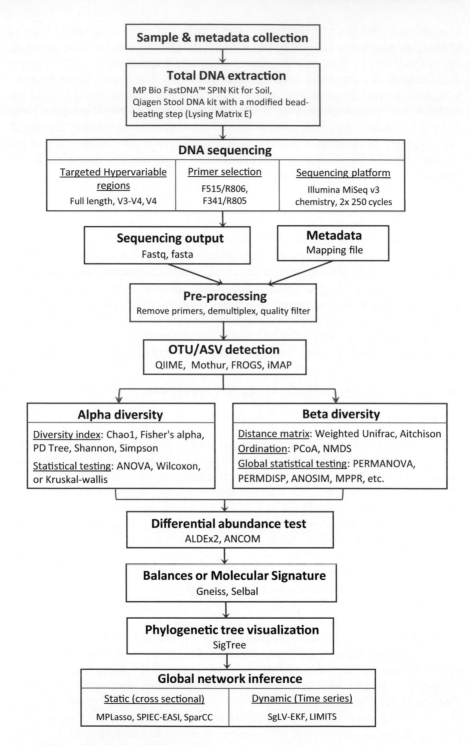

**FIGURE 1.1**    Recommended data analysis pipeline for marker gene-based microbiome studies.

each OTU to represent the whole cluster. The default is to pick the most abundant sequence from a cluster as its representative, as these sequences are less likely to represent sequencing errors. When uclust or usearch is selected, the cluster seed is used as the representative sequence. The QIIME team also recommends the addition of chimera checking after OTU picking by UCHIME to exclude chimera in downstream analyses. The subsequent step in the pipeline includes assigning taxonomy to representative sequences. The latest Greengenes database is used as the default. The sequence alignment and phylogeny construction can then be performed with Python Nearest Alignment Space Termination (PyNAST) and FastTree by default, respectively. An OTU table is finally generated in the Biological Observation Matrix (BIOM) format. For downstream analyses, OTU tables and phylogenetic trees generated from upstream analysis and corresponding mapping files are used. A second-level quality filtering can be done to reduce the problem of spurious OTUs, followed by a rarefaction step at a user-defined subsampling depth. After that, the OTU table is collapsed into taxa to be summarized at each taxonomic level. A series of plots including bar, pie, and area graphs can be generated and then visualized via a web interface. QIIME pipeline integrates two diversity analyses, alpha and beta diversity. Three alpha diversity metrics, phylogenetic diversity (PD)_whole_tree, Chao1, and observed_OTU, are the default outputs. Dozens of other metrics are optional in *alpha_diversity.py* script, for example, Simpson and Shannon indices. QIIME recommends Unifrac (Lozupone and Knight, 2005) for beta diversity analysis and generates weighted and unweighted Unifrac to analyze community differences. Additionally, interactive diversity graphs, such as rarefaction curves based on alpha diversity metrics and principal coordinate analysis (PCoA) based on community beta diversity distance can be accessed through the output HTML documents. Further statistical analysis of taxa and diversities can be performed within QIIME or with external methods. In addition to common t-tests, QIIME also offers multivariate analyses in the script *compare_categories.py*, including analysis of similarities (ANOSIM) and Adonis, to examine beta diversity. OTU network analysis is also integrated in QIIME.

Since 2017, the QIIME team has reengineered and developed a new system, QIIME 2 (Bolyen et al., 2019). As a result, the conventional QIIME or QIIME 1 is no longer officially supported. QIIME 2 also integrates third-party tools in the form of plugins to allow others to contribute to its function. QIIME 2 provides better support for paired-sample and time series analyses. Although several features in QIIME 1 are retained, QIIME 2 offers several key improvements over QIIME 1. One critical aspect of QIIME 2 is using ASV instead of OTU as microbial features. The recommended demultiplexing and denoising workflow in QIIME 2 for AVS identification is the DADA2 algorithm. Deblur is also used as an optional denoising method to combine q2-Vsearch to join reads before proceeding. Specifically, these denoising methods exclude noisy sequences, correct marginal sequence errors (in DADA2), perform chimera removal and singleton removal, join denounced paired-end reads (in DADA2), and perform sequence dereplication. Both DADA2 and Deblur contain internal chimera removal methods and abundance filtering during the denoising process. However, QIIME 2 still keeps three OTU-picking options, similar to QIIME 1. UCHIME and Vectorized search (Vsearch) are used to remove chimera sequences and perform OTU picking, respectively. In addition to the common downstream analysis tools in QIIME 1, QIIME 2 implements several recently released tools, such as q2-ALDEx2, q2-Gneiss, and q2-PICRUSt2, to enable multidimensional analysis. Other new features include a retrospective data tracking system that records all parameters and steps used during data generation. Furthermore, QIIME 2 adds a new interactive visualization method (qiime2 view https://view.qiime2.org) that allows data sharing and interaction without installing QIIME 2. Moreover, QIIME 2 develops a graphical user interface, QIIME 2 Studio (q2studio), and a Python 3 application programmer interface, the artifact Application Programming Interface (API), to suit the needs of both beginners and advanced users.

## MOTHUR

mothur is another widely used data pipeline for amplicon-based microbial community analysis. As a comprehensive pipeline, mothur integrates several preexisting tools and incorporates additional features to process raw community sequencing data (Schloss et al., 2009).

Supporting documents and a discussion forum that contain procedures to process sequence data generated from Sanger, PacBio, Ion Torrent, 454, and Illumina platforms and provide corresponding standard operating procedures are available for mothur users and developers. For example, the MiSeq standard operating procedure contains the procedures for raw sequence demultiplexing, quality control, chimera removal, taxonomic classification, OTU clustering, diversity analysis, and phylogeny-based analysis (Kozich et al., 2013). mothur merges forward and reverse reads to make contigs and removes ambiguous sequences. Unique sequences are then identified and aligned to the reference. mothur provides several alignment databases containing 16S and 18S gene sequences compatible with the Greengenes or SILVA alignments. mothur removes chimeras using the Vsearch algorithm and identifies nonbacterial lineages, such as those related to chloroplasts and mitochondria. Multiple algorithms are available for sequence clustering, including Opticlust (default), Vsearch distance-based greedy clustering, Vsearch abundance-based greedy clustering, furthest neighbor, average neighbor, nearest neighbor, and Unique. The pipeline also performs rarefaction and microbial diversity analyses. A numbers of diversity metrics, such as ACE, Chao1, observed OTU, Simpson, and Shannon, can be calculated. Distance metrics, such as weighted complete lineage, unweighted Unifrac, and Jaccard, are optional with various commands. mothur also contains tools for ordination analysis using PCoA and nonmetric dimensional scaling (NMDS). The diversity results can be statistically tested within mothur using correlation measurements of the relative abundance of each OTU or analysis of molecular variance. Additionally, mothur implements nonparametric analysis tools—Metastats and linear discriminant analysis (LDA) effect size (LEfSe)—to examine if there are significantly different OTUs between groups of interest. mothur workflows are also available in Galaxy.

Both QIIME and mothur share numerous functional features in sequence data preprocessing, OTU clustering, and diversity index extraction, as well as the generation of OTU or feature tables. The major difference lies in interactive visualizations.

QIIME 2 offers several newly developed interactive visualization tools, whereas mothur focuses on generating results that can be easily imported and visualized with other tools. Additionally, unlike QIIME that wraps some third-party tools in a python environment, the mothur team translates many packages in C++ and makes them open source for other contributors to modify and improve (Bolyen et al., 2019; Schloss et al., 2009). A recent study compared the analysis results of QIIME and mothur on a rumen microbiome dataset. The conclusion is that for the most abundant genera, there are no statistical differences between the two pipelines, no matter which reference databases are used (SILVA or Greengenes). However, for microbes in low abundance, mothur is more sensitive than QIIME, but this difference is diminished, and the results become more consistent when SILVA is chosen as the reference database in both pipelines (López-García et al., 2018).

## FROGS

Find, Rapidly, OTUs with Galaxy Solution (FROGS) is a recently developed Galaxy-supported pipeline that aims to analyze large sets of amplicon sequences (Escudié et al., 2017). The pipeline includes a variety of functions, such as preprocessing, clustering, chimera removal, filtering, and taxonomic or phylogenetic affiliation assignment, visualization, and tree construction. FROGS handles both single and paired-end data from the Illumina platform and those generated using 454. The pipeline merges paired-end reads using Flash with 10% mismatch tolerance and ambiguous reads removal. Dereplication is also achieved in this step, and a graphical report is generated for posterior cleaned sequences. The pipeline then uses Swarm for sequence clustering and Vsearch with *de novo* UCHIME to remove chimeras. Notably, an innovative cross-sample validation process is applied to validate the chimeric status on all samples. In each sample, chimeras are first identified separately, but in the end, this sequence is considered chimeric only if it is marked as a chimera in all samples where it exists. This is different from mothur, where only the redundant chimera sequences are removed. FROGS also applies an abundance filter to screen clusters and optionally delete clusters not present in all replications. Taxonomy can be assigned up to the species level with the implemented RDP Classifier or BLASTn+. Common SSU marker gene databases, such as Greengenes, SILVA, and EzBioCloud, can be selected as the reference database. One unique characteristic of FROGS is that it considers conflicting affiliations with BLASTn+, and if affiliation results find multiple hits with different taxonomy, the first level of confliction and lower taxonomies are denoted as "multi-affiliation" in the final OTU table. Because of its modular design, which allows users to choose their tools of preference or processing order, FROGS is a fast, scalable, and parallelizable pipeline (Escudié et al., 2017).

FROGS allows in-depth analyses not only of 16S, 18S, and 23S rRNA genes but also of amplicons from functional genes, such as dsrB. The latest version of FROGS can also be used to analyze ITS data. The entire pipeline can be run in either command line or in Galaxy platform, which is user friendly for those without much bioinformatic experience. FROGS has the advantage of using Swarm and its adaptive sequence agglomeration instead of using a global similarity threshold. Additionally, FROGS has a rigorous step of removing chimera and explicitly considers conflicting affiliations. Compared with QIIME, mothur, and UPARSE, FROGS performs better than mothur and is more conservative than QIIME on the V4 region and better on V3/V4 regions for *in silico* datasets. Furthermore, it performs relatively better for staggered abundances and worse for uniform ones and produces less spurious OTUs than other pipelines on real datasets (Escudié et al., 2017).

## iMAP

The Integrated Microbiome Analysis Pipeline (iMAP) is a very recent development that provides the research community with a user-friendly and portable tool that integrates bioinformatics analysis and data visualization (Buza et al., 2019). The pipeline includes bundles of commands wrapped individually in driver scripts for performing various analyses and data visualization. It requires data files (sample metadata and raw sequences), software, and reference databases to be in place before execution via either a command line interface or from a Docker container command line interface. Outputs from major steps can be conveniently transformed, visualized, and summarized into a progress report. The default reference databases are up-to-date SILVA seed or Greengenes for mothur and QIIME, respectively.

One of the interesting features of iMAP is that it allows exploratory analysis of sample metadata or experimental/environmental variables. iMAP uses seqkit for the general inspection of raw sequences, FastQC for base quality assessment, and BBDuk for trimming and filtering low-quality or control reads. iMAP uses standard approaches in mothur (default) and QIIME 2 for sequence processing and classification. Moreover, it applies additional quality control and removes all undesirable matches including the unknown and any sequences classified to nonbacterial lineages, such as archaea, chloroplasts, eukaryotes, mitochondria, and viruses.

iMAP uses a fairly unique approach for OTU clustering and taxonomy assignment. It relies on a combination of phylotype, OTU-based, and phylogeny methods to assign conserved taxonomy to OTUs. Merged quality sequences are binned into known phylotypes up to the genus level. All sequences are binned into clusters of OTUs based on their similarity at ≥97% identity, and precision and the false discovery rate (FDR) are then calculated using Opticlust, a default mothur function for assigning OTUs. In the phylogeny method, a tree that displays consensus taxonomy for each node is generated. The output from all three methods—phylotype, OTU-based, and phylogeny—is manually reviewed, deduplicated, and integrated to form a complete OTU taxonomy output.

The pipeline uses the R package for microbial diversity analysis. At least three ordination methods—principal component analysis (PCA), PCoA, and NMDS—are provided. Furthermore, phylogenetic annotation is done using Interactive Tree Of Life (iTOL) tree viewer with the aid of selected annotation files, such as the species richness, diversity, and relative abundances files.

While the iMAP pipeline uses an integrated approach for OTU clustering and taxonomy assignment and demonstrates improvements over some widely used pipelines, such as mothur and QIIME, it offers limited solutions for downstream analysis beyond microbial diversity and a phylogenetic tree view, such as the identification of differential abundant taxa and biomarker discovery using advanced statistical algorithms and inference of microbial interaction networks in both static (cross-sectional) and time series data. Furthermore, while using Docker images is the first step, the pipeline is still in a preliminary phase, and much effort is needed to address data reproducibility concerns in relation to modern microbiome data workflows.

## RECENT ADVANCES IN COMPUTATIONAL TOOL DEVELOPMENT

### UNIQUENESS OF MARKER GENE SURVEY DATASETS

Unlike species abundance data obtained in macroecology, OTU or ASV tables generated for the marker gene–based microbiome study have some unique challenges. The absolute count data in the OTU table are largely dependent on sequencing depth and are not a good proxy for the original abundance of microorganisms in a microbial community. As a result, the relative abundance or proportion is more biologically relevant than absolute counts. Data, such as those in the OTU table, that are naturally described as proportions or probabilities or as having a constant or irrelevant fixed sum (for example, 1.0) are referred to as compositional (Gloor et al., 2017). The compositional data pose special challenges for downstream statistical analyses and have been discussed in detail (Aitchison, 1982; Fernandes et al., 2014). These challenges include total value constraints, strong correlation with OTU or ASV, and subcompositional incoherence.

The second salient feature about the taxon (OTU) sample matrix is sparseness. Only a small number of OTUs are detectable in all biological samples collected, and a typical OTU table contains numerous zeros. These zeros include both structural zeros (i.e., those representing the true or absolute absence of a taxon from a given sample, regardless of sequencing depth) and technical or rounded zeros (Kaul et al., 2017) that result from insufficient sampling or sequencing depth. The high frequency of both types of zeros in the dataset requires special consideration. Consequently, several methods have been developed for zero replacement (Brill et al., 2019; Quinn et al., 2019; Rivera-Pinto et al., 2018).

The 16S dataset or OTU sample matrix is often multidimensional in nature, typically including a few thousand OTUs and up to a few hundred samples. Furthermore, there may exist a correlation structure in 16S datasets, and a strong correlation between OTUs negatively affects the performance of subsequent statistical testing (Hawinkel et al., 2017). Several recent studies have clearly demonstrated that dealing with compositionality in the 16S dataset is not optional (Gloor et al., 2017; Mandal et al., 2015), and statistical tests ignoring these unique characteristics of 16S data often fail to control the FDR (Hawinkel et al., 2017).

### STATISTICAL TESTING AND DIFFERENTIALLY ABUNDANT TAXON IDENTIFICATION

One of the key areas of interest in microbiome studies is to detect features (taxa or ASV) displaying a statistically significant difference in relative abundance between two groups of interest or pathophysiological conditions. These significant taxa or features can be readily developed as biomarkers or signatures for therapeutic options (Hawinkel et al., 2017). Over the years, many classical statistical tools have been used to identify significantly different taxa. For example, while t-tests and Analysis of variance (ANOVA) are often used to compare alpha diversity indices between experimental groups, they are also used to detect significant taxa, for example, in a study involving HIV-positive patients with or without antiretroviral therapy and healthy controls (McHardy et al., 2013). Similarly, nonparametric counterparts of these tests, including the Wilcoxon rank sum test and the Kruskal–Wallis test by rank, are also widely used in microbiome studies. LEfSe is an algorithm for high-dimensional biomarker discovery and identification of genomic features such as genes, pathways, or taxa under experimental or pathophysiological conditions (Segata et al., 2011). The algorithm includes three major steps—detecting features (taxa or ASV) significant in relative abundance using the nonparametric Kruskal–Wallis test, investigating biological consistency using the Wilcoxon rank sum test, and using LDA to estimate the effect size of each differentially abundant feature. The method has been widely used for microbiome data analysis, including the discovery of biomarkers or differentially abundant taxa derived from OTU or ASV tables or biological pathway data inferred using PICRUSt (Kageyama et al., 2019; Lo Presti et al., 2019; Puri et al., 2018; Sims et al., 2019). The popularity of the method is partially driven by the implementation of a user-friendly Galaxy version of the algorithm (http://huttenhower.sph.harvard.edu/galaxy/).

In several regards, OTU or ASV count data are similar to gene expression data obtained using microarrays or RNAseq. As a result, many algorithms developed in the early years of the millennium to detect differentially expressed genes, such as DESeq2 and EdgeR, can be readily adapted to analyze marker gene survey data (McMurdie and Holmes, 2014). In 2013, Paulson et al. proposed a novel normalization procedure, cumulative sum scaling normalization, to correct the bias in the assessment of differential abundance introduced by widely used total-sum normalization (Paulson et al., 2013). A zero-inflated Gaussian (ZIG) distribution mixture model that accounts for biases in differential abundance testing resulting from undersampling of the microbial community was also proposed in that paper. Unlike the *ad-hoc* heuristic approach used in LEfSe, ZIG uses linear modeling and has been shown to be more sensitive under simulated conditions. More differentially abundant species can be identified using ZIG than LEfSe in real microbiome datasets (Paulson et al., 2013). However, this method does not address the compositionality issue inherent in marker gene datasets, which poses particular challenges, and traditional statistical tools often become invalid.

In 2014, an algorithm dealing with compositional data typically seen in datasets involving multiple omics approaches was developed. This method, ALDEx2 (Fernandes et al., 2014), includes several straightforward steps. First, the counts are converted to probabilities by Monte Carlo sampling from the Dirichlet distribution with the addition of a uniform prior, usually 1/2. The resultant Monte Carlo Dirichlet instance is then normalized using the centered log-ratio (CLR) approach. The value is the base 2 logarithms of the abundance of the feature in each Dirichlet instance in each sample divided by the geometric mean abundance of the Dirichlet instance of the sample. Significance tests between groups of interest are then conducted using the Welch's t-test and the Wilcoxon rank sum test; $P$ values obtained are corrected using the Benjamini–Hochberg procedure; and the effect size is also estimated. Compared to traditional statistical test tools, such as the widely used LEfSe, ALDEx2 tends to reduce the number of false positives, especially when the sample size is small

(Fernandes et al., 2014). Moreover, the method enables a unified analysis for high-throughput sequencing datasets, including marker gene count tables, RNAseq, and ChIPseq datasets.

Recently, a novel statistical framework called analysis of composition of microbiomes (ANCOM) has been developed to detect taxa differing significantly in two or more populations or experimental groups (Mandal et al., 2015). The framework is based on Aitchison log-ratios without distributional assumptions and is therefore quite flexible. ANCOM uses the W statistic and selects an internal threshold (W values) for significance (no $P$ values provided). One of the limitations of the framework is the assumption that less than 25% of the taxa are changing significantly between two groups, which limits its application when two populations or groups under comparison have drastic differences. Nevertheless, when compared to the conventional t-test and the aforementioned ZIG method, ANCOM can reduce false positives by as much as 68% or even more while improving detection power. Since its advent, the method has become rapidly accepted (Iszatt et al., 2019; Peterson et al., 2019) and is now implemented in the QIIME pipeline.

A detailed comparison of several methods designed for differential abundance detection (originally intended for gene expression count data obtained using microarrays or RNAseq) under various scenarios, including sample size, effect size, and distributional assumptions, has been recently conducted (Hawinkel et al., 2017). For example, the sensitivity of both ANCOM and ALDEx2 is fairly low (<25%) under the negative binomial distribution with or without correlation. Of the methods tested, DESeq2 and SAMseq have modest sensitivity when the sample size is small, while metagenomeSeq is more powerful with a sensitivity > 50% when the sample size is larger than 25. However, all methods fail to control the FDR. Compared to ALDEx2, ANCOM has a much higher FDR under all the scenarios tested, which is in sharp contrast to the original claim that the method has reasonable power to detect differentially abundance log-ratios while controlling the FDR at a nominal level (<0.05). Other studies have also suggested that ANCOM is unable to control the FDR, especially under the global null setting (Brill et al., 2019). Moreover, ANCOM is computationally intensive when used at the OTU level without filtering out very rare features. Weiss et al. (2017) compared several methods along with ANCOM and suggested that ANCOM behaves better in terms of sensitivity and controlling the FDR than those methods not specifically designed for handling compositionality.

During the preparation of this chapter, we conducted a direct comparison of several popular methods using a published 16S rRNA gene dataset (Liu et al., 2019) (Sequence Read Archive (SRA) accession: PRJNA534501). The part of the dataset used for this comparison included two experimental groups, normal control mice ($N = 10$) and colitis mice induced with dextran sulfate sodium (DSS) ($N = 10$). The sample OTU matrix includes $20 \times 1,666$ data points, a typical dataset commonly seen in controlled animal experiments.

The number of significant genera identified by all four non-ANCOM–related methods is 22, whereas the number of significant genera identified by all six methods is 15 (Table 1.2); 15 of the 16 genera identified by ANCOM (v2) are also detected by all other methods. ALDEx2 performs well compared to other methods. For compositional datasets, such as those obtained in marker gene–based microbiome studies, we

**TABLE 1.2**
**The Number of Differentially Abundant Genera Identified by Six Algorithms Tested**

| Version | Method | LEfSe | ANCOM_ v1 | ANCOM_ v2 | Wilcoxon | DESeq2 | ALDEx2 |
|---------|--------|-------|-----------|-----------|----------|--------|--------|
| v1.0 | LEfSe | 35 | 23 | 16 | 31 | 24 | 24 |
| v1.1-3 | ANCOM_v1 | | 23 | 16 | 22 | 21 | 20 |
| v2.0 | ANCOM_v2 | | | 16 | 15 | 15 | 15 |
| v1.0 | Wilcoxon | | | | 31 | 24 | 24 |
| v1.12.4 | DESeq2 | | | | | 25 | 22 |
| v1.4.0 | ALDEx2 | | | | | | 24 |

All algorithm except LEfSe was at a cutoff value of the FDR $< 0.05$. The default cutoff for LEfSe was used (absolute LDA $> 2.0$). The values in off-diagonal entries indicate the number of significant genera identified by both methods.

would recommend ALDEx2 as a default option for detecting taxa with significantly different abundance between groups of interest.

## BALANCES AND MICROBIAL SIGNATURE IDENTIFICATION

Although changes in the relative abundance of individual taxa or ASV induced by treatments or alterations in pathophysiological status can be compared using the statistical methods discussed above, the interpretation of compositional data is somewhat more difficult than real vectors in standard analysis (Egozcue and Pawlowsky-Glahn, 2005). Moreover, in the real world, understanding the relationship or balance (log ratio) of two or more features (parts) of the sample composition within a group or between groups becomes more relevant. Recently, the balance concept developed by Egozcue and Pawlowsky-Glahn (2005) has been applied to marker gene–based microbiome analysis (Morton et al., 2017). Morton et al. developed a method called Gneiss to construct balance trees using clustering tools or a phylogenetic tree and isometric log-ratio transformation. Once constructed, balances can be analyzed using standard statistical methods, such as linear regression. Morton et al. (2017) demonstrated that by focusing on subcommunities or groups of taxa instead of individual taxa of a microbial community, the balance tree approach can better yield novel insights into niche differentiation. The open-source software can be accessed at https://github.com/biocore/gneiss. It is also implemented in the QIIME 2 pipeline. A nice video about this software is freely available at https://www.youtube.com/watch?v=HAULM1WQkew.

Examining the treatment effect on individual OTUs or taxa is an important step in microbiome studies. It is of particular interest to identify and visualize branches in a phylogenetic tree whose members (OTUs or taxa) display a significant consensus (overall) abundance response to treatments or changes in conditions. Motivated by this, a new software package called SigTree (Stevens et al., 2017) has been developed.

This software relies on meta-analytic principles and provides tools to use the results of OTU-level significance tests (with meaningful one-sided $P$ values) to identify and visualize branches in a phylogenetic tree that are significantly responsive to experimental interventions or changes in environmental conditions. SigTree uses $P$ values rather than raw data and allows users to select models appropriate for specific study designs, including accounting for study-specific data distribution (Poisson, negative binomial, or nonparametric). The package also provides two multiple testing correction options, the Hommel and Benjamini–Yekutieli corrections. Together, the authors claim these flexible features allow SigTree to be applicable in *any* experimental design and with *any* high-throughput technology. Compared to Gneiss, which does not include convenient tree-level visualization tools, SigTree provides better tree visualization. Moreover, SigTree does not have the constraints typically associated with the isometric log-ratio transformation used in Gneiss, including issues with zero replacement.

A novel approach superficially similar to Gneiss has been proposed to identify balances or microbial signatures, a group of taxa that can better predict treatment outcomes or a phenotype of interest (Rivera-Pinto et al., 2018). This package, selbal, uses a greedy stepwise algorithm for the selection of balances that preserves the principles of compositional data analysis. The process of balance identification by selbal includes two steps, modeling the response variable and identifying the smallest number of taxa with the highest prediction or classification accuracy. The software also provides several choices for zero replacement, including the default geometric Bayesian multiplicative replacement method. The variables can be categorical (dichotomous) or numerical (continuous). To demonstrate its utilities, we analyzed the aforementioned dataset (Liu et al., 2019) (SRA accession: PRJNA534501) using selbal with default parameters. Three variables are considered, treatment (dichotomous, normal, or DSS), spleen weight (g, numerical), and colon length (cm, numerical). The selbal algorithm selects 20 variables (genera) with good classification accuracy that are compatible with the 24 genera identified using ALDEx2. As Figure 1.2a shows, a microbial signature consisting of the balance (log ratio) of *Streptococcus* (numerator) to an unclassified genus in the family Peptostreptococcaceae (denominator) can readily distinguish between DSS-induced colitis mice and normal control mice. The balance value for DSS mice is negative, suggesting that the relative abundance of the unclassified genus in Peptostreptococcaceae is much higher than that of *Streptococcus*. The cross-validation data indicate that this global balance is very robust and is selected 62% of the time during the validation. Moreover, a balance, consisting of four genera, an unclassified genus in the family Clostridiaceae and the genus *Clostridium* (numerator) and *Streptococcus* and [*Clostridium*] in the family Peptostreptococcaceae, has a strong predictive power for the spleen weight ($R^2 = 0.818$) with a very low mean squared error of 0.0041 (Figure 1.2b). Two of the four genera, *Clostridium* and *Streptococcus*, are included in balance selection more than 60% of the time, further indicating that the selected global balance is robust. In addition, the algorithm also identifies a microbial signature for the colon length, but the association is modest with $R^2 = 0.47$.

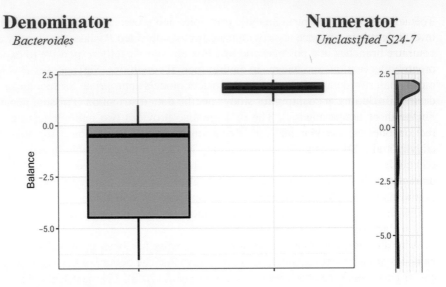

**FIGURE 1.2A**   A microbial signature consisting of the balance (log ratio) of Streptococcus (numerator) to an unclassified genus in the family Peptostreptococcaceae (denominator).

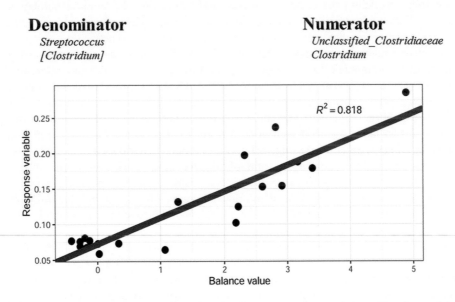

**FIGURE 1.2B**   Regression Analysis of the microbial signature in association with spleen weight.

## TOOLS FOR NETWORK ANALYSIS AND THEIR APPLICATIONS

Detecting robust microbial associations or interactions and identifying microbial co-occurrence patterns or keystone species is one of the essential steps in understanding the structure and function of the gut microbiome. Network algorithms are able to encode the interactions between the components in complex systems. Microbial interaction network inference based on network theory and practice provides system-level insight into potential ecological relationships of microorganisms in a microbial community. For example, modularity, the extent to which microbial interactions are organized into modules or subnetworks in a global network, may reflect habitat heterogeneity or phylogenetic clustering of closely related microbes, and modules with closed-linked species may represent some key coevolution units (Olesen et al., 2007). Furthermore, knowledge of interaction networks forms the foundation to predictively model the interplay between environmental factors and microbial populations (Kurtz et al., 2015) and may hold keys to the development of efficacious probiotics and antibiotic therapeutics. Ultimately, the knowledge obtained by modeling microbial interactions should facilitate microbial community engineering via the targeted elimination and expansion of keystone species in a network. Motivated by these lofty goals, dozens of algorithms have been developed to infer microbial co-occurrence patterns and model microbial interaction network dynamics (Barberán et al., 2012; Faust et al., 2012; Freilich et al., 2010; Ruan et al., 2006). For example, a meta-network framework has recently been proposed to decipher microbial interactions and construct more meaningful networks with biologically important clusters and hubs (Yang et al., 2019). The framework starts with a loose definition strategy to recover more correlations before correlation calculation. While direct relationships are discovered, association rule mining is subsequently applied to detect complex forms of correlations, including indirect correlations using Functional Similarity Weight (FS-weight) and nonlinear correlations using the part mutual information adjusted by path consistency algorithm, which enables the detection of interactions that are often missed using they Pearson and Spearman approaches.

Habitat filtering, the co-occurrence of microbes due to habitats rather than biological interactions being sampled, can induce apparent correlations, resulting in a network dominated by habitat effects and the masking of true correlations of biological interest (Berry and Widder, 2014). The phenomenon can confound microbial interaction network inference when samples from different habitats are combined. To overcome this issue, a novel algorithm to correct for habitat filtering effects has been proposed (Brisson et al., 2019). This algorithm significantly improves correlation detection accuracy compared to Spearman and Pearson correlations, thus enabling the construction of consensus correlation networks from datasets combining multiple habitats.

Weiss et al. (2016) conducted a comprehensive benchmarking comparison analysis of the performance of eight microbial network inference methods. Commonly used network inference tools are based on a broad range of underlying methodologies, such as correlation and regression-based tools (Compositionality Corrected by REnormalizaion and PErmutation (CCREPE), Sparse Correlations for Compositional data (SparCC), Random Matrix Theory (RMT)), graphical model inference tools (Sparse Inverse Covariance Estimation for Ecological Association Inference [SPIEC-EASI]), extended local similarity analysis (eLSA), and mutual information-based tools (Mutual Information Clustering (MIC)). Weiss et al. (2016) concluded that while different tools have various strengths and weaknesses in response to the diverse challenges presented by microbiome data, all tools result in a high false-positive rate. An ensemble approach, including CoNet, SparCC, and Spearman and Pearson methods, tends to enhance the precision of detection. While paired with

Pearson correlation, the RMT approach (Molecular ecological network analyses (MENA)) also significantly improves precision. Furthermore, dataset characteristics and desired ecological relationship discovery determine the selection of the better tool. While datasets have high compositionality, SparCC is better at inferring linear relationships with high precision. While sparsity is < 50% (after filtering to remove very rare OTUs), local similarity analysis (LSA) is good for both time series (longitudinal) and cross-sectional studies, while MIC is good for cross-sectional studies. Otherwise, ensemble approaches tend to increase precision. Nevertheless, nonlinear relationships are very difficult to detect using these tools.

To address compositionality and dimensionality challenges in the microbiome data during network inference, Friedman and Alm (2012) pioneered the development of SparCC, which is capable of estimating linear Pearson correlation values from compositional data using CLR transformation. Since its advent, this popular algorithm has been widely applied to microbiome studies and is subject to many benchmarking comparisons (Deshpande et al., 2018; Friedman and Alm, 2012; Jackson et al., 2018; Wang et al., 2018). However, SparCC does not consider the influence of errors in compositional data, which may reduce the correlation estimation accuracy. Moreover, the $P$ value estimator used by SparCC may lead to bias and overestimating significance. The limitations of SparCC have been discussed by Fang et al. (2015). Recently, a fast and parallelizable implementation of the SparCC algorithm with an unbiased $P$ value estimator was published (Watts et al., 2018). This implementation significantly reduces run time and memory consumption while maintaining performance equivalent to the original SparCC. A novel strategy called SPIEC-EASI was later developed to address some of the issues associated with SparCC (Kurtz et al., 2015). SPIEC-EASI network inference consists of two steps. First, a CLR log transformation is applied. Second, SPIEC-EASI estimates the interaction graph from the transformed data using one of the methods, neighborhood selection (Meinshausen and Bühlmann (MB) method) and sparse inverse covariance selection or graphical Least Absolute Shrinkage and Selection Operator (LASSO). Unlike empirical correlation or covariance estimation used in SparCC and CCREPE, SPIEC-EASI infers an underlying graphical model using the concept of conditional independence. Under various simulated scenarios, SPIEC-EASI, especially with neighborhood covariance selection, outperforms SparCC and CCREPE in terms of network recovery. All compositionality-based methods tested—SPIEC-EASI, SparCC, and CCREPE—are better than the Pearson correlation method in detecting global network topology features. Furthermore, the networks inferred by SPIEC-EASI are more reproducible than those obtained by SparCC and CCREPE. SPIEC-EASI infers considerably sparser model networks than the other two methods.

A novel framework called Microbial Prior LASSO (MPLasso) has been recently proposed (Lo and Marculescu, 2017). In their study, Lo and Marculescu use the graphical LASSO algorithm to infer the microbial association network. The uniqueness of the method is that the authors are among the first to integrate text mining results from the scientific literature (i.e., experimentally verified biological information) as prior knowledge to infer the microbial graph structure. To acquire experimentally verified microbial associations, the PubMed database is searched via two routes, microbial co-occurrence data in the literature are examined and compared to by chance alone and the machine learning–based is the method (Lim et al., 2016) to extract the interaction information. MPLasso outperforms all methods tested, including the aforementioned SPIEC-EASI, SparCC, and CCREPE, as well as Correlation Inference for Compositional Data through Lasso (CCLasso) and regularized estimation of the basis covariance based on compositional data (REBACCA) in terms of area under the precision-recall curve and the accuracy (ACC) of network association prediction in synthetic datasets. In the presence of prior knowledge, MPLasso can achieve remarkably high accuracy in terms of the edge recovery rate, up to 95%. Moreover, MPLasso can robustly and accurately estimate microbial interactions, with reproducibility up to 90% in real microbiome datasets.

Microbial communities are dynamic in nature. The abundance of community members fluctuates temporally or in response to environmental factors or perturbations. Similarity-based network inferring tools (Bray–Curtis, Pearson, Spearman, or LSA) treat time series data as a static snapshot and ignore their temporal dependencies (Alshawaqfeh et al., 2017) and are generally unable to infer nonlinear relationships, especially those with multispecies complex interactions. The Lotka–Volterra equations, a pair of first-order nonlinear differential equations, have been frequently used to describe the dynamics of biological systems in traditional macroecology. Recently, the role of dynamic systems theory in understanding microbial community dynamics, especially the utility of generalized Lotka–Volterra models, has been extensively discussed (Gao et al., 2018; Gonze et al., 2018). For example, using generalized Lotka Volterra dynamics modeling, Berry and Widder (2014) found that co occurrence networks can recapitulate interaction networks under certain conditions, but they lose interpretability when the effects of habitat filtering become significant (Berry and Widder, 2014). In particular, networks suffer from local hot spots of spurious correlation in the neighborhood of keystone or hub species that engage in many interactions. Recently, a new approach called Learning Interactions from Microbial Time Series (LIMITS) has been developed (Fisher and Mehta, 2014). LIMITS uses sparse linear regression with bootstrap aggregation to infer a discrete-time Lotka–Volterra model for microbial dynamics and overcome some of the obstacles commonly encountered while inferring microbial interactions. The obstacles include the observations that a correlation in the abundance between two microbial species does not necessarily imply their actual interaction and that it is difficult to infer parameters in time series data due to the sum constraint on the relative abundance (compositionality) in typical microbiome datasets. When applied to real microbiome datasets, LIMITS is able to successfully detect interaction networks dominated by distinct keystone species.

Alshawaqfeh et al. (2017) proposed a stochastic generalized Lotka–Volterra dynamic model that adopts the extended Kalman filter (SgLV-EKF) algorithm to model the microbial interaction network dynamics (Alshawaqfeh et al., 2017). The proposed stochastic model accounts for the uncertainty in the model by adding a noise term in the dynamic equation, while extended Kalman filter, due to its ability to estimate the parameters of nonlinear interactions from a limited number of observations, is used for the first time to estimate the abundance level of microbes and their interactions. SgLV-EKF is also compared to five other algorithms, including two similarity-based (Pearson correlation coefficient and LSA), one integral-based

(Nelder and Mead, 1965), and two regression-based (Stein's and LIMITS) algorithms using both synthetic and real datasets. SgLV-EKF outperforms the other five algorithms in identifying the structure of the interaction network. Moreover, SgLV-EKF provides robust and reliable performance against the uncertainty in the dynamic model at an accuracy level higher than 75% and that is also higher than that of LIMITS, which provides reliable results with consistent accuracy of approximately 60%. Nelder's algorithm generates results similar to those of SgLV-EKF under varying measurement noise levels but fails to compensate for randomness in the dynamic system and is computationally intensive. Stein's algorithm fails to detect the majority of the interactions and exhibits very low sensitivity, while the two similarity-based algorithms show a significant reduction in their accuracy due to the increase in the process noise power. Moreover, the latter two algorithms lack mathematical modeling of the microbial community and are unable to predict network dynamics.

## WEB-BASED TOOLS FOR MARKER GENE SURVEY DATA

In addition to the pipelines discussed above, such as iMAP, numerous resources and tools have recently been developed and have become widely available to the research community. For example, the mothur and FROGS pipelines are also implemented in the Galaxy and are available online. Moreover, a complete workflow for 16S microbiome data analysis consisting of various R packages, such as DADA2, phyloseq, DESeq2, ggplot2, structSSI, and vegan, has provided good examples of how to use abundant resources in R to conduct analyses from raw read filtering to community-level analyses, including supervised analyses using Random Forest and nonparametric testing using community networks (http://web.stanford.edu/class/bios221/MicrobiomeWorkflowII. html). Several powerful platforms, such as MEtaGenome Analyzer (MEGAN) (Mitra et al., 2011), the metagenomics Rapid Annotation using Subsystems Technology server (MG-RAST) (https://www.mg-rast.org), and Visualization and Analysis of Microbial Population Structures (VAMPS) (https://vamps2.mbl.edu), have been widely used to visualize and analyze raw sequence data for microbial population structures and distributions. While these platforms provide good tools for data preprocessing, including filtering, normalization, and taxonomic profiling, they generally do not contain sophisticated algorithms for the identification of differentially abundant taxa and the discovery of potential biomarkers and microbial co-occurrence patterns.

Next, we introduce several recent web-based tool suites for in-depth analyses of marker gene–based microbiome data. MicrobiomeAnalyst (https://www.microbiomeanalyst.ca) is a web-based tool suite for the comprehensive statistical, visual, and meta-analysis of microbiome data (Dhariwal et al., 2017). The suite contains four modules, the Marker Data Profiling (MDP) module, the Shotgun Data Profiling module, the Taxon Set Enrichment Analysis module, and the Projection with Public Data module. Both MDP and Projection with Public Data module are specially designed for 16S rRNA maker gene survey data and will be discussed in detail. The input file for MDP is count tables (OTUs or ASV) of various origin, including both a tab delimited text (.txt) or in comma separated values (.csv) and BIOM files from QIIME and mothur pipelines. MDP includes dozens of tools organized in five categories—visual exploration, community profiling, clustering and correlation, comparison and classification, and functional prediction. The tool suite offers multiple choices for data scaling and normalization, including CLR transformation. For visualization, the module provides standard methods for stacked bar or area plots, interactive pie charts, rarefaction curves, and a phylogenetic tree view. Moreover, the module provides a heat tree analysis based on the MetaCoder algorithm (Foster et al., 2017). This unique feature uses the hierarchical structure of taxonomic classifications to quantitatively and statistically depict taxonomic differences between microbial communities of interest. Under the community profiling, the suite enables the generation of six alpha diversity indices—Abundance-based (ACE), Fisher's Alpha, Chao1, observed taxa, Shannon, and Simpson. For beta diversity evaluation, the suite allows two popular ordination methods, PCoA and NMDS, based on five distance matrixes, Bray–Curtis dissimilarity, Jensen–Shannon Divergence, Jaccard Index, unweighted Unifrac measures, and weighted Unifrac measures. Moreover, three algorithms, Permutational multivariate analysis of variance (PERMANOVA), ANOSIM, and distance-based tests for homogeneity of multivariate dispersions (Permutational analysis of multivariate dispersions (PERMDISP)), are provided for global significance testing.

Under the comparative analysis category, multiple algorithms are provided for users to identify taxa that are significantly different between groups of interest and to discover potential biomarkers. In addition to classical univariate analysis (such as t-tests and ANOVA) and nonparametric tests (such as the Mann–Whitney U test or the Kruskal–Wallis rank sum test), MDP also offers metagenomeSeq, edgeR, DESeq2, LEfSe, and Random Forest.

The MDP module also provides two useful tools that enable functional prediction from 16S rRNA count tables, PICRUSt for the Greengene database, and Tax4Fun for the SILVA database. The result is a table containing relative abundance levels of Kyoto Encyclopedia of Genes and Genomes Orthology. The Kyoto Encyclopedia of Genes and Genomes Orthology profiles obtained from predictions can be used for functional diversity profiling based on Kyoto Encyclopedia of Genes and Genomes pathway or Clusters of Orthologous Groups annotation systems. Because one Kyoto Encyclopedia of Genes and Genomes Orthology or Clusters of Orthologous Groups can be assigned to multiple functional groups, MicrobiomeAnalyst offers different approaches to deal with this issue, including simple sum, normalized sum, and weighted sum methods. The results are presented as a stacked area plot organized by experimental factors to help visualize patterns of variations across different conditions. The underlying abundance table is available for downloading. A nice feature of the MicrobiomeAnalyst suite is that R command line history is shown along with the data in the browser.

One of the unique features of the MicrobiomeAnalyst suite is that it contains a module for meta-analysis. The Projection with Public Data module allows users to visually explore their datasets within the context of a compatible public dataset for context reference and pattern discovery using an interactive 3D PCoA plot. While there is still room for improvement, the MicrobiomeAnalyst suite is a very user-friendly online toolbox that enables comprehensive visualization and statistical testing for both marker gene– and whole genome shotgun–based microbiome datasets.

Calypso is a recently developed web application with a powerful yet user-friendly tool suite for the comprehensive analysis of bacterial, archaeal, viral, and eukaryotic communities (Zakrzewski et al., 2017). The package uses count data, metadata, and an optional matrix of pair-wise community distances (such as Unifrac) as input files to mine and visualize microbiome environment interactions. The suite emphasizes multivariate analysis for hypothesis testing, which is one of its key strengths.

The package supports various formats of count data, either a .txt, .csv, or BIOM file, with taxonomic assignments from phylum to OTU levels. Output files from several popular pipelines, such as QIIME (Caporaso et al., 2010), mothur (Schloss et al., 2009), MG-RAST (Meyer et al., 2008), and MetaPhlAn (Segata et al., 2012), can be directly uploaded. The metadata file consists of a simple text file in either .txt or.csv format and contains meta information for each sample, such as sample unique identifiers, sample groups, sample include/exclude options, and optional explanatory or environmental variables, such as control vs. treated, disease status, and physiological parameters. Both numeric and categorical variables are supported.

Calypso provides various tools for data filtering, rarefying, scaling, and transformation, such as asinh, cumulative sum scaling, log, quantile normalization, square root, and total sum of squares (TSS). It also recommends the default choice of either TSS combined with square root transformation or cumulative sum scaling + log2 transformation. Of note, Calypso also provides a CLR transformation, which is one of the most widely used transformations designed for compositional data.

Calypso provides many graphical tools for data visualization, including bubble plot, heatmap, interactive hierarchical tree, Krona plot, and standard bar charts, box plots, and strip charts. Users can exclude samples, select colors, and change figure resolution and dimensions. Output files include data tables in either .csv or .txt formats and publication-quality images in PNG, PDF, or SVG formats.

Calypso allows users to calculate up to eight alpha diversity indices, such as ACE, Chao1, Fisher's Alpha, Evenness, Richness, Shannon, and Simpson. These alpha diversity measures can be viewed using various bar charts, strip charts, box plots, scatter plots, dot plots, and interactive boxplots. The significance can be tested using ANOVA or nonparametric Wilcoxon and Kruskal–Wallis rank sum tests. Complex associations between microbial diversity and multiple explanatory variables can be identified by multiple linear regression. Calypso also supports diversity analysis using mcpHill (Pallmann et al., 2012), which simultaneously investigates several diversity measures by unifying them in the same mathematical family of indices. The advantage of mcpHill is that it may provide biological insights that would remain hidden when only examining one arbitrary or *a priori* committed measure of diversity.

Calypso emphasizes multivariate analysis and provides a broad range of ordination methods for beta diversity, including unsupervised, such as PCA, PCoA, detrended correspondence analysis, and NMDS, and supervised methods, such as redundancy analysis and canonical correspondence analysis, using several distance matrixes. Moreover, the package offers several methods of global significance testing. For example, associations between microbial community composition and a single environmental variable can be identified by PERMDISP2 or by comparing intragroup and intergroup community distances using ANOSIM. More complex environment–microbiome associations can be identified and tested using redundancy analysis, correspondence analysis, and PERMANOVA (or Adonis). These methods test if variance in community composition can be explained by variance in multiple explanatory or environmental variables. The package also has strong graphical capability. For example, PCoA can be viewed in three ways, 2D, 3D, and interactive. Furthermore, two different hierarchical clustering tools and a correlation heatmap are provided.

Calypso offers a dozen tools for identifying taxa or features with significantly different abundance between groups of interest. The relative abundance can be compared using ANOVA (one-way, two-way, and nested) and *t*-tests (regular, paired, and Bayesian) or nonparametric tests, such as the Wilcoxon rank test and the Kruskal–Wallis rank sum test. Of particular interest is that the package offers two recent algorithms specifically developed to handle compositional data, ALDEx2 (Fernandes et al., 2014) and ANCOM (Mandal et al., 2015). No other web-based tool suites offer these tools designed for compositionality. Calypso also provides mixed effect regression and machine learning tools, such as Random Forest. All $P$ values are further adjusted for multiple testing corrections, including, Bonferroni and FDR corrections.

Calypso offers four methods for feature or biomarker discovery, LEfSe, stepwise regression, LASSO regularized regression, and Random Forest, more than other similar web-based tools. Features or taxa selected by stepwise or LASSO regularized regression are presented as bar charts that depict the importance of each taxa. Random Forest results are also presented as bar charts, indicating the relative importance of taxa, as estimated by random permutation. Under the advanced section, Calypso offers mixMC, a multivariate framework that takes into account the sparsity and compositionality of microbiome count data (Lê Cao et al., 2016). The framework enables a holistic understanding of microbial communities through insightful graphical output and highlighting features or taxa with discriminative differences between environmental variables. When emphasizing repeated-measures design with a multilevel variance decomposition, mixMC can be used in a more general case to compare phenotypes or disease outcomes.

Calypso also includes several tools for the identification of co-occurrence patterns using network analysis. Five algorithms are provided in Calypso for network inference, including those based on Pearson's correlation or Spearman's rho and weighted gene correlation network analysis (Langfelder and Horvath, 2008). Moreover, the LASSO regression-based approach involves the abundance of each taxon regressing on all remaining taxa iteratively until the most relevant associations are identified. However, an ensemble-based approach is based on multiple similarity measures combining Bray–Curtis dissimilarities with Pearson correlation and Spearman's rho. For each similarity/dissimilarity measure, the significance of the correlation is computed. $P$ values for Bray–Curtis dissimilarities are computed with permutation. $P$ values are further corrected using multiple testing by the FDR. Table 1.3 summarizes some of the major features offered in three popular web-based tool suites, the two discussed above and METAGENassist (Arndt et al., 2012).

Overall, Calypso is an easy-to-use web-based toolbox packed with many sophisticated statistical algorithms for microbiome studies. It allows a scientist without any programming skills to produce a rapid, robust, and comprehensive analysis of compositional data.

**TABLE 1.3**

**Summarization of Feature Categories of Three Major Web-Based Tools for Marker Gene Studies.**

| Category | METAGEN-Assist | MicrobiomeAnalyst | Calypso |
|---|---|---|---|
| Web-based Implementation | Yes | Yes | Yes |
| Version | | | v8.84 |
| URL | http://www. metagenassist.ca | https://www. microbiomeanalyst.ca/ | http://cgenome.net/calypso/ |
| Data input | OTU table, BIOM file | OTU/ASV table, BIOM file | OTU/ASV table, BIOM file |
| Data processing | Scaling, transformation | Rarefying, scaling, transformation | Rarefying, scaling, transformation |
| Quantitative visualization | Bar chart, pie chart | Bar chart, pie chart, phylogenetic tree, heat tree | Bar chart, bubble plot, heatmap, scatterplot, strichart |
| Clustering | Dendrogram, heatmaps, SOM | Dendrogram, heatmaps | Dendrogram, heatmaps, SOM |
| Hierarchical tree | No | Yes | Yes |
| Alpha diversity | No | 6 indices | 8 indices |
| Beta diversity | | | |
| Distance matrix | Yes | Yes | Yes |
| Ordination/ multivariate analysis | PCA, PSL-DA | PCoA, NMDS | PCA, PCoA, PLS, RDA, CCA, DCA, NMDS |
| Global significance testing | No | ANOSIM, PERMANOVA, PERMDISP | ANOSIM, PERMANOVA, PERMDISP |
| Univaraite analysis | *T*-test, ANOVA, Wilcoxon, Kruskal–Wallis | *T*-test, ANOVA, Wilcoxon, Kruskal–Wallis, edgeR, DESeq2, MicrobiomeSeq | *T*-test, ANOVA, Wilcoxon, Kruskal–Wallis, DESeq2, ANCOM, ALDEx2 |
| Feature/biomarker discovery | Random Forest, SVM | LEfSe, Random Forest | LEfSe, Random Forest, LASSO, stepwise regression, SVM |
| Functional prediction | No | PICRUSt and Tax4Fun | PICRUSt |
| Correlation analysis | Pearson, Spearman, Kendall | Pearson, Spearman, Kendall, SparCC | Pearson, Spearman, Kendall, WGCNA, network analysis, factor analysis |
| Multiple testing correction | No | Yes | Yes |
| Regression | No | Yes | Yes |

RDA: redundancy analysis; DCA: detrended correspondence analysis; CCA: canonical correspondence analysis; WGCNA: Weighted correlation network analysis; PLS: Partial least squares; SVM: Support Vector Machines.

## CONCLUSIONS

The advent of high-throughput sequencing technologies and the rapid development of user-friendly bioinformatic algorithms have enabled a renaissance of marker gene–based studies. Freely accessible reference databases have rapidly expanded. Several user-friendly pipelines, such as QIIME, mothur, and FROGS, have been developed. Numerous algorithms and sophisticated statistical testing, including machine learning, have been proposed to detect differentially abundant taxa, identify biomarkers and taxa correlated with environmental variables, and infer microbial interaction networks. Easy-to-use web-based tool suites for data analysis have also become available. However, microbial network inference is still in its infancy, and biological interpretation and validation of inferred microbial interactions are still extremely difficult. There are no public databases available for microbial interactions. While many challenges remain, we strongly believe that knowledge of microbial association and co-occurrence patterns will establish a foundation to predictively model the interplay between environmental factors and microbial populations (Kurtz et al., 2015). This knowledge will ultimately facilitate the development of microbial community engineering by targeted elimination and/or expansion of keystone species in a microbial community and hold keys to efficacious synbiotic and antibiotic therapeutics.

## ACKNOWLEDGMENTS

Mention of trade names or commercial products in this publication is solely for the purpose of providing specific information and does not imply recommendation or endorsement by the US Department of Agriculture. The US Department of Agriculture is an equal opportunity provider and employer.

## REFERENCES

Abarenkov, K., Somervuo, P., Nilsson, R.H., Kirk, P.M., Huotari, T., Abrego, N., Ovaskainen, O., 2018. Protax-fungi: a web-based tool for probabilistic taxonomic placement of fungal internal transcribed spacer sequences. *New Phytologist* 220, 517–525.

Abbas, A., He, X., Niu, J., Zhou, B., Zhu, G., Ma, T., Song, J., Gao, J., Zhang, M.Q., Zeng, J., 2019. Integrating Hi-C and FISH data for modeling of the 3D organization of chromosomes. *Nature Communications* 10, 2049.

Aitchison, J., 1982. The Statistical Analysis of Compositional Data. *Journal of the Royal Statistical Society Series B (Methodological)* 44, 139–177.

Alshawaqfeh, M., Serpedin, E., Younes, A.B., 2017. Inferring microbial interaction networks from metagenomic data using SgLV-EKF algorithm. *BMC Genomics* 18, 228–228.

Ambardar, S., Gupta, R., Trakroo, D., Lal, R., Vakhlu, J., 2016. High throughput sequencing: an overview of sequencing chemistry. *Indian Journal of Microbiology* 56, 394–404.

Arndt, D., Xia, J., Liu, Y., Zhou, Y., Guo, A.C., Cruz, J.A., Sinelnikov, I., Budwill, K., Nesbo, C.L., Wishart, D.S., 2012. METAGENassist: a comprehensive web server for comparative metagenomics. *Nucleic Acids Research* 40, W88–95.

Baker, P.I., Love, D.R., Ferguson, L.R., 2009. Role of gut microbiota in Crohn's disease. *Expert Review of Gastroenterology & Hepatology* 3, 535–546.

Balvočiūtė, M., Huson, D.H., 2017. SILVA, RDP, Greengenes, NCBI and OTT — how do these taxonomies compare? *BMC Genomics* 18, 114.

Barberán, A., Bates, S.T., Casamayor, E.O., Fierer, N., 2012. Using network analysis to explore co-occurrence patterns in soil microbial communities. *ISME Journal* 6, 343–351.

Bauman, J.G.J., Wiegant, J., Borst, P., van Duijn, P., 1980. A new method for fluorescence microscopical localization of specific DNA sequences by in situ hybridization of fluorochrome-labelled RNA. *Experimental Cell Research* 128, 485–490.

Bentley, D.R., Balasubramanian, S., Swerdlow, H.P., Smith, G.P., Milton, J., Brown, C.G., Hall, K.P., Evers, D.J., Barnes, C.L., Bignell, H.R., 2008. Accurate whole human genome sequencing using reversible terminator chemistry. *Nature* 456, 53.

Berry, D., Widder, S., 2014. Deciphering microbial interactions and detecting keystone species with co-occurrence networks. *Frontiers in Microbiology* 5, 219.

Besser, J., Carleton, H.A., Gerner-Smidt, P., Lindsey, R.L., Trees, E., 2018. Next-generation sequencing technologies and their application to the study and control of bacterial infections. *Clinical Microbiology and Infection* 24, 335–341.

Bolyen, E., Rideout, J.R., Dillon, M.R., Bokulich, N.A., Abnet, C.C., Al-Ghalith, G.A., Alexander, H., Alm, E.J., Arumugam, M., Asnicar, F., Bai, Y., Bisanz, J.E., Bittinger, K., Brejnrod, A., Brislawn, C.J., Brown, C.T., Callahan, B.J., Caraballo-Rodríguez, A.M., Chase, J., Cope, E.K., Da Silva, R., Diener, C., Dorrestein, P.C., Douglas, G.M., Durall, D.M., Duvallet, C., Edwardson, C.F., Ernst, M., Estaki, M., Fouquier, J., Gauglitz, J.M., Gibbons, S.M., Gibson, D.L., Gonzalez, A., Gorlick, K., Guo, J., Hillmann, B., Holmes, S., Holste, H., Huttenhower, C., Huttley, G.A., Janssen, S., Jarmusch, A.K., Jiang, L., Kaehler, B.D., Kang, K.B., Keefe, C.R., Keim, P., Kelley, S.T., Knights, D., Koester, I., Kosciolek, T., Kreps, J., Langille, M.G.I., Lee, J., Ley, R., Liu, Y.-X., Loftfield, E., Lozupone, C., Maher, M., Marotz, C., Martin, B.D., McDonald, D., McIver, L.J., Melnik, A.V., Metcalf, J.L., Morgan, S.C., Morton, J.T., Naimey, A.T., Navas-Molina, J.A., Nothias, L.F., Orchanian, S.B., Pearson, T., Peoples, S.L., Petras, D., Preuss, M.L., Pruesse, E., Rasmussen, L.B., Rivers, A., Robeson, M.S., Rosenthal, P., Segata, N., Shaffer, M., Shiffer, A., Sinha, R., Song, S.J., Spear, J.R., Swafford, A.D., Thompson, L.R., Torres, P.J., Trinh, P., Tripathi, A., Turnbaugh, P.J., Ul-Hasan, S., van der Hooft, J.J.J., Vargas, F., Vázquez-Baeza, Y., Vogtmann, E., von Hippel, M., Walters, W., Wan, Y., Wang, M., Warren, J., Weber, K.C., Williamson, C.H.D., Willis, A.D., Xu, Z.Z., Zaneveld, J.R., Zhang, Y., Zhu, Q., Knight, R., Caporaso, J.G., 2019. Reproducible, interactive, scalable and extensible microbiome data science using QIIME 2. *Nature Biotechnology* 37, 852–857.

Branton, D., Deamer, D.W., Marziali, A., Bayley, H., Benner, S.A., Butler, T., Di Ventra, M., Garaj, S., Hibbs, A., Huang, X., Jovanovich, S.B., Krstic, P.S., Lindsay, S., Ling, X.S., Mastrangelo, C.H., Meller, A., Oliver, J.S., Pershin, Y.V., Ramsey, J.M., Riehn, R., Soni, G.V., Tabard-Cossa, V., Wanunu, M., Wiggin, M., and Schloss, J.A., 2008. The potential and challenges of nanopore sequencing. *Nature Biotechnology* 26, 1146–1153.

Brill, B., Amir, A., Heller, R., 2019. Testing for differential abundance in compositional counts data, with application to microbiome studies. arXiv preprint arXiv:1904.08937.

Brisson, V., Schmidt, J., Northen, T.R., Vogel, J.P., Gaudin, A., 2019. A new method to correct for habitat filtering in microbial correlation networks. *Frontiers in Microbiology* 10, 585.

Buza, T.M., Tonui, T., Stomeo, F., Tiambo, C., Katani, R., Schilling, M., Lyimo, B., Gwakisa, P., Cattadori, I.M., Buza, J., 2019. iMAP: an integrated bioinformatics and visualization pipeline for microbiome data analysis. *BMC Bioinformatics* 20, 1–18.

Callahan, B.J., Wong, J., Heiner, C., Oh, S., Theriot, C.M., Gulati, A.S., McGill, S.K., Dougherty, M.K., 2019. High-throughput amplicon sequencing of the full-length 16S rRNA gene with single-nucleotide resolution. BioRxiv, 392332.

Cani, P.D., Delzenne, N.M., 2011. The gut microbiome as therapeutic target. *Pharmacology & Therapeutics* 130, 202–212.

Caporaso, J.G., Kuczynski, J., Stombaugh, J., Bittinger, K., Bushman, F.D., Costello, E.K., Fierer, N., Pena, A.G., Goodrich, J.K., Gordon, J.I., 2010. QIIME allows analysis of high-throughput community sequencing data. *Nature Methods* 7, 335.

Case, R. J., Boucher, Y., Dahllöf, I., Holmström, C., Doolittle, W. F., & Kjelleberg, S., 2007. Use of 16S rRNA and rpoB genes as molecular markers for microbial ecology studies. *Applied and Environmental Microbiology* 73, 278–288.

Chakravorty, S., Helb, D., Burday, M., Connell, N., Alland, D., 2007. A detailed analysis of 16S ribosomal RNA gene segments for the diagnosis of pathogenic bacteria. *Journal of Microbiological Methods* 69, 330–339.

Cole, J.R., Wang, Q., Cardenas, E., Fish, J., Chai, B., Farris, R.J., Kulam-Syed-Mohideen, A.S., McGarrell, D.M., Marsh, T., Garrity, G.M., Tiedje, J.M., 2009. The Ribosomal Database Project: improved alignments and new tools for rRNA analysis. *Nucleic Acids Research* 37, D141–D145.

Cole, J.R., Wang, Q., Fish, J.A., Chai, B., McGarrell, D.M., Sun, Y., Brown, C.T., Porras-Alfaro, A., Kuske, C.R., Tiedje, J.M., 2013. Ribosomal Database Project: data and tools for high throughput rRNA analysis. *Nucleic Acids Research* 42, D633–D642.

Crocetti, G.R., Hugenholtz, P., Bond, P.L., Schuler, A., Keller, J., Jenkins, D., Blackall, L.L., 2000. Identification of polyphosphate-accumulating organisms and design of 16S rRNA-directed probes for their detection and quantitation. *Applied and Environmental Microbiology* 66, 1175–1182.

Culman, S.W., Bukowski, R., Gauch, H.G., Cadillo-Quiroz, H., Buckley, D.H., 2009. T-REX: software for the processing and analysis of T-RFLP data. *BMC Bioinformatics* 10, 171.

D'Amore, R., Ijaz, U.Z., Schirmer, M., Kenny, J.G., Gregory, R., Darby, A.C., Shakya, M., Podar, M., Quince, C., Hall, N., 2016. A comprehensive benchmarking study of protocols and sequencing platforms for 16S rRNA community profiling. *BMC Genomics* 17, 55.

DeSantis, T.Z., Brodie, E.L., Moberg, J.P., Zubieta, I.X., Piceno, Y.M., Andersen, G.L., 2007. High-density universal 16S rRNA microarray analysis reveals broader diversity than typical clone library when sampling the environment. *Microbial Ecology* 53, 371–383.

DeSantis, T.Z., Hugenholtz, P., Larsen, N., Rojas, M., Brodie, E.L., Keller, K., Huber, T., Dalevi, D., Hu, P., Andersen, G.L., 2006. Greengenes, a chimera-checked 16S rRNA gene database and workbench compatible with ARB. *Applied and Environmental Microbiology* 72, 5069–5072.

Deshpande, N.P., Riordan, S.M., Castaño-Rodríguez, N., Wilkins, M.R., Kaakoush, N.O., 2018. Signatures within the esophageal microbiome are associated with host genetics, age, and disease. *Microbiome* 6, 227.

Dhariwal, A., Chong, J., Habib, S., King, I.L., Agellon, L.B., Xia, J., 2017. MicrobiomeAnalyst: a web-based tool for comprehensive statistical, visual and meta-analysis of microbiome data. *Nucleic Acids Research* 45, W180–w188.

Duerkop, B.A., Vaishnava, S., Hooper, L.V., 2009. Immune responses to the microbiota at the intestinal mucosal surface. *Immunity* 31, 368–376.

Earl, J.P., Adappa, N.D., Krol, J., Bhat, A.S., Balashov, S., Ehrlich, R.L., Palmer, J.N., Workman, A.D., Blasetti, M., Sen, B., 2018. Species-level bacterial community profiling of the healthy sinonasal microbiome using Pacific Biosciences sequencing of full-length 16S rRNA genes. *Microbiome* 6, 190.

Egozcue, J.J., Pawlowsky-Glahn, V., 2005. Groups of Parts and Their Balances in Compositional Data Analysis. *Mathematical Geology* 37, 795–828.

El Aidy, S., Van Baarlen, P., Derrien, M., Lindenbergh-Kortleve, D.J., Hooiveld, G., Levenez, F., Doré, J., Dekker, J., Samsom, J.N., Nieuwenhuis, E.E., 2012. Temporal and spatial interplay of microbiota and intestinal mucosa drive establishment of immune homeostasis in conventionalized mice. *Mucosal Immunology* 5, 567.

Ellis, C.L., Ma, Z.-M., Mann, S.K., Li, C.-S., Wu, J., Knight, T.H., Yotter, T., Hayes, T.L., Maniar, A.H., Troia-Cancio, P.V., 2011. Molecular characterization of stool microbiota in HIV-infected subjects by panbacterial and order-level 16S ribosomal DNA (rDNA) quantification and correlations with immune activation. *Journal of Acquired Immune Deficiency Syndromes (1999)* 57, 363.

Escudié, F., Auer, L., Bernard, M., Mariadassou, M., Cauquil, L., Vidal, K., Maman, S., Hernandez-Raquet, G., Combes, S., Pascal, G., 2017. FROGS: find, rapidly, OTUs with galaxy solution. *Bioinformatics* 34, 1287–1294.

Fang, H., Huang, C., Zhao, H., Deng, M., 2015. CCLasso: correlation inference for compositional data through Lasso. *Bioinformatics* 31, 3172–3180.

Faust, K., Sathirapongsasuti, J.F., Izard, J., Segata, N., Gevers, D., Raes, J., Huttenhower, C., 2012. Microbial co-occurrence relationships in the human microbiome. *PLoS Computational Biology* 8, e1002606.

Fernandes, A.D., Reid, J.N.S., Macklaim, J.M., McMurrough, T.A., Edgell, D.R., Gloor, G.B., 2014. Unifying the analysis of high-throughput sequencing datasets: characterizing RNA-seq, 16S rRNA gene sequencing and selective growth experiments by compositional data analysis. *Microbiome* 2, 15.

Finstad, K.M., Probst, A.J., Thomas, B.C., Andersen, G.L., Demergasso, C., Echeverría, A., Amundson, R.G., Banfield, J.F., 2017. Microbial community structure and the persistence of cyanobacterial populations in salt crusts of the Hyperarid Atacama Desert from genome-resolved metagenomics. *Frontiers in Microbiology* 8, 1435.

Fisher, C.K., Mehta, P., 2014. Identifying keystone species in the human gut microbiome from metagenomic timeseries using sparse linear regression. *PLoS One* 9, e102451.

Foster, Z.S.L., Sharpton, T.J., Grünwald, N.J., 2017. Metacoder: an R package for visualization and manipulation of community taxonomic diversity data. *PLOS Computational Biology* 13, e1005404.

Fox, J.G., Feng, Y., Theve, E.J., Raczynski, A., Fiala, J.L., Doernte, A.L., Williams, M., McFaline, J., Essigmann, J., Schauer, D., 2010. Gut microbes define liver cancer risk in mice exposed to chemical and viral transgenic hepatocarcinogens. *Gut* 59, 88–97.

Fredriksson, N.J., Hermansson, M., Wilén, B.-M., 2014. Tools for T-RFLP data analysis using Excel. *BMC Bioinformatics* 15, 361.

Freilich, S., Kreimer, A., Meilijson, I., Gophna, U., Sharan, R., Ruppin, E., 2010. The large-scale organization of the bacterial network of ecological co-occurrence interactions. *Nucleic Acids Research* 38, 3857–3868.

Friedman, J., Alm, E.J., 2012. Inferring correlation networks from genomic survey data. *PLoS Computational Biology* 8, e1002687.

Gao, X., Huynh, B.-T., Guillemot, D., Glaser, P., Opatowski, L., 2018. Inference of significant microbial interactions from longitudinal metagenomics data. *Frontiers in Microbiology* 9, 2319.

Ginige, M.P., Hugenholtz, P., Daims, H., Wagner, M., Keller, J., Blackall, L.L., 2004. Use of stable-isotope probing, full-cycle rRNA analysis, and fluorescence in situ hybridization-microautoradiography to study a methanol-fed denitrifying microbial community. *Applied and Environmental Microbiology* 70, 588–596.

Gloor, G.B., Hummelen, R., Macklaim, J.M., Dickson, R.J., Fernandes, A.D., MacPhee, R., Reid, G., 2010. Microbiome profiling by illumina sequencing of combinatorial sequence-tagged PCR products. *PLoS One* 5, e15406.

Gloor, G.B., Macklaim, J.M., Pawlowsky-Glahn, V., Egozcue, J.J., 2017. Microbiome datasets are compositional: and this is not optional. *Frontiers in Microbiology* 8, 2224.

Gonze, D., Coyte, K.Z., Lahti, L., Faust, K., 2018. Microbial communities as dynamical systems. *Current Opinion in Microbiology* 44, 41–49.

Green, M.R., Sambrook, J., 2012. *Molecular cloning. A laboratory manual 4th.* Cold Spring Harbor Laboratory Press, New York.

Guillamön, J.M., Sabaté, J., Barrio, E., Cano, J., Querol, A., 1998. Rapid identification of wine yeast species based on RFLP analysis of the ribosomal internal transcribed spacer (ITS) region. *Archives of Microbiology* 169, 387–392.

Guillou, L., Bachar, D., Audic, S., Bass, D., Berney, C., Bittner, L., Boutte, C., Burgaud, G., de Vargas, C., Decelle, J., Del Campo, J., Dolan, J.R., Dunthorn, M., Edvardsen, B., Holzmann, M., Kooistra, W.H., Lara, E., Le Bescot, N., Logares, R., Mahe, F., Massana, R., Montresor, M., Morard, R., Not, F., Pawlowski, J., Probert, I., Sauvadet, A.L., Siano, R., Stoeck, T., Vaulot, D., Zimmermann, P., Christen, R., 2013. The Protist Ribosomal Reference database (PR2): a catalog of unicellular eukaryote small sub-unit rRNA sequences with curated taxonomy. *Nucleic Acids Research* 41, D597–604.

Gužvić, M., 2013. The history of DNA sequencing/ISTORIJAT SEKVENCIRANJA DNK. *Journal of Medical Biochemistry* 32, 301–312.

Hawinkel, S., Mattiello, F., Bijnens, L., Thas, O., 2017. A broken promise: microbiome differential abundance methods do not control the false discovery rate. *Briefings in Bioinformatics* 20, 210–221.

Heintz-Buschart, A., Wilmes, P., 2018. Human gut microbiome: function matters. *Trends in Microbiology* 26, 563–574.

Hugenholtz, P., Tyson, G.W., Blackall, L.L., 2002. *Design and evaluation of 16S rRNA-targeted oligonucleotide probes for fluorescence in situ hybridization, Gene probes.* Humana Press, Totowa, NJ, pp. 29–42.

Iszatt, N., Janssen, S., Lenters, V., Dahl, C., Stigum, H., Knight, R., Mandal, S., Peddada, S., González, A., Midtvedt, T., Eggesbø, M., 2019. Environmental toxicants in breast milk of Norwegian mothers and gut bacteria composition and metabolites in their infants at 1 month. *Microbiome* 7, 34.

Jackson, M.A., Bonder, M.J., Kuncheva, Z., Zierer, J., Fu, J., Kurilshikov, A., Wijmenga, C., Zhernakova, A., Bell, J.T., Spector, T.D., 2018. Detection of stable community structures within gut microbiota co-occurrence networks from different human populations. *PeerJournal* 6, e4303.

Joossens, M., Huys, G., Cnockaert, M., De Preter, V., Verbeke, K., Rutgeerts, P., Vandamme, P., Vermeire, S., 2011. Dysbiosis of the faecal microbiota in patients with Crohn's disease and their unaffected relatives. *Gut* 60, 631–637.

Kageyama, S., Takeshita, T., Takeuchi, K., Asakawa, M., Matsumi, R., Furuta, M., Shibata, Y., Nagai, K., Ikebe, M., Morita, M., Masuda, M., Toh, Y., Kiyohara, Y., Ninomiya, T., Yamashita, Y., 2019. Characteristics of the salivary microbiota in patients with various digestive tract cancers. *Frontiers in Microbiology* 10, 1780.

Kaul, A., Mandal, S., Davidov, O., Peddada, S.D., 2017. Analysis of microbiome data in the presence of excess zeros. *Frontiers in Microbiology* 8, 2114–2114.

Klindworth, A., Pruesse, E., Schweer, T., Peplies, J., Quast, C., Horn, M., Glöckner, F.O., 2012. Evaluation of general 16S ribosomal RNA gene PCR primers for classical and next-generation sequencing-based diversity studies. *Nucleic Acids Research* 41, e1.

Koskinen, K., Pausan, M.R., Perras, A.K., Beck, M., Bang, C., Mora, M., Schilhabel, A., Schmitz, R., Moissl-Eichinger, C., 2017. First insights into the diverse human archaeome: specific detection of archaea in the gastrointestinal tract, lung, and nose and on skin. *MBio* 8, e00824-17.

Kozich, J.J., Westcott, S.L., Baxter, N.T., Highlander, S.K., Schloss, P.D., 2013. Development of a dual-index sequencing strategy and curation pipeline for analyzing amplicon sequence data on the MiSeq Illumina sequencing platform. *Applied and Environmental Microbiology* 79, 5112–5120.

Kuperman, A.A., Zimmerman, A., Hamadia, S., Ziv, O., Gurevich, V., Fichtman, B., Gavert, N., Straussman, R., Rechnitzer, H., Barzilay, M., 2019. Deep microbial analysis of multiple placentas shows no evidence for a placental microbiome. *BJOG: An International Journal of Obstetrics & Gynaecology* 127, 159–169.

Kurtz, Z.D., Müller, C.L., Miraldi, E.R., Littman, D.R., Blaser, M.J., Bonneau, R.A., 2015. Sparse and Compositionally Robust Inference of Microbial Ecological Networks. *PLoS Computational Biology* 11, e1004226.

Lam, H.Y., Clark, M.J., Chen, R., Chen, R., Natsoulis, G., O'huallachain, M., Dewey, F.E., Habegger, L., Ashley, E.A., Gerstein, M.B., 2012. Performance comparison of whole-genome sequencing platforms. *Nature Biotechnology* 30, 78.

Langfelder, P., Horvath, S., 2008. WGCNA: an R package for weighted correlation network analysis. *BMC Bioinformatics* 9, 559.

Langille, M.G.I., Zaneveld, J., Caporaso, J.G., McDonald, D., Knights, D., Reyes, J.A., Clemente, J.C., Burkepile, D.E., Vega Thurber, R.L., Knight, R., Beiko, R.G., Huttenhower, C., 2013. Predictive functional profiling of microbial communities using 16S rRNA marker gene sequences. *Nature Biotechnology* 31, 814–821.

Lê Cao, K.-A., Costello, M.-E., Lakis, V.A., Bartolo, F., Chua, X.-Y., Brazeilles, R., Rondeau, P., 2016. MixMC: a multivariate statistical framework to gain insight into microbial communities. *PLoS One* 11, e0160169.

Leaw, S.N., Chang, H.C., Sun, H.F., Barton, R., Bouchara, J.-P., Chang, T.C., 2006. Identification of medically important yeast species by sequence analysis of the internal transcribed spacer regions. *Journal of Clinical Microbiology* 44, 693–699.

LeBlanc, J.G., Milani, C., de Giori, G.S., Sesma, F., van Sinderen, D., Ventura, M., 2013. Bacteria as vitamin suppliers to their host: a gut microbiota perspective. *Current Opinion in Biotechnology* 24, 160–168.

Lee, I., Ouk Kim, Y., Park, S.C., Chun, J., 2016. OrthoANI: An improved algorithm and software for calculating average nucleotide identity. *International Journal of System and Evolutionary Microbiology* 66, 1100–1103.

Ley, R.E., 2010. Obesity and the human microbiome. *Current Opinion in Gastroenterology* 26, 5–11.

Li, R.W., Wu, S., Vi, R.L.B., Li, W., Li, C., 2012. Perturbation dynamics of the rumen microbiota in response to exogenous butyrate. *PloS One* 7, e29392.

Lim, K.M.K., Li, C., Chng, K.R., Nagarajan, N., 2016. @ MInter: automated text-mining of microbial interactions. *Bioinformatics* 32, 2981–2987.

Liu, F., Wang, T.T.Y., Tang, Q., Xue, C., Li, R.W., Wu, V.C.H., 2019. Malvidin 3-glucoside modulated gut microbial dysbiosis and global metabolome disrupted in a murine colitis model induced by dextran sulfate sodium. *Molecular Nutrition & Food Research* 63, e1900455.

Lo, C., Marculescu, R., 2017. MPLasso: inferring microbial association networks using prior microbial knowledge. *PLoS Computational Biology* 13, e1005915.

Lo Presti, A., Zorzi, F., Del Chierico, F., Altomare, A., Cocca, S., Avola, A., De Biasio, F., Russo, A., Cella, E., Reddel, S., Calabrese, E., Biancone, L., Monteleone, G., Cicala, M., Angeletti, S., Ciccozzi, M., Putignani, L., Guarino, M.P.L., 2019. Fecal and mucosal microbiota profiling in irritable bowel syndrome and inflammatory bowel disease. *Frontiers in Microbiology* 10, 1655.

López-García, A., Pineda-Quiroga, C., Atxaerandio, R., Pérez, A., Hernández, I., García-Rodríguez, A., González-Recio, O., 2018. Comparison of mothur and QIIME for the analysis of rumen microbiota composition based on 16S rRNA amplicon sequences. *Frontiers in Microbiology* 9, 3010.

Lozupone, C., Knight, R., 2005. UniFrac: a new phylogenetic method for comparing microbial communities. *Applied and Environmental Microbiology* 71, 8228–8235.

Mandal, S., Van Treuren, W., White, R.A., Eggesbø, M., Knight, R., Peddada, S.D., 2015. Analysis of composition of microbiomes: a novel method for studying microbial composition. *Microbial Ecology in Health and Disease* 26, 27663.

Marchesi, J.R., Ravel, J., 2015. The vocabulary of microbiome research: a proposal. *Microbiome* 3, 1–3.

Marsh, T.L., 1999. Terminal restriction fragment length polymorphism (T-RFLP): an emerging method for characterizing diversity among homologous populations of amplification products. *Current Opinion in Microbiology* 2, 323–327.

McDonald, D., Price, M.N., Goodrich, J., Nawrocki, E.P., DeSantis, T.Z., Probst, A., Andersen, G.L., Knight, R., Hugenholtz, P., 2012. An improved Greengenes taxonomy with explicit ranks for ecological and evolutionary analyses of bacteria and archaea. *ISME Journal* 6, 610.

McHardy, I.H., Li, X., Tong, M., Ruegger, P., Jacobs, J., Borneman, J., Anton, P., Braun, J., 2013. HIV Infection is associated with compositional and functional shifts in the rectal mucosal microbiota. *Microbiome* 1, 26.

McMurdie, P.J., Holmes, S., 2014. Waste not, want not: why rarefying microbiome data is inadmissible. *PLOS Computational Biology* 10, e1003531.

Meyer, F., Paarmann, D., D'Souza, M., Olson, R., Glass, E.M., Kubal, M., Paczian, T., Rodriguez, A., Stevens, R., Wilke, A., Wilkening, J., Edwards, R.A., 2008. The metagenomics RAST server – a public resource for the automatic phylogenetic and functional analysis of metagenomes. *BMC Bioinformatics* 9, 386.

Mitra, S., Stärk, M., Huson, D.H., 2011. Analysis of 16S rRNA environmental sequences using MEGAN. *BMC Genomics* 12, S17.

Morton, J.T., Sanders, J., Quinn, R.A., McDonald, D., Gonzalez, A., Vázquez-Baeza, Y., Navas-Molina, J.A., Song, S.J., Metcalf, J.L., Hyde, E.R., Lladser, M., Dorrestein, P.C., Knight, R., 2017. Balance trees reveal microbial niche differentiation. *MSystems* 2, e00162-16.

Muyzer, G., De Waal, E.C., Uitterlinden, A.G., 1993. Profiling of complex microbial populations by denaturing gradient gel electrophoresis analysis of polymerase chain reaction-amplified genes coding for 16S rRNA. *Applied and Environmental Microbiology* 59, 695–700.

Muyzer, G., Smalla, K., 1998. Application of denaturing gradient gel electrophoresis (DGGE) and temperature gradient gel electrophoresis (TGGE) in microbial ecology. *Antonie van Leeuwenhoek* 73, 127–141.

Nakano, Y., Takeshita, T., Yamashita, Y., 2006. TRFMA: a web-based tool for terminal restriction fragment length polymorphism analysis based on molecular weight. *Bioinformatics* 22, 1788–1789.

Nelder, J.A., Mead, R., 1965. A simplex method for function minimization. *The Computer Journal* 7, 308–313.

Nilsson, R.H., Larsson, K.-H., Taylor, A.F S., Bengtsson-Palme, J., Jeppesen, T.S., Schigel, D., Kennedy, P., Picard, K., Glöckner, F.O., Tedersoo, L., Saar, I., Kõljalg, U., Abarenkov, K., 2018. The UNITE database for molecular identification of fungi: handling dark taxa and parallel taxonomic classifications. *Nucleic Acids Research* 47, D259–D264.

Olesen, J.M., Bascompte, J., Dupont, Y.L., Jordano, P., 2007. The modularity of pollination networks. *Proceedings of the National Academy of Sciences of the United States of America* 104, 19891–19896.

Oliver, J.D., 2005. The viable but nonculturable state in bacteria. *The Journal of Microbiology* 43, 93–100.

Osborn, A.M., Moore, E.R., Timmis, K.N., 2000. An evaluation of terminal-restriction fragment length polymorphism (T-RFLP) analysis for the study of microbial community structure and dynamics. *Environmental Microbiology* 2, 39–50.

Pace, N.R., Stahl, D.A., Lane, D.J., Olsen, G.J., 1986. The analysis of natural microbial populations by ribosomal RNA sequences. In: Marshall, K.C. (eds) *Advances in microbial ecology*. Springer, Boston, MA, pp. 1–55.

Pallmann, P., Schaarschmidt, F., Hothorn, L.A., Fischer, C., Nacke, H., Priesnitz, K.U., Schork, N.J., 2012. Assessing group differences in biodiversity by simultaneously testing a user-defined selection of diversity indices. *Molecular Ecology Resources* 12, 1068–1078.

Paulson, J.N., Stine, O.C., Bravo, H.C., Pop, M., 2013. Differential abundance analysis for microbial marker-gene surveys. *Nature Methods* 10, 1200–1202.

Peterson, C.T., Sharma, V., Iablokov, S.N., Albayrak, L., Khanipov, K., Uchitel, S., Chopra, D., Mills, P.J., Fofanov, Y., Rodionov, D.A., Peterson, S.N., 2019. 16S rRNA gene profiling and genome reconstruction reveal community metabolic interactions and prebiotic potential of medicinal herbs used in neurodegenerative disease and as nootropics. *PLoS One* 14, e0213869.

Pruesse, E., Quast, C., Knittel, K., Fuchs, B.M., Ludwig, W., Peplies, J., Glöckner, F.O., 2007. SILVA: a comprehensive online resource for quality checked and aligned ribosomal RNA sequence data compatible with ARB. *Nucleic Acids Research* 35, 7188–7196.

Puri, P., Liangpunsakul, S., Christensen, J.E., Shah, V.H., Kamath, P.S., Gores, G.J., Walker, S., Comerford, M., Katz, B., Borst, A., Yu, Q., Kumar, D.P., Mirshahi, F., Radaeva, S., Chalasani, N.P., Crabb, D.W., Sanyal, A.J., 2018. The circulating microbiome signature and inferred functional metagenomics in alcoholic hepatitis. *Hepatology* 67, 1284–1302.

Quast, C., Pruesse, E., Yilmaz, P., Gerken, J., Schweer, T., Yarza, P., Peplies, J., Glöckner, F.O., 2012. The SILVA ribosomal RNA gene database project: improved data processing and web-based tools. *Nucleic Acids Research* 41, D590–D596.

Quinn, T.P., Erb, I., Gloor, G., Notredame, C., Richardson, M.F., Crowley, T.M., 2019. A field guide for the compositional analysis of any-omics data. *GigaScience* 8, giz107.

Rhoads, A., Au, K.F., 2015. PacBio sequencing and its applications. *Genomics, Proteomics & Bioinformatics* 13, 278–289.

Rivera-Pinto, J., Egozcue, J.J., Pawlowsky-Glahn, V., Paredes, R., Noguera-Julian, M., Calle, M.L., 2018. Balances: a new perspective for microbiome analysis. *MSystems* 3, e00053-00018.

Rooks, M.G., Garrett, W.S., 2016. Gut microbiota, metabolites and host immunity. *Nature Reviews Immunology* 16, 341–352.

Ruan, Q., Dutta, D., Schwalbach, M.S., Steele, J.A., Fuhrman, J.A., Sun, F., 2006. Local similarity analysis reveals unique associations among marine bacterioplankton species and environmental factors. *Bioinformatics* 22, 2532–2538.

Salipante, S. J., Kawashima, T., Rosenthal, C., Hoogestraat, D. R., Cummings, L. A., Sengupta, D. J., Harkins, T. T., Cookson, B. T., & Hoffman, N. G., 2014. Performance comparison of Illumina and ion torrent next-generation sequencing platforms for 16S rRNA-based bacterial community profiling. *Applied and environmental microbiology* 80, 7583–7591.

Sansonetti, P.J., Di Santo, J.P., 2007. Debugging how bacteria manipulate the immune response. *Immunity* 26, 149–161.

Schaechter, M., 2015. A brief history of bacterial growth physiology. *Frontiers in Microbiology* 6, 289–289.

Schloss, P.D., Westcott, S.L., Ryabin, T., Hall, J.R., Hartmann, M., Hollister, E.B., Lesniewski, R.A., Oakley, B.B., Parks, D.H., Robinson, C.J., 2009. Introducing mothur: open-source, platform-independent, community-supported software for describing and comparing microbial communities. *Applied and Environmental Microbiology* 75, 7537–7541.

Schoch, C.L., Seifert, K.A., Huhndorf, S., Robert, V., Spouge, J.L., Levesque, C.A., Chen, W., Fungal Barcoding, C., Fungal Barcoding Consortium Author List, 2012. Nuclear ribosomal internal transcribed spacer (ITS) region as a universal DNA barcode marker for fungi. *Proceedings of the National Academy of Sciences of the United States of America* 109, 6241–6246.

Schwiertz, A., Jacobi, M., Frick, J.-S., Richter, M., Rusch, K., Köhler, H., 2010. Microbiota in pediatric inflammatory bowel disease. *The Journal of Pediatrics* 157, 240–244.

Segata, N., Izard, J., Waldron, L., Gevers, D., Miropolsky, L., Garrett, W.S., Huttenhower, C., 2011. Metagenomic biomarker discovery and explanation. *Genome Biology* 12, R60.

Segata, N., Waldron, L., Ballarini, A., Narasimhan, V., Jousson, O., Huttenhower, C., 2012. Metagenomic microbial community profiling using unique clade-specific marker genes. *Nat Methods* 9, 811–814.

Sender, R., Fuchs, S., Milo, R., 2016. Revised estimates for the number of human and bacteria cells in the body. *PLoS Biolgy* 14, e1002533–e1002533.

Shin, J., Lee, S., Go, M.-J., Lee, S.Y., Kim, S.C., Lee, C.-H., Cho, B.-K., 2016. Analysis of the mouse gut microbiome using full-length 16S rRNA amplicon sequencing. *Scientific Reports* 6, 29681.

Sims, T.T., Colbert, L.E., Zheng, J., Delgado Medrano, A.Y., Hoffman, K.L., Ramondetta, L., Jazaeri, A., Jhingran, A., Schmeler, K.M., Daniel, C.R., Klopp, A., 2019. Gut microbial diversity and genus-level differences identified in cervical cancer patients versus healthy controls. *Gynecol Oncology* 155, 237–244.

Soergel, D.A., Dey, N., Knight, R., Brenner, S.E., 2012. Selection of primers for optimal taxonomic classification of environmental 16S rRNA gene sequences. *ISME Journal* 6, 1440.

Sommer, F., Bäckhed, F., 2013. The gut microbiota—masters of host development and physiology. *Nature Reviews Microbiology* 11, 227.

Stevens, J.R., Jones, T.R., Lefevre, M., Ganesan, B., Weimer, B.C., 2017. SigTree: a microbial community analysis tool to identify and visualize significantly responsive branches in a phylogenetic tree. *Computational and Structural Biotechnology Journal* 15, 372–378.

Stinson, L.F., Boyce, M.C., Payne, M.S., Keelan, J.A., 2019. The not-so-sterile womb: evidence that the human fetus is exposed to bacteria prior to birth. *Frontiers in Microbiology* 10, 1124.

Theis, K.R., Romero, R., Winters, A.D., Greenberg, J.M., Gomez-Lopez, N., Alhousseini, A., Bieda, J., Maymon, E., Pacora, P., Fettweis, J.M., 2019. Does the human placenta delivered at term have a microbiota? Results of cultivation, quantitative real-time PCR, 16S rRNA gene sequencing, and metagenomics. *American Journal of Obstetrics and Gynecology* 220, e261–e267.

Thijs, S., Op De Beeck, M., Beckers, B., Truyens, S., Stevens, V., Van Hamme, J.D., Weyens, N., Vangronsveld, J., 2017. Comparative evaluation of four bacteria-specific primer pairs for 16S rRNA gene surveys. *Frontiers in Microbiology* 8, 494.

Tringe, S.G., Hugenholtz, P., 2008. A renaissance for the pioneering 16S rRNA gene. *Current Opinion in Microbiology* 11, 442–446.

Trussart, M., Yus, E., Martinez, S., Baù, D., Tahara, Y.O., Pengo, T., Widjaja, M., Kretschmer, S., Swoger, J., Djordjevic, S., Turnbull, L., Whitchurch, C., Miyata, M., Marti-Renom, M.A., Lluch-Senar, M., Serrano, L., 2017. Defined chromosome structure in the genome-reduced bacterium mycoplasma pneumoniae. *Nature Communications* 8, 14665.

Voelkerding, K.V., Dames, S.A., Durtschi, J.D., 2009. Next-generation sequencing: from basic research to diagnostics. *Clinical Chemistry* 55, 641–658.

v. Wintzingerode, F., Göbel, U.B., Stackebrandt, E., 1997. Determination of microbial diversity in environmental samples: pitfalls of PCR-based rRNA analysis. *FEMS Microbiology Reviews* 21, 213–229.

Wang, J., Zheng, J., Shi, W., Du, N., Xu, X., Zhang, Y., Ji, P., Zhang, F., Jia, Z., Wang, Y., 2018. Dysbiosis of maternal and neonatal microbiota associated with gestational diabetes mellitus. *Gut* 67, 1614–1625.

Watts, S.C., Ritchie, S.C., Inouye, M., Holt, K.E., 2018. FastSpar: rapid and scalable correlation estimation for compositional data. *Bioinformatics* 35, 1064–1066.

Weiss, S., Van Treuren, W., Lozupone, C., Faust, K., Friedman, J., Deng, Y., Xia, L.C., Xu, Z.Z., Ursell, L., Alm, E.J., Birmingham, A., Cram, J.A., Fuhrman, J.A., Raes, J., Sun, F., Zhou, J., Knight, R., 2016. Correlation detection strategies in microbial data sets vary widely in sensitivity and precision. *ISME Journal* 10, 1669–1681.

Weiss, S., Xu, Z.Z., Peddada, S., Amir, A., Bittinger, K., Gonzalez, A., Lozupone, C., Zaneveld, J.R., Vázquez-Baeza, Y., Birmingham, A., Hyde, E.R., Knight, R., 2017. Normalization and microbial differential abundance strategies depend upon data characteristics. *Microbiome* 5, 27.

Whitman, W.B., Coleman, D.C., Wiebe, W.J., 1998. Prokaryotes: the unseen majority. *Proceedings of the National Academy of Sciences* 95, 6578–6583.

Wilks, J., Golovkina, T., 2012. Influence of microbiota on viral infections. *PLoS Pathogens* 8, e1002681.

Woese, C.R., 1987. Bacterial evolution. *Microbiological Reviews* 51, 221.

Woese, C.R., Fox, G.E., 1977. Phylogenetic structure of the prokaryotic domain: the primary kingdoms. *Proceedings of the National Academy of Sciences* 74, 5088–5090.

Woese, C.R., Kandler, O., Wheelis, M.L., 1990. Towards a natural system of organisms: proposal for the domains archaea, bacteria, and eucarya. *Proceedings of the National Academy of Sciences* 87, 4576–4579.

Wu, I., Kim, H.S., Ben-Yehezkel, T., 2019. A single-molecule long-read survey of human transcriptomes using LoopSeq synthetic long read sequencing. bioRxiv, 532135.

Yang, P., Yu, S., Cheng, L., Ning, K., 2019. Meta-network: optimized species-species network analysis for microbial communities. *BMC Genomics* 20, 187.

Yoon, S.-H., Ha, S.-M., Kwon, S., Lim, J., Kim, Y., Seo, H., Chun, J., 2017. Introducing EzBioCloud: a taxonomically united database of 16S rRNA gene sequences and whole-genome assemblies. *International Journal of Systematic and Evolutionary Microbiology* 67, 1613.

Zakrzewski, M., Proietti, C., Ellis, J.J., Hasan, S., Brion, M.-J., Berger, B., Krause, L., 2017. Calypso: a user-friendly web-server for mining and visualizing microbiome–environment interactions. *Bioinformatics* 33, 782–783.

# 2 Phageome in Gut Microbiome

*Yujie Zhang, Yen-Te Liao, Logan Tom,*
*Somanshu Sharma, and Vivian C.H. Wu*
United States Department of Agriculture

## CONTENTS

## THE ORIGINS AND ROLES OF PHAGES, PHAGEOME, AND ITS COMPOSITION IN HUMAN GUT MICROBIOTA

Bacteriophages (phages) are viruses that infect bacteria and are the most abundant biological entities in the biosphere, with estimated $10^{31}$ virions (Mushegian, 2020). They are found wherever bacteria live, including soil, water, and the human body, and for instance, approximately 140,000 phage sequences were found to reside in the human intestines (Camarillo-Guerrero et al., 2021; Dalmasso et al., 2014; Roux et al., 2016; Trubl et al., 2018). Within phage populations, there is an amazing diversity of protein structure, genome, and host ranges, and researchers continue to reform the understanding of phages (Hsu et al., 2019). Bacteriophages were first discovered by British bacteriologist Frederick Twort in 1915 when he observed plaques of dead bacteria on plates of bacterial lawns. In 1917, Felix d'Herelle reported an increase of phages in the stools of recovering *Shigella* dysentery patients, paving the way for phage therapy (Letarov, 2020). Although overshadowed by the discovery and widespread use of penicillin antibiotics in 1942, phages have been used extensively in Russia and Georgia to combat bacterial infections in humans. In addtion, bacteriophages have been useful instruments in numerous biological discoveries, such as the mechanisms of translation and DNA replication (Keen, 2015).

DOI: 10.1201/b22970-3

Phages infect bacteria through a lytic or lysogenic life cycle (Howard-Varona et al., 2017; Hsu et al., 2019). Lytic phages (or virulent phages) inject their viral genome into a host bacterium and use host's cellular machinery to replicate their genome and produce viral proteins that can form progeny. Eventually, the host cell is lysed open to release the viral progeny, which goes on to infect more bacteria (Manrique et al., 2017). Lysogenic phages (or temperate phages) insert their genome into a host cell and integrate their DNA into the bacterial host's genome as a prophage or present as a free plasmid called phagemid; thereby, in the lysogenic life cycle, the phage replicates whenever the cell does, without producing progeny (Howard-Varona et al., 2017). After integration of the phage genome, the lytic cycle can be activated via prophage induction from a number of triggers, such as antibiotic stress that is commonly related to the gut environments for disease treatment (Allen et al., 2011; Grif et al., 1998; Sutcliffe et al., 2021; Zhang et al., 2020).

In certain microbiota, phages do not simply live with and infect bacteria, but they play dynamic roles to shape their surroundings. The community of phages (also known as the phageome) in the gut has positive and negative impacts on gastrointestinal fitness and impacts the bacterial community. Specifically, in the human gut, phages in the gastrointestinal (GI) tract affect the microbiota composition by lysing bacteria depending on the density of bacterial species; this drives microbial diversity and evolution and stabilizes the microbial population. Phages can benefit from any viable host bacteria in the gut, where a slight increase in bacteria can quickly lead to a large bloom in phages (Manrique et al., 2017). Some lysogenic phages can transport important genes, such as those involved in anaerobic respiration and macromolecule biosynthesis, between different host cells through transduction, which contributes to the gut microbiota's ecological role (Kieft et al., 2021; Sutcliffe et al., 2021). Furthermore, phages can affect the gut microbiota by removing gut bacteria. A study conducted by Sutcliffe et al. reported that common oral medication, such as nonsteroidal anti-inflammatory drugs (NSAID), inhibited the growth of bacteria in the human gut microbiota by inducing prophages in a species-specific manner, increasing the phage population, and changing the composition of the gut microbiota. However, the mechanisms of functions of NSAIDS are yet to be studied with the gut microbiota (Sutcliffe et al., 2021). The dynamics of phages in the gastrointestinal (GI) tract were further observed by Zuo et al. when researchers collected fecal samples from COVID-19 patients of varying disease severity and used shotgun metagenomics to characterize the gut RNA and DNA viromes (Zuo et al., 2021). COVID-19 patients were shown to have a significant decrease in multiple viruses, including phages, compared to non-COVID-19 patients. Viruses found in COVID-19 patients contained more inflammation- and virulence-associated genes, which affected the metabolism and virulence of bacterial hosts and may contribute to the gastrointestinal symptoms seen in COVID-19 patients. These viruses, including phages, were also inversely correlated with proinflammatory proteins and leukocytes in the blood, which means that phages affect host body immunity. The imbalance of the gut virome in COVID-19 patients again highlights that the proper healthy gut phageome (HGP) is a balanced steady state in the body.

The diversity and abundance of the gut microbiota are not simply present at birth, but in humans, it develops in a newborn's first 2–3 years of life and stabilizes over adult years. The microbiota colonizes within the first 1–4 days of life, where the diversity of the phage community is initially high, but a further steady decrease in overall viral diversity in the first 2.5 years of life leads to a rise in microbial populations and diversity. This eventually revives the viral population through prophage induction, and these induced prophages in the human microbiota become a crucial source of phages in the gut (Manrique et al., 2017). Adult phage communities are relatively stable, and most phages at this time contain dsDNA or ssDNA. A larger *Microviridae* to *Caudovirales* ratio has been correlated with healthier adults, and most are temperate phages (Townsend et al., 2021). At the point of development, the phage virome is also highly varied and sensitive to the individual host gut microbiota, and for each individual, multiple different phages are intertwined and play vital roles in the gut, which cannot be replicated in other individual adults because of diet, environment, and maternal lineages (Hallowell et al., 2021). Although the gut phage composition is mostly unique to the individual, there does exist a reservoir of common phages, notably one example being crAssphage, which was isolated in 73% of 450 global fecal metagenomes. Out of 4,301 phages isolated from two study individuals, 23 "core phages" were found in more than 50% of healthy individuals around the world, questioning the composition of these core phages in the HGP and the role they play in health; it even has been proposed that some of the core phages might play more impactful roles in human health (Norman et al., 2015). In addition, it is still debated whether common phages occur among people in the same environment, such as household members, or among unrelated individuals, and evidence exists to support each view. The details of the HGP are still poorly understood, but partially through predator–prey relationships and lytic–lysogenic balances, an active phageome is key to a healthy and functional gut ecosystem (Manrique et al., 2016).

Ogilvie et al. studied a human gut-specific phage named φB124-14, and phage φB124-14's genome was compared with 611 other human gut phages and 48 chromosomal sequences from its host *Bacteroides fragilis*, which is a normal gut microbe that is essential to healthy GI function (Ogilvie et al., 2012). Although its role in the gut was not precisely defined, researchers found both phages and bacteria in the gut are closely related in their genomes, possibly due to horizontal gene transfer. Therefore, phages and microbes in the gut likely share a very similar ecological niche. In addition, phage φB124-14 still plays a specialized role through its thymidylate synthase gene, which is rare in gut viral genomes and possibly helps with the fitness and function of *B. fragilis* through lysogeny. Since *B. fragilis* is important in human mucosal immunity and nutrition, the findings indicated that phage φB124-1 facilitates this healthy role of gut microbes in the body by transferring essential genes between host cells. The finding by Stern et al. supported the concept that specific phages or taxa of phages in a common phage reservoir in the human population are correlated with human health. Researchers identified 991 phages from the gut microbiota of 124 individuals using sequences found in bacterial CRISPR genes, and 78% of these phages were present in two or more individuals (Stern et al., 2012). In his study, Stern et al. also observed varying ratios of phages and bacteria, some individuals showing dominance in phages or host bacteria, and although temperate phages dominate the phage reservoirs, there are even different ratios of lytic and lysogenic phages, suggesting that the HGP changes over a lifetime and varies among individuals. These findings provide a glimpse into the complex ecology of gut microbiota, and more research is required to fully understand the effect of phages.

The GI tract is a heterogeneous ecosystem that not only contains diverse organisms but also distinguished sub-environments. Different locations in the gut respond differently to food macromolecules, microorganisms, and pathogens, and each organ in the tract is structured differently to fit its role in the digestive system. As a result, distinct microbial communities can grow in different locations in the GI tract (Bushman and Liang, 2021). Because most of the phage genome is still unknown and the gut microbiota is naturally individualized, it is difficult to sample and characterize phages in detail across the GI tract. Therefore, not many studies on the locations of phages in the human gut exist. However, through animal models, several studies have provided an overall profile of phages in the gut to shed more light and provide trends in mammalian gut microbiota. Looft et al. compared the intestinal metagenomes of pigs and found that the ileum displays a significant abundance of phages and phage-related genes, and these numbers remained stable over the month-long study, suggesting that phages are concentrated and consistent in the ileum (Looft et al., 2014). Ileal bacteria, mostly consisting of facultative anaerobes like *Streptococcaceae*, and nutrients that are absorbed in the ileum, such as vitamin $B_{12}$, can make the ileum a more comfortable location for phages to settle, compared to the colon (Hsu et al., 2021). Because of physical barriers in the GI tract, such as the ileocecal valve, the phage profile among organs can be different; despite sharing common phages, the virome of the small intestine and the virome of the large intestine and rectum are ultimately unique, which lends caution to the bias of fecal samples to study the gut virome (Guerin and Hill, 2020).

Phages are also present at high numbers in the mucosa, which lines the epithelial layer of the GI tract, and this limits pathogen colonization in the body. Bao et al. added 8 log PFU/mL of phage PA13076 (isolated from chicken feces) or BP96115 (induced from *Salmonella* Pullorum Spu-109) into mouse models for 31 days to track phages throughout the GI tract; they observed that phages gradually increase toward the end of the GI tract in mice, with the highest phage titer (close to 6.5 log PFU/g) present in feces (Bao et al., 2020). In their study, lytic phages are dormant from the stomach to the jejunum and begin to increase in the ileum and colon reaching their peak in feces, while lysogenic phages maintain relatively higher titers from the stomach to the colon but are highest in feces and the cecum. Generally, phages do not settle in the location of the GI tract that is the active site of digestion, such as the stomach and duodenum, because of the hydrochloric acid and proteolytic enzymes present, respectively. Overall, the specific profile of the phage gut community in various GI organs still requires research, but studies already show that phages inhabit distinct areas in the gut based on their structures and function in the body.

## HOW DO PHAGES SHAPE THE HUMAN GUT MICROBIOTA

Phages play an active and important role in the human gut microbiota and the overall human body; and the longitudinal spread of phages in the GI tract points to phages' dominance in the body. Their composition and population across virtually every organ and layer of the GI tract, especially epithelial tissue, suggest an important role in humans (Townsend et al., 2021). Scanlan et al. observed lytic phages playing an ecological role in the gut of phage cocktail-treated mice (Scanlan, 2020). After analyzing the populations of host bacteria and phages, the gut bacteria exhibited a source–sink ecological dynamic, where bacteria would move between different areas of the gut, based on overpopulation, nutrient availability, and population support. Here, because of phages' density-dependent lysis, phages may contribute to the habitat quality, thus fluctuating where gut microbes reside and how many there are. Other observed dynamics with gut microbiota add to this role (Figure 2.1). For example, phages and bacteria can illustrate the Red Queen dynamics, named from Lewis Carroll's *Through the Looking-Glass* when the Red Queen describes the Looking-Glass Land to Alice and says, "Now, here, you see, it takes all the running you can do, to keep in the same place." In the Red Queen dynamics, there is a continual coevolution between bacterial host and phage to defend and counter-defend, each species running to keep up with the other. Phages can also display the kill-the-winner dynamics, which include phages lysing common, susceptible cells and preventing bacterial dominance, or exhibit piggyback-the-winner dynamics, where

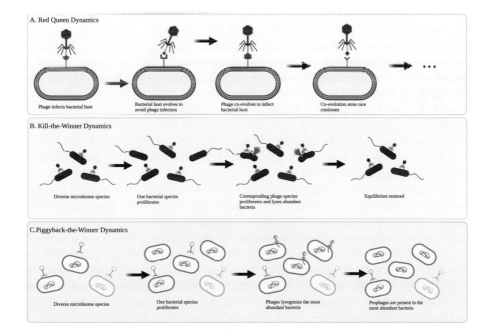

**FIGURE 2.1** Phage–bacteria dynamics in the gut.

lysogenic phages allow for coexistence by integrating with their host (Townsend et al., 2021). The piggyback-the-winner dynamic is predominant in the absence of pathogens and plays a crucial role in the genetic exchange. Prophages have shown up to 5% of the functions in the human gut microbiota by sharing metabolism genes that contribute to nutrient cycling and community stability, thus regulating cell growth and competition (Oh et al., 2019b). Shkoporov and Hill reported the large titer of lysogenic phages in human guts compared with lytic phages. Even in a high concentration of hosts, phages will choose to replicate with bacterial hosts (Shkoporov and Hill, 2019). The gut microbiota abundantly adheres to the top mucin layer in the GI tract where more temperate phages are found and piggyback-the-winner is favored. Despite the risk of lysis, the gut microbiota benefits from phages in the GI tract through lysogeny and regulation of colonization, and phages have formed an important ecological niche with GI microbes.

From the discovery of core phages, such as crAssphage, different phages have been correlated with healthy and ill individuals, posing the existence of the HGP, a gut virome significantly correlated to human health. The disruption of this core virome from equilibrium is either the cause or result of disease, so more investigation is required. Studying phages in relation to human health and gut microbiota requires an overarching view of the GI ecosystem, which is still not well understood (Garmaeva et al., 2019). One angle to this problem is studying the immune system. To the human body, phages are foreign nonself entities that cross the gut epithelium via transcytosis or phagocytosis and come into contact with innate immune cells, such as macrophages and dendritic cells, eventually inducing an antiphage antibody response in lymph nodes (Carroll-Portillo and Lin, 2019). The questions arise when these interactions induce inflammation and immune signaling seen in responses triggered by animal viruses; whether the interactions are beneficial or harmful to the gut microbiota, it is yet clear that the ecological role of phages is tied to human health. A phage-induced immune response can fight off a bacterial infection, subsequently disrupting gut microbes. Phages in the mucosal layers modulate the immune system likely through activating anti-inflammatory cytokines in the lamina propria and suppressing inflammation in the gut, thus stabilizing the intestinal environment and inhibiting nonspecific immune responses present in autoimmunity, hypersensitivity, and infection in the GI tract (Carroll-Portillo and Lin, 2019; Łusiak-Szelachowska et al., 2017).

Changes in the gut phageome have also been associated with diet, and it is well established that diet has a large influence on gut microbiota. Food macromolecules, such as proteins and digestible and nondigestible carbohydrates, induce shifts in the gut microbiota, and subsequently affect overall diversity of gut microbiota (Singh et al., 2017). A study conducted by Townsend et al. had shown that diet also impacts the structure and composition of the gut phageome (Townsend et al., 2021). differences in diet linked with gut phageome differences have been observed over the development of an individual human. Breast milk is high in fats, and studies with mouse models with high-fat diets show increased *Microviridae* to *Siphoviridae* ratios in the gut (Schulfer et al., 2020). As babies wean and eat solid foods, phage composition continues to alter, and an increase in *Pectobacterium* phages and a decrease in *Lactobacillus* phages and *Streptococcus* phages are seen in adulthood. In addition, certain foods are richer sources of phages; fresh meats and fermented foods, such as cheese, soybeans, and sauerkraut, are rich source of phages, so diets concerning these foods may contribute to a wider and larger gut phageome (Chukeatirote et al., 2018). Malnourishment, especially in infancy, significantly disrupts a healthy phageome, which suggests that infancy is a crucial period for phageome development. Malnourished youth contain a phageome that is correlated with individuals with growth stunts and various gut illnesses (Reyes et al., 2015).

Once the phageome stabilizes in adulthood, the individual diet has less of an effect on gut phages; however, the diets from geographical communities and ethnic cultures begin to play a larger role. Zuo et al. studied the gut phage DNA virome in 930 healthy individuals in Hong Kong and Yunnan, China, who spanned various ethnicities and residencies, and geography played the most significant role in shaping both individual's gut virome and bacteriome (Zuo et al., 2020). It is not clear whether the virome affects the bacteriome or vice versa, and geography is impacted by many factors, such as available food sources and region-specific food preparations. However, certain diets in these regions that have been ethnically established, such as barley, buttermilk tea, and Pu'er tea, contributed to virome differences. Urban and rural residencies also affect gut virome; variations in personal hygiene and cleanliness in the kitchen were associated with varying levels of viral diversity. Even though the gut phage community and its regulation are still not fully understood, these studies show the significant effect of environmental factors, diet in particular, on the human gut phageome and bacteriome. Specifically, several foods have been shown to have a direct effect on phages in the human gut, and by extension, gut bacteria as well. Oh et al. reported that dietary fructose and short-chain fatty acids (SCFAs) promote the induction of prophages in gut symbiont *Lactobacillus reuteri* in mouse models in a RecA-dependent manner (Oh et al., 2019a). Researchers observed *L. reuteri* reducing fructose from the diet to mannitol, and other gut microbes were able to convert man nitol to SCFA, which leads to prophage induction. This implies that diet affects gut microbes, which alter the phageome; the phageome then alters gut bacteria by lysis of lysogens. In the colon specifically, nutrient starvation was shown to drive phage production. This likely has to be a consequence of changes in the gut microbiota density and competition, possibly linked with the activation of the SOS response. Garmaeva et al. studied phages in the guts of 11 healthy adults on a gluten-free diet (GFD) and found a decrease of crAss-like phages, *Microviridae*, and *Podoviridae* phages in GFD individuals (Garmaeva et al., 2021). Additionally, the comparison of Bray–Curtis distances between the individuals with GFD and gluten-containing diets revealed the change of the gut virome. Whether the addition of gluten can reverse these changes was not studied, but researchers were able to see how changes in the diet result in changes in the phageome. Cronin et al. researched the effects of physical exercise and regular whey protein supplements on the human gut microbiota (Cronin et al., 2018). Out of 90 study individuals, most experiment participants receiving whey protein experienced higher taxonomic richness and β-diversity in their gut virome than control participants. Overall, diet significantly influences the phages and bacteria in the human gut microbiota, although researchers are still trying to understand mechanistic details.

## PHAGE INTERACTION WITH THE IMMUNE SYSTEM

Phages influence bacterial cells in the gut microbiota, subsequently affecting the immune system. Gut microbes expose the body to a chronically low level of pathogen-associated molecular patterns (PAMPs), which stimulates the body with IgA and CD4/CD8 T cells for future infections. Also, some gut bacteria, such as various *Clostridia* species, induce regulatory T cells and IL-10 production, which suppress immune responses and prevent inappropriate inflammation (Sinha and Maurice, 2019). However, phages can also negatively affect health by causing autoimmune diseases or hypersensitivity when phages cause an inappropriate immune response. Activated prophages from the gut microbiota can play a part in this when phages are released from bacterial cells and access immune cells to elicit a response (Carroll-Portillo and Lin, 2019). The lysing of bacterial host cells by phages would upset immune signals from gut microbes in the gut and disrupt the balance of immunity. In addition, the lysing of bacterial cells releases many PAMPs, including DNA and endotoxins, that can activate the immune system, which can inflame and damage the GI tract. Through transduction, phages could hypothetically carry virulence factors from pathogens to any bacterial cell in the gut microbiota. However, because phages usually have specific host ranges, this hypothesis still desires research to explain the expansion of virulence (Carroll-Portillo and Lin, 2019; Sinha and Maurice, 2019).

Phages have been associated with various illnesses, which further describes phages' dynamic role in human health. Seth et al. studied the gut virome in Gulf War illness (GWI) patients, who experienced bowel inflammation, headaches, neuroinflammation, and other unexplained symptoms (Seth et al., 2019). Increases in gut viral populations and diversity, specifically in dsDNA phages, are observed in GWI patients and animal models. The changes of virome have been positively correlated with gut bacterial dysbiosis and the loosening of GI epithelial tight junctions, such as the activation of Toll-like receptor (TLR)- 6 and TLR-9 pathways, increasing permeability inside the body. Increases in phages have also been associated with increases in proinflammatory cytokines, such as IL-6. Whether or not changes in the gut phageome or the bacteriome-caused symptoms in GWI could not be concluded, and there may be independent or cumulative causes at play. However, in mouse GWI models, the broad-spectrum antiviral ribavirin and the induction of gut sterility by antibiotics both improved symptoms, and therapeutics for GWI can possibly target the gut virome or bacteriome. On the other hand, phage therapy can change gut microbiota to treat diseases. Febvre et al. studied the use of phages against general GI inflammatory symptoms, and $10^6$ PFU per dose of a commercial four-phage cocktail, PreforPro, that targets *E. coli* was orally administered to patients over 28 days (Febvre et al., 2019). Most patients experienced symptom alleviation after the end of the trial, and the phage cocktail additionally did not disturb the overall diversity and richness of the gut microbiota. *E. coil* was generally reduced in the gut. Reductions in *Clostridium perfringens* and increases in the genus *Eubacterium* were observed; because *Eubacterium* spp. produced butyrate, this could lead to a decrease in inflammation and clinical improvement in the patients. The detailed interaction between gut phageome and human disease was further discussed in a later section.

## PHAGEOME AND HEALTH AND DISEASE

The gut microbiota can be characterized as the community of microorganisms that live in the gastrointestinal tracts. This community plays a vital role in the regulation and maintenance of human health and is established prenatally with the transmission of microorganisms from mother to fetus. Several properties of these gut-residing microbes play an imperative role in the homeostasis of the body, and deviations or disruptions in the ecology of the gut microbiota have been implicated in the emergence of several diseases and metabolic disorders.

Gut microbiota diversity and interactions with hosts have been linked to energy homeostasis and the emergence of conditions such as obesity (Bäckhed et al., 2004; Ley et al., 2005; Ridaura et al., 2013). A study conducted by Bäckhed et al. discovered a connection between the gut microbiome and fat storage with subsequent adipose tissue accumulation in humans (Bäckhed et al., 2004). The results showed that microbiota in the gut could lead to the suppression of fasting-induced adipocyte factor (Fiaf) protein, thus promoting fat storage, which, in excess, can lead to obesity. While obesity is certainly a major health outcome following the disruption of gut microbiota ecology, dysbiosis (harmful changes in gut flora) can also lead to other significant health disorders (Cheng et al., 2020; Zhu et al., 2018). One of these diseases is inflammatory bowel disease (IBD), which occurs when there are regions of excessive inflammation along the gastrointestinal tract. Frank et al. compared the GI tract tissue samples from patients with two IBDs: Crohn's disease (CD) and ulcerative colitis (UC), as well as non-IBD controls to determine changes in gut microbiomes; they found that IBD was correlated with lower diversity of gut microbiota and lower levels of microbiota from the *Firmicutes* and *Bacteroidetes* phyla (Frank et al., 2007). In addition, recent studies showcase that the microbiome can actually affect the cardiovascular system and even influence mental processes via the microbiota–gut–brain (MGB) axis. There are limited case studies showing this link in humans, but several animal studies have corroborated and emphasized the connection between gut microbiota and non-gastrointestinal disease (Fröhlich et al., 2016; Gan et al., 2014; Gaykema et al., 2004; Kelly et al., 2016). A study by Lam et al. investigated the effect of antibiotic-induced dysbiosis treatments on cardiovascular health in rats and showed that both treatments led to a reduction in myocardial infarction rate by 27% and 29%, respectively (Lam et al., 2016). The antibiotics help eliminate harmful bacteria in the gut that could potentially increase the severity of myocardial infarction, thus showcasing that reducing certain species of bacteria can help reduce the risk of myocardial infarction. Work by Sudo et al. suggests a link between the gut microbiome and neurodevelopmental pathways (Sudo et al., 2004). These researchers tested neural development and stress response in germ-free (GF) mice, specific pathogen-free (SPF) mice, and gnotobiotic mice. The results showcased that the GF mice had an exaggerated hypothalamic–pituitary–adrenal stress response phenotype, which could be rescued when these mice were transplanted with fecal microbiota from SPF mice. Collectively, these studies demonstrated that the gut microbiome plays a vital role in the proper functions and development of the human body.

As previously described, phageome is a crucial part of shaping the gut micro-biota and it plays a major role in the maintenance and defense of the healthy gut microbiome. The effect of phages on the health of the gut microbiome was studied by Duerkop et al., who performed experiments on mammalian intestinal bacterial *Enterococcus faecalis* (Duerkop et al., 2012). The research found that an isolated *E. faecalis* strain V583 revealed that this bacterial strain created a composite phage φV1/7, which is derived from two prophages: φV1 and φV7. Moreover, a link between bacteriophages and the health of the gut microbiome was observed since the infection with φV1/7 likely rendered V583 bacterial strains a competitive advantage over other strains in both *in vitro* and *in vivo* models. Thus, the dependence of the gut micro-biota on production and infection by bacteriophages is evident. These viruses that reside in the gut microbiota are also highly diverse and have many unique properties and life cycles. Reyes et al. explored the diversity of viruses in the gut microbiome by analyzing fecal samples during 1 year at three different time points from female monozygotic twins and their mothers (Reyes et al., 2010). The results demonstrated that the co-twins and mothers exhibited a significantly higher degree of virome simi-larity compared to unrelated individuals. Additionally, Reyes et al. discovered that even though there were large differences in intestinal viral content between different people, the viral content within an individual often was stable over time; greater than 95% of the virotypes in individuals were retained over the one-year period of the study. This is in stark contrast to the parasitic and competitive nature of bacteria–phage dynamics observed in other ecological systems. Thus, the implication of these results reveals that healthy gut microbiomes maintain a stable and diverse viral popu-lation, which can benefit the bacterial species residing in the gastrointestinal tract.

Phages have been associated with various illnesses (Table 2.1). For example, a study by Zuo et al. compared the virome data from rectal mucosa samples of both patients with ulcerative colitis and healthy controls (Zuo et al., 2019). The results showed that compared to healthy controls, in patients with ulcerative colitis, there was an expansion of mucosa phages as well as a decrease in diversity and richness of phages from the *Caudovirales*, whereas there was also an increase in *Escherichia* phage and *Enterobacteria* phage populations in patients with ulcerative colitis family. Notably, the ulcerative colitis patients also demonstrated a markedly increased num-ber of diverse viral function defects and yet higher expression of phage genes related to bacterial pathogenicity and bacterial host fitness. The phageome is not only related to ulcerative colitis but can also play a role in other human diseases, such as diabetes. A study by Tetz et al. revealed that there was an association between decreasing levels of amyloid-producing *Escherichia coli* abundance in the gut and the emergence of type I diabetes (Tetz et al., 2019). Furthermore, the researchers noted an increase in the *E. coli* phage/*E. coli* ratio prior to the decreasing levels of *E. coli*; this phenom-enon revealed that prophage induction was responsible for the depletion of the gut's amyloid-producing *E. coli* populations and thus the emergence of type 1 diabetes in the patients. The enteric phageome also plays a role in diseases related to the immune system. Particularly, an acquired immunodeficiency syndrome (AIDS), caused by the human immunodeficiency virus (HIV), is linked to the gut virome in many ways. Monaco et al. investigated both HIV-infected and HIV-uninfected Ugandan patients to determine a link between certain viruses of the gut and AIDS and found that there

**TABLE 2.1**
**Relationship between Gut Phageome and Human Diseases**

| Diseases | Changes in the Gut Phageome | Example References |
|---|---|---|
| Ulcerative colitis | A decrease in diversity and richness of *Caudovirales* phages; an increase in abundance of *Caudovirales* phages and *Enterobacteria* phages in particular | Zuo et al. (2019) |
| | Each disease type and cohort have unique bacteriophages; decreased bacterial diversity and richness was inversely correlated to gut phageome changes | Norman et al. (2015) |
| Crohn's disease | A significant expansion of *Caudovirales* bacteriophages | Norman et al. (2015) |
| | Temperate bacteriophages dominate the gut virome | Clooney et al. (2019) |
| | Decreased prevalence of core bacteriophages (phages preset in more than 20% of healthy individuals) | Manrique et al. (2016) |
| | Largest abundance of phages in CD ileum tissue and CD gut wash sample | Wagner et al. (2013) |
| Type 1 diabetes | Increase in the *E. coli* phage/*E. coli* ratio due to prophage induction | Tetz et al. 2019 |
| | Evenness of two major phage groups, *Myoviridae* and *Podoviridae*, was lower; diversity of intestinal *E. coli* phages is significantly higher | Townsend et al. (2021) |
| Type 2 diabetes | The relative numbers of the *Myoviridae*, *Podoviridae*, *Siphoviridae*, and unclassified *Caudovirales* families increased significantly | Ma et al. (2018) |
| | Abundance of phages specific to *Enterobacteriaceae* hosts increased significantly | Chen et al. (2021) |
| Acquired immunodeficiency syndrome (AIDS) | Increase in adenoviruses and viruses from the *Anelloviridae* | Monaco et al. (2016) |
| Stunting | Lower phage diversity; a decrease in temperate phages | Mirzaei et al. (2020) |

was an increase in adenoviruses and viruses from the *Anelloviridae* that were associated with the HIV infection (Monaco et al., 2016). These studies thus solidify the link between the gut phageome and the emergence of a variety of diseases.

Importantly, while there is limited information on the gut phageome, several studies indicated that most viral populations could not be assigned taxonomy and were kept unknown as the viral "dark matter". Finkbeiner et al. studied diarrhea samples from 12 children and employed a novel "micro-mass sequencing" technique to detect the presence of both known and unknown viruses in the samples (Finkbeiner et al., 2008). The results showed that there were several known viruses in these samples, such as rotaviruses, caliciviruses, astroviruses, and adenoviruses. Additionally, the samples revealed the presence of several unknown viruses, which held very little sequence similarity to viromes in the GenBank database. What this study shows is that viruses are highly interconnected to gastrointestinal health, and understanding and characterizing viral genomes can help lead to a broader understanding of both causes and treatments of prevalent diseases. Recently, several studies investigated different techniques to explore this viral dark matter (Fitzgerald et al., 2021). For instance, Benler et al. discussed their search for unknown human gut phages using phage hallmark genes. Their studies led them to discover 3,738 complete phage genomes from 451 different genera, thus illustrating how vast and unknown the human gut phageome truly is (Benler et al., 2021). In the future, further studies and techniques are needed to help explore this unknown gut phageome.

## PHAGE-BASED THERAPY FOR HUMAN GUT-RELATED DISEASE IS A PROMISING APPROACH TO CONTROL/PREVENT HUMAN DISEASE

It is clear that a diverse set of phages play an important role in human health and disease. In addition, infection with foreign viruses has been implicated in causing a variety of gastrointestinal diseases. The application of phage benchwork can help provide a useful framework for better understanding and diagnosing pathogens of the human gut microbiome. One such phage benchwork technique is virome metagenomics. The field of virome metagenomics involves collecting and characterizing the genomic sequences of viruses from a community of organisms. The application of virome metagenomics in the context of the gut microbiome can help researchers determine the causative factors of various gut-related diseases and understand the microbiome of the gut in greater detail. Fernandes et al. studied the fecal viromes of children with ulcerative colitis (UC), Crohn's disease (CD), and healthy controls to understand the pathogenesis of inflammatory bowel disease via virome metagenomics (Fernandes et al., 2019). The results showed that a higher number of *Caudovirales* phages was found in patients with CD but not UC. Additionally, compared to healthy controls, children with CD had a lower richness of phages from *Microviridae*. These findings indicate that virome metagenomics is a powerful tool in understanding the makeup and composition of the gut microbiome and changes in this composition that lead to different diseases. Virome metagenomics has also helped expand the study of the pathogenesis of autoimmune diseases. In particular, classifying gut viromes can help determine what kinds of bacteria host may be responsible for triggering the immune system to target the host's own body. Kim et al. collected 182 fecal and plasma samples from case children with islet autoimmunity and healthy controls (Kim et al., 2019). The researchers were able to detect a total of 129 viruses that were statistically significantly different between the case and control samples using metagenomics analysis. Additionally, five enterovirus A species were detected at significantly higher levels in the islet autoimmune samples than controls. These results highlight a potential causal link between enterovirus A species and the emergence of islet autoimmunity in children. Furthermore, the results underscore the effectiveness of gut virome metagenomics as a laboratory technique to analyze the pathogenicity of diseases. The use of virome metagenomics and its relation to bacterial species of the gut can also help understand nutritional disorders. This topic is the focus of research by Reyes et al., who investigated severe acute malnutrition (SAM) in children and its connection to the gut microbiome (Reyes et al., 2015). The researchers analyzed metagenomes of virus-like particles (VLPs) from fecal samples of Malawian twin infants who were either concordant for healthy growth or discordant for severe acute malnutrition. They discovered that phages from the *Anelloviridae* and

*Circoviridae* families were present at significantly different levels in the discordant from concordant health pairs. Virome metagenomics has also been a useful technique in identifying previously unknown etiological agents responsible for gastrointestinal disorders or health problems. For example, while several pathogenic substances and metabolic conditions could cause diarrhea, there was a rise in unexplained severe diarrhea in children in Turkey in 2015. Altay et al. examined stool samples from the Turkish children with diarrhea using virome metagenomic analyses to investigate the possible etiological agents responsible for the disease (Altay et al., 2015). The authors found that there was bufavirus (a type of parvovirus) DNA present in about 1.4% of the diarrhea samples but in none of the healthy samples (Altay et al., 2015). Additionally, further analysis of this bufavirus showed that children with this virus had more severe diarrhea compared to other children; the specific type of bufavirus responsible for this diarrhea was bufavirus genotype 3. Another study also elucidated the importance of virome metagenomics to identify etiological viruses responsible for diarrhea (Yinda et al., 2019). These researchers analyzed the fecal samples from 221 Cameroonians with symptoms of gastroenteritis via virome metagenomic sequencing. The results showcased that there was an abundance of viruses belonging to the families of *Adenoviridae*, *Astroviridae*, *Caliciviridae*, *Picornaviridae*, and *Reoviridae* among these samples. Additionally, orthoreovirus, picobirnavirus, and smacovirus were also all found in the samples and showed a genetic similarity to viruses in fecal samples from bats and other animals. Thus, these results highlight not only the importance of virome metagenomics in determining the cause of diseases such as diarrhea but also underscore viral metagenomics being potentially used to trace back the source of these etiological viruses to other animal hosts.

The use of genetically engineered phages holds promising therapeutic applications. Phage therapy is an emerging field that uses bacteriophages to target and eliminate specific pathogenic bacteria. As described earlier, dysbiosis (disruptions in the microbiome) in the gut, through the imbalance of bacterial species, can lead to various health problems. Thus, the selective elimination of these harmful bacteria through phage therapy can be a major breakthrough in controlling several health disorders. This novel approach also has its advantage over traditional antibiotics, which are often not specific to harmful bacteria and can thus cause the side effect of eliminating beneficial gut bacteria as well. The specificity and efficiency of phage-based therapy can potentially make this the dominant medical procedure for curing gastrointestinal diseases. While phage-based therapy certainly has its advantages, there are definite disadvantages of this procedure in a medical setting. Excessive use of phage therapy can lead to the potential evolution of pathogenic bacteria to become phage-resistant. Thus, this would mean that in the future, stronger or more complicated phage treatments, such as using more virulent phages or phage cocktails, may be needed for therapeutic benefit. Additionally, errors in the engineering of phages for phage therapy could also lead to disastrous health consequences, such as virulence against the healthy gut microbiota or off-target effects. To overcome these barriers, several studies have tested the efficacy of phage-based therapy in controlling and preventing human gut-related diseases. Phage-based therapy is still a new and emerging field, so most of these studies are *in vitro* and animal model studies with potential future applications in human medicine.

Contemporary phage therapy has relied on lytic phages and usually involves multiple types of phages to create "phage cocktails" for greater efficacy. As of today, according to a review by Lin et al., phage therapy products have not been approved for human use in the EU or the USA (Lin et al., 2017). However, phage therapy has been approved and widely used in the biocontrol of foodborne pathogens by the food industry (Kazi and Annapure, 2016; Niu et al., 2009). Research in the field of phage therapy is still persistent, and the medical potential of phage therapy as an antibacterial treatment is being studied globally. Work by Maura et al. tested the efficacy of a three-phage cocktail (CLB_P1, CLB_P2, and CLB_P3) in eliminating enteroaggregative *Escherichia coli* (EAEC) O104:H4 55989Str strain using mouse models (Maura et al., 2012). The results showcased that after 24 hours, the bacteriophage treatment led to significantly lower concentrations of 55989Str in the ileum of the mice and slightly lower concentrations in the fecal matter. Thus, the efficacy and potential application of phages in eliminating pathogenic bacteria in the gut are evident. These decreases were only transient but with a return to baseline concentrations of 55989Str 3 days after treatment. The results of bacterial regrowth after 3 days highlight the limitations of contemporary phage therapy, indicating that more research is needed to design long-lasting treatments against bacterial pathogens. On the other hand, phage therapy has the potential as a supplemental treatment to aid other therapeutic procedures. One of the primary medical areas that phage-based therapy has been tested on is cancer. Particularly, phage therapy has been explored to use in combination with other conventional cancer therapies, like chemotherapy. Research conducted by Zheng et al. studied mouse models with colorectal cancer to test the ability of phages to aid chemotherapy in treating cancer (Zheng et al., 2019). The bacteria *Fusobacterium nucleatum* tends to promote tumors along the gastrointestinal tract, leading to colorectal cancer. Thus, the researchers used irinotecan-loaded dextran nanoparticles covalently linked to azide-modified phages to selectively eliminate harmful *Fusobacterium nucleatum* in the gut. Their results revealed that this phage-based treatment led to significantly more successful first-line chemotherapy treatments in mice compared to controls. Additionally, the authors repeated the treatment in piglets and found that there were no significant changes in hemocyte counts, immunoglobulin and histamine levels, and liver and renal functions. The finding suggests that phage-based therapy can potentially be used as a supplemental treatment for colorectal cancer with little to no side effects.

In addition, there has been an interest in using phage therapy to deliver CRISPR-Cas9 systems to the gut in order to make genomic edits for the microbiome. Lam et al. used mouse models to study the effects of using engineered bacteriophages as vehicles for CRISPR delivery into the gut (Lam et al., 2021). The researchers engineered the filamentous bacteriophage M13 to deliver exogenous CRISPR-Cas9 DNA to *Escherichia coli* populations of the mouse GI tract. The results reported that using phages as a delivery mechanism for CRISPR systems induced chromosomal deletions in the selected bacteria in both *in vitro* and *in vivo* settings. However, some conclusions showcased potential drawbacks of this technique, including bacterial deletion of the CRISPR DNA to escape targeting. This study provides a proof of concept for future studies and suggests that manipulating the gut microbiome is possible by using a phage delivery system.

Yet another important benchwork tool for phage therapy applications to the human gut is fecal viral transplants. Fecal viral transplants involve screening and obtaining viral populations of stool samples from one healthy individual and transplanting the viruses into the colon of another recipient individual (Bojanova and Bordenstein, 2016). Essentially, it allows the microbiota of the healthy individual to repopulate the gut of the sick individual. This technique has been proposed as a therapeutic treatment for gastrointestinal diseases, given the connection between gut microbiota and human health and the role that phages play in this connection. One of the primary advantages of using fecal viral transplants is preventing and treating bacterial infections of the gut. As described earlier, numerous pathogenic bacterial species can disrupt the healthy gut microbiome and cause dysbiosis. Thus, it is important to eliminate these pathogenic agents to restore a healthy gut. The use of bacteriophages emerges as a possible solution. Zuo et al. compared the virome and bacterial microbiome changes in *Clostridium difficile* infection (CDI) of the gut subjects treated with fecal microbiota transplantation (FMT) or with vancomycin (Zuo et al., 2018). The results showed that the FMT treatment significantly decreased *Caudovirales* DNA in subjects with CDI. Additionally, FMT resulted in changes in both bacterial microbiota and virome in the gut, while the vancomycin treatment only changed the bacterial composition of the gut. These findings suggest that FMT may be a beneficial way to treat bacterial infection of the gut. Some applications of fecal viral transplantation are still being tested in animal models. One such application is the use of fecal viral transplantation in improving the restoration of the normal bacterial gut microbiota after antibiotic treatment. Draper et al. disrupted the mice's gut microbiome using a combination of penicillin and streptomycin (Draper et al., 2020). After that, the bacteriome of mice from either fecal viral transplants or fecal viral transplants with heat and nuclease treatment (both of which killed the bacteriophages as controls) was observed. The results indicated that the fecal viral transplanted mice showcased a higher degree of resemblance to the pre-antibiotic treatment bacteriome. Moreover, analysis of the gut viromes of both groups of mice demonstrated that the fecal viral transplanted mice maintained the phages used in the transplantation over time, suggesting long-term benefits. Thus, the results of this study suggest the role of fecal viral transplantation is not only a primary treatment but also a way to mitigate side effects and improve recovery after other medical treatments, such as antibiotics.

## THE CHALLENGES OF PHAGEOME IN HUMAN GUT MICROBIOME, PERSPECTIVES, AND FUTURE DIRECTIONS

As phage research continues to develop, phage therapy remains a safe and effective therapeutic approach to bacterial infections and inflammatory illnesses associated with the GI tract. Theoretically, phages are not dangerous to human tissue because phages are viruses that specifically infect bacterial cells without affecting eukaryotic cells. Phages' host ranges target specific bacterial species or serotypes, so other cells, including natural microbiota, are not infected (Lewis and Hill, 2020). Phages have already been successfully used in medicine in several studies. Clarke et al. collected clinical reports regarding 277 patients who received phage therapy for joint and bone infections by various bacterial species from 1933 to 2020; over 95% of patients received significant clinical improvement, even total resolution of the infection (Clarke et al., 2020). Although localized pain and swelling were found in some patients, researchers concluded that the phages were contaminated with endotoxins from raw phage lysates. Beatrix and Domingo-Calap reviewed similar results concerning phage therapy clinical trials in GI diseases (Gutiérrez and Domingo-Calap, 2020). Based on a randomized, double-blind, placebo-controlled trial treating chronic diarrhea patients with a four-phage cocktail, patients experienced alleviated symptoms after 28 days of oral treatment. This was correlated with reduced proinflammatory *E. coli* and reductions in inflammatory cytokines and enzymes, such as aminotransferases. Alpha and beta diversity parameters were maintained, also meaning the phages did not disrupt the gut microbiota. Phage therapy has been successfully administered throughout clinical experiences, likely indicating the safety and efficacy of phage therapy against GI diseases caused by pathogenic bacteria.

When studying phages in the human gut microbiota, there are still research gaps and challenges. In general, some phage genomes are unknown and share little homology with known phage sequences. Unknown and hypothetical viral sequences are continually prevalent in phage research that often force current genomic and taxonomic systems to think instead of seeing current data in a new light (Shkoporov and Hill, 2019). Phages are constantly evolving, and the diversity of viral genomes also hinders how well researchers can align phages with references. Metagenomic approaches have successfully facilitated the characterization of different phages in the environment and closely linked the gut virome and bacteriome; however, at this time, pure genomic studies are not able to detail specific phage–host interactions. As genomic and sequence-based tools become more popular, researchers will be losing whole picture if the information from *in vitro* and *in vivo* studies is missing. This would create a methodological bias that does not account for phage biology and evolutionary history and low sensitivity toward small DNA yields from phages. Moreover, unlike bacteria, phages lack universal phylogenetic markers, and thus, it is very complicated to gather large quantities of viral genetic material within metagenomic data without contamination of bacterial sequences based on current protocols (Garmaeva et al., 2019).

When utilizing phages in therapy or application, the stability of phages is also a challenge because it is frequently variable across phage species and formulations, which makes it difficult for researchers to maintain phage titers through experiments and clinical trials (Garmaeva et al., 2019). If not frozen or cooled down, phages will spontaneously mutate over long periods of storage, which can impair the fitness of phages and research data (Garmaeva et al., 2019). In addition, there is generally a lack of quality and safety guidelines for preparing phages, especially for therapy. Although there are strict regulations for pharmaceutical products, few standards have been addressed specifically for phage research and application. Also, phage research currently lacks a simple, fast, and high-throughput method to screen phages. The techniques, including double-layer agar plates, real-time PCR, and flow cytometry, commonly used for phage research are not easily compatible with all phages while producing quick results (Pires et al., 2020). To efficiently continue phage therapy, it is required to improve experimental methods, including methods in genomics, molecular biology, and microbiology; standards of pharmacokinetics and pharmacodynamics of phages also need to be investigated (Luong et al., 2020). The optimal routes of administration, dosage, and the appropriate diseases for phage therapy are also research gaps. Moreover, the phage resistance has not been currently addressed and remains a barrier to more effective research and phage therapy (Yang et al., 2020). Therefore, there can be uncertainty among researchers, patients, and consumers, regarding the effectiveness of phages and the arms race between phages and their bacterial hosts. As phages in the gut microbiota continue to be studied, there will still be gaps to be investigated in the future, such as the exploration of the viral dark matter.

While understanding the multitude of gastrointestinal diseases and other health disorders that arise from the dysbiosis of the gut microbiota remains a goal for microbiology research, there are still many current and future studies focusing on manipulating the gut microbiome for therapeutic benefit, despite the challenges and research gaps. Since the microbiome is inherently linked to a variety of immune and metabolic responses, ways to manipulate the microbiome by enriching or changing its composition and diversity can hold the key to therapeutic treatments for a variety of health conditions. One of the emerging techniques to use the gut microbiome for therapeutic benefit is fecal microbiota transplantation which has shown successful therapy in IBD clinical trials (Oka and Sartor, 2020). Still, it is not always effective. There have been many documented cases of fecal microbiota transfer failures, where the technique failed to eliminate pathogenic bacterial species or resulted in the recurrence of gastrointestinal problems, like diarrhea (Allegretti et al., 2018). Recent research has been using fecal viral transplants instead of whole fecal microbiota transplants. There have been a few studies recently that have shown proof of the concept of this technique. Of note, Lin et al. researched the effectiveness of transplanting only VLPs, many of which are bacteriophages, in mice compared to performing whole fecal microbiota transplants (Lin et al., 2019). The goal was to test the efficacy of both techniques to treat small intestinal bacterial overgrowth (SIBO). The results revealed that the transplantation of the VLPs was as effective as normal FMT. Using only bacteriophages has several advantages over traditional FMT. First, fecal microbiota transplants have the risk of transferring potentially dangerous pathogenic bacterial species from the donor to the recipient. This risk is eliminated with fecal viral transplants, as no bacteria are transferred during this procedure. Additionally, fecal viral transplants could theoretically lead to higher efficacy than FMT since researchers can carefully select and screen for specific phages or viruses from fecal samples. While fecal viral transplants certainly have their advantages, there are still numerous ways to improve the technique. Future research should focus on improving the selection and isolation of phages from fecal samples to yield the most efficacious results. Additionally, while this technique has been tested in animal models, future studies will need to be conducted with human trials to see whether these results can truly be extrapolated for human therapeutic benefit.

While fecal viral transplants can help add or eliminate bacterial species to the gut microbiome, an emerging field of study focuses on the genetic manipulation of the microbiome to combat diseases. One of the most interesting contemporary examples of this has been using bacteriophages as vehicles to deliver CRISPR-Cas9 systems to the gut, as previously mentioned. Additional research on CRISPR and phages can potentially help revolutionize this field. There are several concerns regarding

CRISPR and gene editing that must be taken into consideration and investigated by future research. For example, one major topic of focus regarding current and future studies is to reduce the off-target effects of the CRISPR-Cas9 system. Improving specificity and screening of bacteriophages to be used as vehicles for the CRISPR systems is also another potential topic for future research.

Overall, while several recent studies have already shown how effective understanding and manipulating the phageome of gut microbiota can be, there are many mysteries in the field that remain to be discovered, as described above. Additionally, there are many potential directions for the future of this expanding field, including establishing core gut viral and genetic databases, studying the evolutionary adaptations of the gut microbiota to changing viral environments, and observing specific changes in host phenotypes in response to alterations in the gut phageome. Future research will hopefully discover the underlying mechanism and interactions of gut microbiota and find more efficient alternatives to these challenges related to human health and diseases.

## REFERENCES

Allegretti, J.R., Allegretti, A.S., Phelps, E., Xu, H., Fischer, M., Kassam, Z., 2018. Classifying fecal microbiota transplantation failure: an observational study examining timing and characteristics of fecal microbiota transplantation failures. *Clin. Gastroenterol. Hepatol.* 16, 1832–1833. https://doi.org/10.1016/J.CGH.2017.10.031

Allen, H.K., Looft, T., Bayles, D.O., Humphrey, S., Levine, U.Y., Alt, D., Stanton, T.B., 2011. Antibiotics in feed induce prophages in swine fecal microbiomes. *MBio* 2(6), e00260-11. https://doi.org/10.1128/MBIO.00260-11/SUPPL_FILE/MBO006111199ST4.DOC

Altay, A., Yahiro, T., Bozdayi, G., Matsumoto, T., Sahin, F., Ozkan, S., Nishizono, A., Söderlund-Venermo, M., Ahmed, K., 2015. Bufavirus Genotype 3 in Turkish children with severe diarrhoea. *Clin. Microbiol. Infect.* 21, 965.e1–965.e4. https://doi.org/10.1016/j.cmi.2015.06.006

Bäckhed, F., Ding, H., Wang, T., Hooper, L. V., Gou, Y.K., Nagy, A., Semenkovich, C.F., Gordon, J.I., 2004. The gut microbiota as an environmental factor that regulates fat storage. *Proc. Natl. Acad. Sci. U. S. A.* 101, 15718. https://doi.org/10.1073/PNAS.0407076101

Bao, H., Zhang, H., Zhou, Y., Zhu, S., Pang, M., Shahin, K., Olaniran, A., Schmidt, S., Wang, R., 2020. Transient carriage and low-level colonization of orally administrated lytic and temperate phages in the gut of mice. *Food Prod. Process. Nutr.* 21(2), 1–8. https://doi.org/10.1186/S43014-020-00029-7

Benler, S., Yutin, N., Antipov, D., Rayko, M., Shmakov, S., Gussow, A.B., Pevzner, P., Koonin, E. V., 2021. Thousands of previously unknown phages discovered in whole-community human gut metagenomes. *Microbiome* 9(1), 1–17. https://doi.org/10.1186/S40168-021-01017-W

Bojanova, D.P., Bordenstein, S.R., 2016. Fecal transplants: what is being transferred? *PLoS Biol.* 14(7). https://doi.org/10.1371/JOURNAL.PBIO.1002503

Bushman, F., Liang, G., 2021. Assembly of the virome in newborn human infants. *Curr. Opin. Virol.* 48, 17–22. https://doi.org/10.1016/J.COVIRO.2021.03.004

Camarillo-Guerrero, L.F., Almeida, A., Rangel-Pineros, G., Finn, R.D., Lawley, T.D., 2021. Massive expansion of human gut bacteriophage diversity. *Cell* 184, 1098–1109.e9. https://doi.org/10.1016/J.CELL.2021.01.029

Carroll-Portillo, A., Lin, H.C., 2019. Bacteriophage and the innate immune system: access and signaling. *Microorganisms* 7(12), 625. https://doi.org/10.3390/MICROORGANISMS7120625

Chen, Q., Ma, X., Li, C., Shen, Y., Zhu, W., Zhang, Y., Guo, X., Zhou, J., Liu, C., 2021. Enteric phageome alterations in patients with type 2 diabetes. *Front. Cell. Infect. Microbiol.* 856. https://doi.org/10.3389/fcimb.2020.575084

Cheng, L., Qi, C., Zhuang, H., Fu, T., Zhang, X., 2020. gutMDisorder: a comprehensive database for dysbiosis of the gut microbiota in disorders and interventions. *Nucleic Acids Res.* 48, D554–D560. https://doi.org/10.1093/NAR/GKZ843

Chukeatirote, E., Phongtang, W., Kim, J., Jo, A., Jung, L.S., Ahn, J., 2018. Significance of bacteriophages in fermented soybeans: a review. *Biomol. Concepts* 9, 131–142. https://doi.org/10.1515/BMC-2018-0012

Clarke, A.L., Soir, S. De, Jones, J.D., 2020. The safety and efficacy of phage therapy for bone and joint infections: a systematic review. *Antibiotics* 9, 795. https://doi.org/10.3390/ANTIBIOTICS9110795

Clooney, A.G., Sutton, T.D., Shkoporov, A.N., Holohan, R.K., Daly, K.M., O'Regan, O., Ryan, F.J., Draper, L.A., Plevy, S.E., Ross, R.P., Hill, C., 2019. Whole-virome analysis sheds light on viral dark matter in inflammatory bowel disease. *Cell Host Microbe* 26(6), 764–778. https://doi.org/10.1016/j.chom.2019.10.009

Cronin, O., Barton, W., Skuse, P., Penney, N.C., Garcia-Perez, I., Murphy, E.F., Woods, T., Nugent, H., Fanning, A., Melgar, S., Falvey, E.C., Holmes, E., Cotter, P.D., O'Sullivan, O., Molloy, M.G., Shanahan, F., 2018. A prospective metagenomic and metabolomic analysis of the impact of exercise and/or whey protein supplementation on the gut microbiome of sedentary adults. *MSystems* 3(3), e00044-18. https://doi.org/10.1128/MSYSTEMS.00044-18

Dalmasso, M., Hill, C., Ross, R.P., 2014. Exploiting gut bacteriophages for human health. *Trends Microbiol.* 22, 399–405. https://doi.org/10.1016/J.TIM.2014.02.010

Draper, L.A., Ryan, F.J., Dalmasso, M., Casey, P.G., McCann, A., Velayudhan, V., Ross, R.P., Hill, C., 2020. Autochthonous faecal viral transfer (FVT) impacts the murine microbiome after antibiotic perturbation. *BMC Biol.* 18(1), 1–14. https://doi.org/10.1186/S12915-020-00906-0

Duerkop, B.A., Clements, C.V., Rollins, D., Rodrigues, J.L.M., Hooper, L.V., 2012. A composite bacteriophage alters colonization by an intestinal commensal bacterium. *Proc. Natl. Acad. Sci. U. S. A.* 109, 17621–17626. https://doi.org/10.1073/PNAS.1206136109/-/DCSUPPLEMENTAL

Febvre, H.P., Rao, S., Gindin, M., Goodwin, N.D.M., Finer, E., Vivanco, J.S., Lu, S., Manter, D.K., Wallace, T.C., Weir, T.L., 2019. PHAGE study: effects of supplemental bacteriophage intake on inflammation and gut microbiota in healthy adults. *Nutrients* 11(3), 666. https://doi.org/10.3390/NU11030666

Fernandes, M.A., Verstraete, S.G., Phan, T., Deng, X., Stekol, E., Lamere, B., Lynch, S.V., Heyman, M.B., Delwart, E., 2019. Enteric virome and bacterial microbiota in children with ulcerative colitis and Crohn disease. *J. Pediatr. Gastroenterol. Nutr.* 68, 30–36. https://doi.org/10.1097/MPG.0000000000002140

Finkbeiner, S.R., Allred, A.F., Tarr, P.I., Klein, E.J., Kirkwood, C.D., Wang, D., 2008. Metagenomic analysis of human diarrhea: viral detection and discovery. *PLoS Pathog.* 4(2), e1000011. https://doi.org/10.1371/JOURNAL.PPAT.1000011

Fitzgerald, C.B., Shkoporov, A.N., Upadrasta, A., Khokhlova, E. V., Ross, R.P., Hill, C., 2021. Probing the "Dark Matter" of the human gut phageome: culture assisted metagenomics enables rapid discovery and host-linking for novel bacteriophages. *Front. Cell. Infect. Microbiol.* 100. https://doi.org/10.3389/FCIMB.2021.616918

Frank, D.N., St. Amand, A.L., Feldman, R.A., Boedeker, E.C., Harpaz, N., Pace, N.R., 2007. Molecular-phylogenetic characterization of microbial community imbalances in human inflammatory bowel diseases. *Proc. Natl. Acad. Sci. U. S. A.* 104, 13780–13785. https://doi.org/10.1073/PNAS.0706625104

Fröhlich, E.E., Farzi, A., Mayerhofer, R., Reichmann, F., Jačan, A., Wagner, B., Zinser, E., Bordag, N., Magnes, C., Fröhlich, E., Kashofer, K., Gorkiewicz, G., Holzer, P., 2016. Cognitive impairment by antibiotic-induced gut dysbiosis: analysis of gut microbiota-brain communication. *Brain. Behav. Immun.* 56, 140–155. https://doi.org/10.1016/J.BBI.2016.02.020

Gan, X.T., Ettinger, G., Huang, C.X., Burton, J.P., Haist, J. V., Rajapurohitam, V., Sidaway, J.E., Martin, G., Gloor, G.B., Swann, J.R., Reid, G., Karmazyn, M., 2014. Probiotic administration attenuates myocardial hypertrophy and heart failure after myocardial infarction in the rat. *Circ. Heart Fail.* 7, 491–499. https://doi.org/10.1161/CIRCHEARTFAILURE.113.000978

Garmaeva, S., Gulyaeva, A., Sinha, T., Shkoporov, A.N., Clooney, A.G., Stockdale, S.R., Spreckels, J.E., Sutton, T.D.S., Draper, L.A., Dutilh, B.E., Wijmenga, C., Kurilshikov, A., Fu, J., Hill, C., Zhernakova, A., 2021. Stability of the human gut virome and effect of gluten-free diet. *Cell Rep.* 35(7), 109132. https://doi.org/10.1016/J.CELREP.2021.109132

Garmaeva, S., Sinha, T., Kurilshikov, A., Fu, J., Wijmenga, C., Zhernakova, A., 2019. Studying the gut virome in the metagenomic era: challenges and perspectives. *BMC Biol.* 17(1), 1–14. https://doi.org/10.1186/S12915-019-0704-Y

Gaykema, R.P.A., Goehler, L.E., Lyte, M., 2004. Brain response to cecal infection with Campylobacter jejuni: analysis with Fos immunohistochemistry. *Brain. Behav. Immun.* 18, 238–245. https://doi.org/10.1016/J.BBI.2003.08.002

Grif, K., Dierich, M.P., Karch, H., Allerberger, F., 1998. Strain-specific differences in the amount of Shiga toxin released from enterohemorrhagic *Escherichia coli* O157 following exposure to subinhibitory concentrations of antimicrobial agents. *Eur. J. Clin. Microbiol. Infect. Dis.* 17, 761–766. https://doi.org/10.1007/S100960050181

Guerin, E., Hill, C., 2020. Shining light on human gut bacteriophages. *Front. Cell. Infect. Microbiol.* 481. https://doi.org/10.3389/FCIMB.2020.00481

Gutiérrez, B., Domingo-Calap, P., 2020. Phage therapy in gastrointestinal diseases. *Microorganisms* 8, 1–11. https://doi.org/10.3390/MICROORGANISMS8091420

Hallowell, H.A., Higgins, K. V., Roberts, M., Johnson, R.M., Bayne, J., Maxwell, H.S., Brandebourg, T., Hiltbold Schwartz, E., 2021. Longitudinal analysis of the intestinal microbiota in the obese mangalica pig reveals alterations in bacteria and bacteriophage populations associated with changes in body composition and diet. *Front. Cell. Infect. Microbiol.* 934. https://doi.org/10.3389/FCIMB.2021.698657

Howard-Varona, C., Hargreaves, K.R., Abedon, S.T., Sullivan, M.B., 2017. Lysogeny in nature: Mechanisms, impact and ecology of temperate phages. *ISME Journal.* 11(7), 1511–1520. https://doi.org/10.1038/ismej.2017.16

Hsu, B.B., Gibson, T.E., Yeliseyev, V., Liu, Q., Lyon, L., Bry, L., Silver, P.A., Gerber, G.K., 2019. Dynamic modulation of the gut microbiota and metabolome by bacteriophages in a mouse model. *Cell Host Microbe* 25, 803–814.e5. https://doi.org/10.1016/J.CHOM.2019.05.001

Hsu, C.L., Duan, Y., Fouts, D.E., Schnabl, B., 2021. Intestinal virome and therapeutic potential of bacteriophages in liver disease. *J. Hepatol.* 75, 1465–1475. https://doi.org/10.1016/j.jhep.2021.08.003

Kazi, M., Annapure, U.S., 2016. Bacteriophage biocontrol of foodborne pathogens. *J. Food Sci. Technol.* 53(3), 1355–1362. https://doi.org/10.1007/s13197-015-1996-8

Keen, E.C., 2015. A century of phage research: bacteriophages and the shaping of modern biology. *Bioessays* 37, 6. https://doi.org/10.1002/BIES.201400152

Kelly, J.R., Borre, Y., O' Brien, C., Patterson, E., El Aidy, S., Deane, J., Kennedy, P.J., Beers, S., Scott, K., Moloney, G., Hoban, A.E., Scott, L., Fitzgerald, P., Ross, P., Stanton, C., Clarke, G., Cryan, J.F., Dinan, T.G., 2016. Transferring the blues: depression-associated gut microbiota induces neurobehavioural changes in the rat. *J. Psychiatr. Res.* 82, 109–118. https://doi.org/10.1016/J.JPSYCHIRES.2016.07.019

Kieft, K., Zhou, Z., Anderson, R.E., Buchan, A., Campbell, B.J., Hallam, S.J., Hess, M., Sullivan, M.B., Walsh, D.A., Roux, S., Anantharaman, K., 2021. Ecology of inorganic sulfur auxiliary metabolism in widespread bacteriophages. *Nat. Commun.* 121(12), 1–16. https://doi.org/10.1038/s41467-021-23698-5

Kim, K.W., Horton, J.L., Pang, C.N.I., Jain, K., Leung, P., Isaacs, S.R., Bull, R.A., Luciani, F., Wilkins, M.R., Catteau, J., Lipkin, W.I., Rawlinson, W.D., Briese, T., Craig, M.E., 2019. Higher abundance of enterovirus A species in the gut of children with islet autoimmunity. *Sci. Rep.* 9(1), 1–8. https://doi.org/10.1038/S41598-018-38368-8

Lam, K.N., Spanogiannopoulos, P., Soto-Perez, P., Alexander, M., Nalley, M.J., Bisanz, J.E., Nayak, R.R., Weakley, A.M., Yu, F.B., Turnbaugh, P.J., 2021. Phage-delivered CRISPR-Cas9 for strain-specific depletion and genomic deletions in the gut microbiome. *Cell Rep.* 37(5), 109930. https://doi.org/10.1016/J.CELREP.2021.109930

Lam, V., Su, J., Hsu, A., Gross, G.J., Salzman, N.H., Baker, J.E., 2016. Intestinal microbial metabolites are linked to severity of myocardial infarction in rats. *PLoS One* 11(8), e0160840. https://doi.org/10.1371/JOURNAL.PONE.0160840

Letarov, A.V., 2020. History of early bacteriophage research and emergence of key concepts in virology. *Biochemistry (Mosc.)* 85, 1093–1112. https://doi.org/10.1134/S0006297920090096

Lewis, R., Hill, C., 2020. Overcoming barriers to phage application in food and feed. *Curr. Opin. Biotechnol.* 61, 38–44. https://doi.org/10.1016/j.copbio.2019.09.018

Ley, R.E., Bäckhed, F., Turnbaugh, P., Lozupone, C.A., Knight, R.D., Gordon, J.I., 2005. Obesity alters gut microbial ecology. *Proc. Natl. Acad. Sci. U. S. A.* 102(31), 11070–11075. https://doi.org/10.1073/pnas.0504978102

Lin, D.M., Koskella, B., Lin, H.C., 2017. Phage therapy: an alternative to antibiotics in the age of multi-drug resistance. *World J. Gastrointest. Pharmacol. Ther.* 8, 162. https://doi.org/10.4292/WJGPT.V8.I3.162

Lin, D.M., Koskella, B., Ritz, N.L., Lin, D., Carroll-Portillo, A., Lin, H.C., 2019. Transplanting fecal virus-like particles reduces high-fat diet-induced small intestinal bacterial overgrowth in mice. *Front. Cell. Infect. Microbiol.* 348. https://doi.org/10.3389/FCIMB.2019.00348

Looft, T., Allen, H.K., Cantarel, B.L., Levine, U.Y., Bayles, D.O., Alt, D.P., Henrissat, B., Stanton, T.B., 2014. Bacteria, phages and pigs: the effects of in-feed antibiotics on the microbiome at different gut locations. *ISME J.* 8, 1566–1576. https://doi.org/10.1038/ISMEJ.2014.12

Luong, T., Salabarria, A.C., Roach, D.R., 2020. Phage therapy in the resistance era: where do we stand and where are we going? *Clin. Ther.* 42, 1659–1680. https://doi.org/10.1016/J.CLINTHERA.2020.07.014

Łusiak-Szelachowska, M., Weber-Dąbrowska, B., Jończyk-Matysiak, E., Wojciechowska, R., Górski, A., 2017. Bacteriophages in the gastrointestinal tract and their implications. *Gut Pathog.* 9(1), 1–5. https://doi.org/10.1186/S13099-017-0196-7

Ma, Y., You, X., Mai, G., Tokuyasu, T. and Liu, C., 2018. A human gut phage catalog correlates the gut phageome with type 2 diabetes. *Microbiome* 6(1), 1–12. https://doi.org/10.1186/s40168-018-0410-y

Manrique, P., Bolduc, B., Walk, S.T., Der Van Oost, J., De Vos, W.M., Young, M.J., 2016. Healthy human gut phageome. *Proc. Natl. Acad. Sci. U. S. A.* 113, 10400–10405. https://doi.org/10.1073/PNAS.1601060113

Manrique, P., Dills, M., Young, M.J., 2017. The human gut phage community and its implications for health and disease. *Viruses* 9(6), 141. https://doi.org/10.3390/V9060141

Maura, D., Galtier, M., Le Bouguénec, C., Debarbieux, L., 2012. Virulent bacteriophages can target O104:H4 enteroaggregative *Escherichia coli* in the mouse intestine. *Antimicrob. Agents Chemother.* 56, 6235–6242. https://doi.org/10.1128/AAC.00602-12

Mirzaei, M.K., Khan, M.A.A., Ghosh, P., Taranu, Z.E., Taguer, M., Ru, J., Chowdhury, R., Kabir, M.M., Deng, L., Mondal, D., Maurice, C.F., 2020. Bacteriophages isolated from stunted children can regulate gut bacterial communities in an age-specific manner. *Cell Host Microbe* 27(2), 199–212. https://doi.org/10.1016/j.chom.2020.01.004

Monaco, C.L., Gootenberg, D.B., Zhao, G., Handley, S.A., Ghebremichael, M.S., Lim, E.S., Lankowski, A., Baldridge, M.T., Wilen, C.B., Flagg, M., Norman, J.M., Keller, B.C., Luévano, J.M., Wang, D., Boum, Y., Martin, J.N., Hunt, P.W., Bangsberg, D.R., Siedner, M.J., Kwon, D.S., Virgin, H.W., 2016. Altered virome and bacterial microbiome in human immunodeficiency virus-associated acquired immunodeficiency syndrome. *Cell Host Microbe* 19, 311–322. https://doi.org/10.1016/J.CHOM.2016.02.011

Mushegian, A.R., 2020. Are there $10^{31}$ virus particles on earth, or more, or fewer? *J. Bacteriol.* 202. https://doi.org/10.1128/JB.00052-20

Niu, Y.D., McAllister, T.A., Xu, Y., Johnson, R.P., Stephens, T.P., Stanford, K., 2009. Prevalence and impact of bacteriophages on the presence of Escherichia coli O157:H7 in feedlot cattle and their environment. *Appl. Environ. Microbiol.* 75, 1271–1278. https://doi.org/10.1128/AEM.02100-08

Norman, J.M., Handley, S.A., Baldridge, M.T., Droit, L., Liu, C.Y., Keller, B.C., Kambal, A., Monaco, C.L., Zhao, G., Fleshner, P., Stappenbeck, T.S., McGovern, D.P.B., Keshavarzian, A., Mutlu, E.A., Sauk, J., Gevers, D., Xavier, R.J., Wang, D., Parkes, M., Virgin, H.W., 2015. Disease-specific alterations in the enteric virome in inflammatory bowel disease. *Cell* 160, 447. https://doi.org/10.1016/J.CELL.2015.01.002

Ogilvie, L.A., Caplin, J., Dedi, C., Diston, D., Cheek, E., Bowler, L., Taylor, H., Ebdon, J., Jones, B.V., 2012. Comparative (meta)genomic analysis and ecological profiling of human gut-specific bacteriophage φB124-14. *PLoS One* 7, 35053. https://doi.org/10.1371/JOURNAL.PONE.0035053

Oh, J.H., Alexander, L.M., Pan, M., Schueler, K.L., Keller, M.P., Attie, A.D., Walter, J., van Pijkeren, J.P., 2019a. Dietary fructose and microbiota-derived short-chain fatty acids promote bacteriophage production in the gut symbiont *Lactobacillus reuteri*. *Cell Host Microbe* 25, 273–284.e6. https://doi.org/10.1016/J.CHOM.2018.11.016

Oh, J.H., Lin, X.B., Zhang, S., Tollenaar, S.L., Özçam, M., Dunphy, C., Walter, J., van Pijkeren, J.P., 2019b. Prophages in *Lactobacillus reuteri* are associated with fitness trade-offs but can increase competitiveness in the gut ecosystem. *Appl. Environ. Microbiol.* 86(1), e01922-19. https://doi.org/10.1128/AEM.01922-19

Oka, A., Sartor, R.B., 2020. Microbial-based and microbial-targeted therapies for inflammatory bowel diseases. *Dig. Dis. Sci.* 65, 757–788. https://doi.org/10.1007/S10620-020-06090-Z

Pires, D.P., Costa, A.R., Pinto, G., Meneses, L., Azeredo, J., 2020. Current challenges and future opportunities of phage therapy. *FEMS Microbiol. Rev.* 44, 684–700. https://doi.org/10.1093/FEMSRE/FUAA017

Reyes, A., Blanton, L. V., Cao, S., Zhao, G., Manary, M., Trehan, I., Smith, M.I., Wang, D., Virgin, H.W., Rohwer, F., Gordon, J.I., 2015. Gut DNA viromes of Malawian twins discordant for severe acute malnutrition. *Proc. Natl. Acad. Sci. U. S. A.* 112, 11941–11946. https://doi.org/10.1073/PNAS.1514285112

Reyes, A., Haynes, M., Hanson, N., Angly, F.E., Heath, A.C., Rohwer, F., Gordon, J.I., 2010. Viruses in the faecal microbiota of monozygotic twins and their mothers. *Nature* 466(7304), 334–338. https://doi.org/10.1038/nature09199

Ridaura, V.K., Faith, J.J., Rey, F.E., Cheng, J., Duncan, A.E., Kau, A.L., Griffin, N.W., Lombard, V., Henrissat, B., Bain, J.R., Muehlbauer, M.J., Ilkayeva, O., Semenkovich, C.F., Funai, K., Hayashi, D.K., Lyle, B.J., Martini, M.C., Ursell, L.K., Clemente, J.C., Van Treuren, W., Walters, W.A., Knight, R., Newgard, C.B., Heath, A.C., Gordon, J.I.,

2013. Cultured gut microbiota from twins discordant for obesity modulate adiposity and metabolic phenotypes in mice. *Science* 341(6150), 1241214. https://doi.org/10.1126/SCIENCE.1241214

Roux, S., Brum, J.R., Dutilh, B.E., Sunagawa, S., Duhaime, M.B., Loy, A., Poulos, B.T., Solonenko, N., Lara, E., Poulain, J., Pesant, S., Kandels-Lewis, S., Dimier, C., Picheral, M., Searson, S., Cruaud, C., Alberti, A., Duarte, C.M., Gasol, J.M., Vaqué, D., Bork, P., Acinas, S.G., Wincker, P., Sullivan, M.B., 2016. Ecogenomics and potential biogeochemical impacts of globally abundant ocean viruses. *Nature* 537(7622), 689–693. https://doi.org/10.1038/nature19366

Scanlan, P.D., 2020. Resistance may be futile: gut spatial heterogeneity supports bacteria-phage co-existence. *Cell Host Microbe* 28, 356–358. https://doi.org/10.1016/J.CHOM.2020.08.008

Schulfer, A., Santiago-Rodriguez, T.M., Ly, M., Borin, J.M., Chopyk, J., Blaser, M.J., Pride, D.T., 2020. Fecal viral community responses to high-fat diet in mice. *mSphere* 5(1), e00833-19. https://doi.org/10.1128/MSPHERE.00833-19

Seth, R.K., Maqsood, R., Mondal, A., Bose, D., Kimono, D., Holland, L.A., Lloyd, P.J., Klimas, N., Horner, R.D., Sullivan, K., Lim, E.S., Chatterjee, S., 2019. Gut DNA virome diversity and its association with host bacteria regulate inflammatory phenotype and neuronal immunotoxicity in experimental Gulf War illness. *Viruses* 11(10), 968. https://doi.org/10.3390/V11100968

Shkoporov, A.N., Hill, C., 2019. Bacteriophages of the human gut: the "known unknown" of the microbiome. *Cell Host Microbe* 25, 195–209. https://doi.org/10.1016/J.CHOM.2019.01.017

Singh, R.K., Chang, H.W., Yan, D., Lee, K.M., Ucmak, D., Wong, K., Abrouk, M., Farahnik, B., Nakamura, M., Zhu, T.H., Bhutani, T., Liao, W., 2017. Influence of diet on the gut microbiome and implications for human health. *J. Transl. Med.* 151(1), 1–17. https://doi.org/10.1186/S12967-017-1175-Y

Sinha, A., Maurice, C.F., 2019. Bacteriophages: uncharacterized and dynamic regulators of the immune system. *Mediators Inflamm.* https://doi.org/10.1155/2019/3730519

Stern, A., Mick, E., Tirosh, I., Sagy, O., Sorek, R., 2012. CRISPR targeting reveals a reservoir of common phages associated with the human gut microbiome. *Genome Res.* 22, 1985–1994. https://doi.org/10.1101/GR.138297.112

Sudo, N., Chida, Y., Aiba, Y., Sonoda, J., Oyama, N., Yu, X.N., Kubo, C., Koga, Y., 2004. Postnatal microbial colonization programs the hypothalamic-pituitary-adrenal system for stress response in mice. *J. Physiol.* 558, 263–275. https://doi.org/10.1113/JPHYSIOL.2004.063388

Sutcliffe, S.G., Shamash, M., Hynes, A.P., Maurice, C.F., 2021. Common oral medications lead to prophage induction in bacterial isolates from the human gut. *Viruses* 13, 455. https://doi.org/10.3390/V13030455

Tetz, G., Brown, S.M., Hao, Y., Tetz, V., 2019. Type 1 diabetes: an association between autoimmunity, the dynamics of gut amyloid-producing *E. coli* and their phages. *Sci. Rep.* 9(1), 1–11. https://doi.org/10.1038/S41598-019-46087-X

Townsend, E.M., Kelly, L., Muscatt, G., Box, J.D., Hargraves, N., Lilley, D., Jameson, E., 2021. The human gut phageome: origins and roles in the human gut microbiome. *Front. Cell. Infect. Microbiol.* 498. https://doi.org/10.3389/FCIMB.2021.643214

Trubl, G., Jang, H. Bin, Roux, S., Emerson, J.B., Solonenko, N., Vik, D.R., Solden, L., Ellenbogen, J., Runyon, A.T., Bolduc, B., Woodcroft, B.J., Saleska, S.R., Tyson, G.W., Wrighton, K.C., Sullivan, M.B., Rich, V.I., 2018. Soil viruses are underexplored players in ecosystem carbon processing. *mSystems* 3(5), e00076-18. https://doi.org/10.1128/mSystems.00076-18

Wagner, J., Maksimovic, J., Farries, G., Sim, W.H., Bishop, R.F., Cameron, D.J., Catto-Smith, A.G., Kirkwood, C.D., 2013. Bacteriophages in gut samples from pediatric Crohn's disease patients: metagenomic analysis using 454 pyrosequencing. *Inflamm. Bowel Dis.* 19(8), 1598–1608. https://doi.org/10.1097/MIB.0b013e318292477c

Yang, Y., Shen, W., Zhong, Q., Chen, Q., He, X., Baker, J.L., Xiong, K., Jin, X., Wang, J., Hu, F., Le, S., 2020. Development of a bacteriophage cocktail to constrain the emergence of phage-resistant *Pseudomonas aeruginosa*. *Front. Microbiol.* 11, 327. https://doi.org/10.3389/FMICB.2020.00327

Yinda, C.K., Vanhulle, E., Conceição-Neto, N., Beller, L., Deboutte, W., Shi, C., Ghogomu, S.M., Maes, P., Van Ranst, M., Matthijnssens, J., 2019. Gut virome analysis of cameroonians reveals high diversity of enteric viruses, including potential interspecies transmitted viruses. *mSphere*. 4(1), e00585-18. https://doi.org/10.1128/MSPHERE.00585-18

Zhang, Y., Liao, Y.-T. Te Salvador, A., Sun, X., Wu, V.C.H., 2020. Prediction, diversity, and genomic analysis of temperate phages induced from shiga toxin-producing *Escherichia coli* strains. *Front. Microbiol.* 10, 3093. https://doi.org/10.3389/fmicb.2019.03093

Zheng, D.W., Dong, X., Pan, P., Chen, K.W., Fan, J.X., Cheng, S.X., Zhang, X.Z., 2019. Phage-guided modulation of the gut microbiota of mouse models of colorectal cancer augments their responses to chemotherapy. *Nat. Biomed. Eng.* 39(3), 717–728. https://doi.org/10.1038/s41551-019-0423-2

Zhu, Q., Gao, R., Zhang, Y., Pan, D., Zhu, Y., Zhang, X., Yang, R., Jiang, R., Xu, Y., Qin, H., 2018. Dysbiosis signatures of gut microbiota in coronary artery disease. *Physiol. Genomics* 50, 893–903. https://doi.org/10.1152/physiolgenomics.00070.2018

Zuo, T., Liu, Q., Zhang, F., Yeoh, Y.K., Wan, Y., Zhan, H., Lui, G.C.Y., Chen, Z., Li, A.Y.L., Cheung, C.P., Chen, N., Lv, W., Ng, R.W.Y., Tso, E.Y.K., Fung, K.S.C., Chan, V., Ling, L., Joynt, G., Hui, D.S.C., Chan, F.K.L., Chan, P.K.S., Ng, S.C., 2021. Temporal landscape of human gut RNA and DNA virome in SARS-CoV-2 infection and severity. *Microbiome* 9(1), 1–16. https://doi.org/10.1186/S40168-021-01008-X

Zuo, T., Lu, X.J., Zhang, Y., Cheung, C.P., Lam, S., Zhang, F., Tang, W., Ching, J.Y.L., Zhao, R., Chan, P.K.S., Sung, J.J.Y., Yu, J., Chan, F.K.L., Cao, Q., Sheng, J.Q., Ng, S.C., 2019. Gut mucosal virome alterations in ulcerative colitis. *Gut* 68, 1169–1179. https://doi.org/10.1136/GUTJNL-2018-318131

Zuo, T., Sun, Y., Wan, Y., Yeoh, Y.K., Zhang, F., Cheung, C.P., Chen, N., Luo, J., Wang, W., Sung, J.J.Y., Chan, P.K.S., Wang, K., Chan, F.K.L., Miao, Y., Ng, S.C., 2020. Human-gut-DNA virome variations across geography, ethnicity, and urbanization. *Cell Host Microbe* 28, 741–751.e4. https://doi.org/10.1016/J.CHOM.2020.08.005

Zuo, T., Wong, S.H., Lam, K., Lui, R., Cheung, K., Tang, W., Ching, J.Y.L., Chan, P.K.S., Chan, M.C.W., Wu, J.C.Y., Chan, F.K.L., Yu, J., Sung, J.J.Y., Ng, S.C., 2018. Bacteriophage transfer during faecal microbiota transplantation in *Clostridium difficile* infection is associated with treatment outcome. *Gut* 67, 634–643. https://doi.org/10.1136/GUTJNL-2017-313952

# Section II

---

*T1 Preclinical Animal Studies, and Safety and Efficacy Trial in Humans*

# 3 Microbiome and Nutrition – Why Do We Care?
## Discussing a Complex Relationship

Angelos K. Sikalidis
California Polytechnic State University

## CONTENTS

## INTRODUCTORY REMARKS

The term microbiome arises from the Greek words "μικρο" – micro meaning "small" (in mathematics and sciences designated with the Greek letter μ ($10^{-6}$)) – "βίωμα" – biome meaning "of life", in Greek: "μικροβίωμα". Prior to 2001, the term microbiome was in use, mostly to infer a rather small significantly complex ecological niche incorporating plant and animal life. While the study of what is now known as

DOI: 10.1201/b22970-5

the "human microbiome" can be traced as far back as Antonie van Leeuwenhoek (1632–1723), "I then most always saw, with great wonder, that in the said matter there were many very little living animalcules, very prettily a-moving". Leeuwenhoek, who is known to have made over 500 "microscopes", of which fewer than ten have survived to the present day, was a keen, laborious and systematic observer of the microbial world.

In 2001, the term "microbiome" was re-discovered, re-surfaced and used by Nobel laureate-microbiologist Joshua Lederberg to signify the microbial life in symbiosis (under normal healthy conditions) with the human body (Prescott, 2017). In this context, a fair definition of the microbiome could be: "the full complement of microbes (bacteria, viruses, fungi, and protozoa), their genes, and genomes in or on the human body". Microbiota on the other hand, which is used similar to the term microbiome, refers to an "ecological community of commensal, symbiotic and pathogenic microorganisms found in all multicellular organisms studied to date from plants and animals" (Prescott, 2017; Institute of Medicine, 2013). Hence, the difference between microbiota and microbiome is that the latter could be more encompassing in the sense that it refers not only to the organisms but also to the genome present and the relevant implications.

The notion that something existing in the gut could produce health effects is indeed ancient. Furthermore, the idea that fecal matter contains elements that could alter favorable health outcomes to the recipients was also entertained since the antiquity. The history of fecal microbial transplant (FMT) constitutes a characteristic example: Although it is often considered a "novel" therapeutic strategy (Opritu, 2016), it was being practiced while well-documented, certainly in terms of oral administration, in various European medical crafts ever since ancient Greece. The practice is described in numerous key works of medicine of 16th- and 17th-century Europe (Moore, 2019; Faming et al., 2012), while further it was practiced in China since the Don-jin dynasty (4th century AD) (Faming et al., 2012). FMT rectal delivery was used by American doctor I.O. Wilson in 1910, particularly in the effort to instigate favorable changes in fecal bacterial composition in patients with functional bowel disorders ameliorating symptoms (Woodruff, 1910). Therefore, FMT cannot be considered novel, at least not conceptually, whereas its historical and intercultural ubiquity may in all actuality provide solid support to an emerging scientific model, that of gut microbiome functioning as a human body's essential organ, itself comprised of several organisms which have coevolved with human cells such that they are to some extent "us" and we are "them".

On that basis, Alexander Khoruts, a pioneering researcher studying FMT, made the argument that FTM-Clostridium difficile therapy must be viewed as a "transplant" as opposed to a "drug" (Steve and Khoruts, 2014). Evidence regarding commensal and symbiotic intestinal microbes continuously accumulates and supports such an interpretation (Gray, 2017). Moreover, consistent with accepting the microbial origin of human mitochondria (Gray, 2017), this organelle is another example of coevolution through symbiosis where identifiable structures and unique DNA (mtDNA) are evident (Moore, 2019).

Similarly, to several examples in biological sciences, the "microbiome" has enjoyed significant biohype culminating to what some term a "microbiome zeitgeist"

(Prescott, 2017) leading to a "World microbiome day: June 27th". Even though it is well established and widely known both in the scientific community and in the public that bacteria reside at various locales of the human body especially in the large intestine (colon), the importance of the microbiome has gained significant attention due to a significant body of scientific literature over the past 10–15 years indicating and demonstrating that the size and type of microflora populations in the gut could well influence health outcomes, spanning from immune responses to metabolic syndrome (syndrome X), type 2 diabetes mellitus (T2DM), nonalcoholic steatohepatitis, cardiovascular disease (CVD) and some forms of cancer, particularly of colon (Bashiardes et al., 2018). Thus, the microbiome is deemed integral to human physiology, health and disease, while it arguably constitutes the most intimate connection that humans extend to their external environment, mostly through diet. We typically consider the large intestine (colon) as a site hosting a variety of populations of bacteria that reside in a symbiotic mode at that habitat with the human body. While this is not the only bodily location where bacteria reside, it appears to be a location with probably the highest numbers and diversity of bacterial populations extending a rich variety of metabolic and physiological influences.

The human microbiome, especially that of the gut, is being regarded an "essential organ" (Bashiardes et al., 2018), with roughly 150 times more genes than the whole human genome, while the human body contains at least 1,000 different species of known bacteria. Microbiotic composition and function differ according to variations in location, age, sex, race, and diet of the host (Steve and Khoruts, 2014). Although determining precise numbers is rather challenging and of questionable accuracy, it has been proposed that the number of human cells while at the order of 40 trillion human cells ($4 \times 10^{13}$) in a typical human body is less than that of bacterial $10^{14}$–$10^{15}$ (Sender et al., 2016a, 2016b; Savage, 1977). There are recent estimates updating the total number of bacteria in the 70 kg "reference man" to be $3.8 \times 10^{13}$, while for human cells, same estimates identify the dominant role of the hematopoietic lineage to the total count (90%) and revise past estimates to $3.0 \times 10^{13}$ human cells (Sender et al., 2016a). The same analysis also updates the widely cited 10:1 ratio, showing that the number of bacteria in the body is actually of the same order as the number of human cells (Sender et al., 2016a).

The Human Microbiome Project (HMP) was initiated by the National Institutes of Health (NIH) in 2007, with the majority of funding ($153 million of the $173 million as of 2013 alone) coming from the NIH Common Fund (Institute of Medicine, 2013). The project was initiated aiming to characterize the genomic makeup of all microbes inhabiting the human body. Nonetheless, gradually even more so a growing number of scientists place increasing emphasis on the importance of studying beyond the identification on the microbes present but also the function of those microbes. HMP used sequencing to examine the microbes associated with the human body. HMP's major purpose has been to generate resources for the research community, focusing on building a "healthy cohort" reference database of human–microbiome genome sequences (known as metagenomic sequences), computational tools for complex metagenomic sequences analyses and clinical protocols for human–microbiome sampling (Institute of Medicine, 2013).

## THE HUMAN GUT MICROBIOME

A variety of bacteria, archaea, yeasts, planctomycetes and filamentous fungi and viruses, such as Senegal virus, are examples of human gastrointestinal (GI) residents and evidence of the complexity characterizing the human GI microbiome. While estimates of species numbers in the gut exhibit significant variation, the adult microbiota is generally accepted to consist of over 1,000 species, which in turn are grouped into a few bacterial phyla, with over 7,000 strains (Thakur et al., 2014). Several differentiating ecological habitats comprise the GI tract, while foods typically provide microbes even after gastric treatment. Despite the reduction in the microbial load after gastric emptying, significant populations remain in the chyme found in the stomach, the small and later large intestine (Mondot and Lepage, 2016).

The most prominent phyla out of the several detected in the stomach are as follows: Firmicutes, Bacteroidetes, Proteobacteria, Actinobacteria and Fusobacteria. Cultivable species mainly belong to the genera Streptococcus, Neisseria and Lactobacillus, and very high interindividual variation is observed in the gastric microbiome at the genus level. The bile and pancreatic secretions in the small intestine together with peristalsis maintain low levels of the bacterial population compared to that of colon. Respective to levels of bacterial population, intestinal contents range from duodenum to the ileocecal segment as $10^4$ to $10^6$–$10^7$ CFU/g, respectively (Mondot and Lepage, 2016). Small intestine microbiota is mainly composed of facultative aerobic–anaerobic species (Streptococcus, Lactobacillus, Enterobacteriaceae) but also strict anaerobes (Clostridium and Veillonella). Fecal microflora samples, while they may provide a view on the dominant intestinal microbiota composition, only partially describe the distal colonic microbiota (Mondot and Lepage, 2016).

The colonic microbiota is characterized by the presence of four major phyla: Firmicutes, Bacteroidetes, Actinobacteria and Proteobacteria, with Firmicutes and Bacteroidetes accounting for over 90% of the total bacteria in the ecosystem. The Firmicutes often dominate and are divided into two major classes of Gram-positive bacteria in the gut: Clostridia (mainly Clostridium cluster IV and Clostridium XIVa) and Bacilli (Bacillales and Lactobacillales). The phylum Bacteroidetes includes most Gram-negative bacteria, is less diverse with respect to species and is subdivided into three predominant genera: Bacteroides, Prevotella and Porphyromonas (Mondot and Lepage, 2016).

To study microbial communities in a variety of environments, culture-independent methods have been developed. These methods typically entail the use of small subunit ribosomal RNA gene (16S rRNA) of the environmental microorganisms, thus providing information on microbial diversity in the gut. In a mere decade of use, these methods have described several species that significantly exceeds that of the cultivated species. More specifically, out of over 1,200 microbes described in the gut, only 12% were detected by the application of both a molecular approach and a culture, while the vast majority (roughly 75%) were observed only via 16S rRNA gene sequencing (Institute of Medicine, 2013; Mondot and Lepage, 2016).

Genes involved in immunity, nutrient absorption, energy metabolism and intestinal barrier function are modulated by the gut microbiota in, as demonstrated, both humans and mouse models (Thakur et al., 2014; Sarkar et al., 2016). Moreover, there are several factors implicated to extending higher or lower degrees of influence to gut microbiota composition, including genetics, health status, mode of delivery at birth and environmental exposures.

## THE METABOLOME AND MICROBIOME CONNECTION

Personalized health approaches require integrative, systems-level tactics considering human biocomplexity. In this context, microbiome research aligns powerfully with this paradigm. When considering the gene–diet–microbial axis, genome is merely one of the components that ultimately comprise the human "mega system". Therefore, even though genome-wide association studies (GWASs) are commonly performed, they do not necessarily enlighten as revealingly since links are rarely deterministic, while, moreover, statistical significance often times does not translate at all, or at least equally powerfully, to biological significance of function. There are several such examples of weak biological connections between the mere genetic association and the actual biological phenotype as per metabolic profiles and functions.

For instance, researchers reported that the 32 statistically significant body mass index (BMI)-associated genes identified accounted for a thin 1.47% of actual BMI value variation (Speliotes et al., 2010). Other researchers have actually revealed an association between obesity and microbiome (Ley et al., 2006; Turnbaugh et al., 2006). This is just an example of the highly controversial and consensus-lacking obesity–microbiome connection. While most of the scientific community recognizes the possibility for a connection, it is rather difficult to determine what the relationship is, what the underlying mechanism is and finally what is the order of events (i.e., obesity informs the microbiome or is it the other way around? While if there is a cross talk, how does such dynamic evolve?). Some investigators propose that the main underlying cause for inconsistencies that lead to controversial and conflicting results regarding the obesity–microbiome relationship stems from the fact that there are significant differences regarding the level of phylogeny as well as the design of the experiments conducted. These include lack of concise measures, models and translation to clinical environment. Nonetheless, there seems to be no agreement as to standardization and/ or best practices regarding those types of approaches (Institute of Medicine, 2013). Systems-level approach has shown that a tremendous number of human diseases are genetically connected, which is biologically plausible, with oftentimes the same gene or groups of genes implicated in different disorders. However, understanding the human genome in itself is not enough toward personalized/precision health care. The microbiome represents yet another new level of complexity and genetic link (Institute of Medicine, 2013).

Beyond the varying degrees of disease risk that complex interactions between the microbiome and its host generate, diverse metabolic phenotypes in turn associated with pathologies are also observed (Holmes et al., 2008). Actually, while disease risk levels and metabolic phenotypes are biologically and statistically associated in such manner, measurement of metabolite levels (biomarkers) can assess disease risk. The idea that changes in metabolic products are an indication of disease is certainly not new. However, as new high-throughput technologies are used to produce a rather extensive bulk of information on metabolites and construct detailed metabolic profiles, the complexity of such information generated is significant primarily due to the fact that not only are all human cells producing metabolites (with more than 500 functionally distinct cell types), but so do all microbial cells (Nicholson et al., 2005) which may well add exponentially to the metabolite pools.

Microbes produce short-chain fatty acids (SCFAs), bile acids and related oxysterols, vasoactive (aromatic) amines, cresols and aromatic acids, endocannabinoids, and a host of other compounds (Hussein et al., 2022). Moreover, several microbial metabolites participate in human metabolism. For example, bile acids, which are critically important host signaling molecules, are cometabolized by microbes, with significant implications for liver and colonic disease risk (Nicholson et al., 2005). Bile acids are biosynthesized hepatically daily, stored in the gallbladder, released as needed into the mammalian gut, used as emulsifiers to drive lipid absorption and recycled via the enterohepatic circulation thereby returning to the liver. However, as enterohepatic circulation is not 100% efficient, there is always a smaller or larger portion of the overall produced bile that will result in the colon where it will be deconjugated into cholic acid by Lactobacillus and other gut-residing bacteria. The cholic acid, in turn, can be dehydroxylated by yet other microbes into deoxycholic acid which is both hepatoxic and carcinogenic. Furthermore, microbial cometabolism of bile acids may also negatively impact lipid bioavailability (Nicholson et al., 2010).

Additional to its potential toward contributing to personalized medicine, metabolic phenotyping carries potential for applications at the entire population level. Holmes and coworkers (2008) introduced the concept of metabolome-wide association studies, the metabolic equivalent of GWAS, and demonstrated significant geographic variation in metabolic phenotypes. Similar concept has been entertained by Yap and colleagues, while comparable metabolic variation has been associated with varying risks of cardiovascular as well as other diseases (Yap et al., 2010). Hence, it seems that there is mounting evidence to suggest that as humans coevolve with their natural/geographic environment, part of such coevolution is the evolution of their microbiome as well as their metabolic profile and ensuing risk for certain diseases of metabolic background.

## HOST–GUT MICROBIOME METABOLIC INTERACTIONS

While typically the consensus was that microbes were thought as from dangerous to undesirable at best, the communities both scientific and lay do appreciate the various aspects that the microbiome entails along with the beneficial ones that are health promoting. Furthermore, it is increasingly more appreciated that it is in fact more accurate to consider microbial communities (oftentimes diverse and in a dynamic state) as opposed to microbes as units *per se*.

The development of a highly complex gut ecosystem in the human host begins at or possibly even prior to birth, while the intestinal microbiota early colonization depends on various environmental exposures. The taxa colonizing the otherways relatively "sterile" newborn intestine are largely determined by the mode of delivery. Newborn intestinal colonization in the case of vaginal birth initiates while the neonate passes through the birth canal. Neonatal's ingestion of microorganisms induces the gut microbiome and initiates its development. Moreover, infant feeding depending on whether it is breastfeeding or formula-feeding further informs the manner in which the intestinal microbiota will develop both in terms of quality and quantity and overall bacterial demography. The early species are placed in the neonatal intestines through maternal feeding. Breastfeeding providing maternal milk carbohydrates naturally selected to feed mutualist microbes in the infant's microbiota provides significant support in the microbial growth. Beyond its nutritive value both fort the infant and its intestinal microbiome, breastfeeding is further credited with reducing infant mortality and limiting the risk of chronic diseases later in life. Breastfed infants exhibit a Bifidobacteria-dominated microbiome inducing a tolerogenic immune response in the gut, hence reducing the risk of pathogen colonization, infection and overall gut inflammation (Wasielewski et al., 2016).

Human milk oligosaccharides (HMOs), the second most abundant milk carbohydrate after lactose, provide 5%–6% of milk's energy content. Gut Bifidobacteria's growth is primarily supported by this type of carbohydrates. Interestingly, since HMOs cannot be digested by humans, it requires microbial fermentation to produce utilizable energy fuel for the host (i.e., human) in the form of SCFAs. Moreover, since breast milk's sialylated oligosaccharides prevent pathogen adhesion to epithelial cells, they contribute significantly to infection prevention. Additionally, breast milk's lipid fraction further contributes to milk's antipathogen properties. Breast milk's triglycerides are converted to antimicrobial fatty acids and monoglycerides by specific lipases produced by the infant, which extend antiviral, -bacterial and -protozoan pathogen properties, creating a hostile environment unsupportive of harmful microbe growth (Wasielewski et al., 2016). Finally, breast milk is significantly advantageous in the sense that is significantly enriched by a variety of antibodies reflective of mother's immunological profile as informed both by innate and by adaptive immunity.

Host-provided glycans are characterized by structural similarities with HMOs and similar antimicrobial properties, offering an alternative to breast milk support route for desirable microbes. The gel-like mucosal structure coating the intestinal epithelium consists of proteins and O-glycosylated carbohydrate chains. This mucosal structure feeds the specific commensal bacteria, which in turn produce SCFAs, while the host can capture the energy from SCFAs, thus contributing toward the energy balance for manufacturing the mucus structure. This mutualistic relationship results in benefit for the host because microbes occupy the glycan-binding sites, thereby preventing pathogen crossing of the mucus layer which would cause inflammation and ultimately infection (Wasielewski et al., 2016).

The symbiotic relationships between microbiota and host stem as a result of a dynamically balanced habitat of symbionts and pathobionts. Perturbations affecting the afore-described delicate balance leading to disturbance in the composition of microbial communities, termed dysbiosis, typically result in disfavorable interactions between the microbiome and the host, leading to increased disease susceptibility. Various studies have demonstrated associations between intestinal dysbiosis and chronic low-grade inflammation and metabolic dysfunctions. Thus, metabolic syndrome, obesity and diabetes may be negatively impacted from changes in the gut microbiome (Hemarajata and Versalovic, 2013; Thakur et al., 2014).

The gut microbiome may be affected by dietary alterations, infections and exposure to antibiotics. Throughout infancy and early childhood, the aforementioned factors can alter the microbial balance in the individual's gut. The infant's intestinal microbiota is characterized by instability and relatively low degree of diversity. Nevertheless, by the toddler years, the intestinal microbiota is similar in diversity and stability to that of adults (Albenberg and Wu, 2014). In adulthood, the equivalent of approximately 2 kg of microbes (yielding a number approximation of about 30 trillion) reside in the human body, with the majority residing in the gut, mostly in the colon. The immune system can generally tolerate high density of microbes in the distal gut, while comparable density in the small intestine causes severe illness. However, in the event of microbial infection where microbes enter circulation, even at low amounts, can cause cardiac collapse and death (Wasielewski et al., 2016).

Defending intestinal homeostasis and host health is achieved via cooperative action of various functional microbial groups. By means of deploying an array of glycoside hydrolases and polysaccharide lyases, the gut microbiome produces essential amino acids and some vitamins, thus facilitating the utilization of nondigestible food compounds, while saccharide fermentation by gut microbiome is a major source of energy for intestinal epithelial cells. Moreover, the bacterial metabolism of dietary fiber to SCFAs can constitute a significant energy source for humans (Thakur et al., 2014). Microbial de-polymerization of complex carbohydrates and proteins leads to the production of a large variety of mono- and oligo-meric compounds, subsequently fermented into SCFAs and ultimately to carbon dioxide and molecular hydrogen. Interestingly, carbohydrate fermentation and SCFA production significantly improve the absorption of calcium, magnesium and phosphorus (Thakur et al., 2014), hence contributing to the nutritive efficiency of diet.

## MICROBIOME – DIET INTERACTIONS

Intestinal microbiota functions as a metabolic organ that influences nutrient uptake, bioavailability, metabolic signaling, energy balance, weight and disease risk in a dynamic manner (Figure 3.1). Unfavorable nutritional environment for the microbiome can lead to intestinal permeability, resulting in low-grade inflammation as well as obesity, and associated chronic metabolic diseases such as nonalcoholic fatty liver disease, dyslipidemia and insulin resistance. Thus, there is a special and rather significant relationship between the type and the amount of nutrients becoming available to the microbiome in the gut, and how the microbiome changes in response to such exposure to the nutrients in terms of its type, numbers and subsequent function and metabolic signaling. This implies a series of events that will ultimately impact metabolism of the host and finally risk for chronic diseases. More specifically, diet exerts a major influence upon host immune function and the GI microbiota. Although components of the human diet (including carbohydrates, fats and proteins) are essential sources of nutrition for the host, they also influence immune function directly through interaction with innate and cell-mediated immune regulatory mechanisms (Heras et al., 2022). Gut microbiome extends influences over many endocrine functions such as adrenal steroidogenesis, thyroid function, sexual hormones, IGF-1 pathway and peptides produced in the GI system. It is fundamental in glycemic control and obesity, while also exerting an important function in modulating the immune system and associated inflammatory disease. The result of this cross talk in gut mucosa is the formation of the intestinal immunological niche (Rossella et al., 2022).

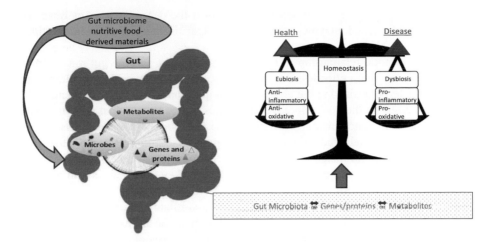

**FIGURE 3.1** Conceptual scheme: microbiome – diet interactions can lead to metabolic signaling, energetics and disease risk modulation. (Adapted from: Sikalidis and Maykish, 2020.)

## THE GUT MICROBIOME AND CARBOHYDRATE METABOLISM

### GENERAL CONSIDERATIONS

Carbohydrates constitute a key nutritional component for mammals and the mammalian microbiome, including that of the gut, typically conferring the majority of energy fuel. In humans, carbohydrates are the most important food energy provider among the macronutrients (between 40% and 80% of total energy intake). Mammals can directly absorb simple sugars, fructose, galactose and glucose, in the proximal jejunum via specialized transmembrane transporter proteins. Mammalian enzymes hydrolyze disaccharides (sucrose, lactose, maltose) and starches to constituent absorbable monomeric units (monosaccharides), but possess rather limited abilities to hydrolyze other polysaccharides. Consequently, on a regular basis and depending on the diet consumed, a significant bulk of undigested plant polysaccharides (cellulose, xylan and pectin) as well as partially digested starch reach the colonic lumen where microbial communities reside. By hosting a vibrant and metabolically active microbiome well able to hydrolyze complex carbohydrates, mammals are not required to invest significant energy, time and resources as well as genetic capital toward the evolution/development and production of complex enzymes that are required to catabolize the numerous polysaccharides in the diet. Microbes, by contrast, possess a plethora of genes encoding various carbohydrate-active enzymes (CAZymes) in the human microbiome (Devaraj et al., 2013; Cantarel et al., 2012). Microbial CAZymes, which comprise a typical mammalian host repertoire, include glycoside hydrolases, carbohydrate esterases, glycosyl transferases and polysaccharide lyases (Cantarel et al., 2012). Approximately 40 g of dietary carbohydrates reach the colon daily, escaping digestion by host enzymes. The main categories are resistant starch, nonstarch polysaccharides and oligosaccharides, although some di- and monosaccharides (e.g., sugar alcohols) may also reach the colon. The human gut microbiota is particularly well adapted to perform the degradation of polysaccharides: 10,000 bacterial enzymes implicated in sugar digestion have been identified (Arnone et al., 2021).

In the symbiotic relationship formed between the host and the gut microbiome, the gut microbes gain effortless direct access to abundant readily fermentable carbon sources to be utilized in the absence of competition, which would otherwise be wasted excreted by the host. Moreover, microbes by the same token may use those complex carbohydrate substrates to support viable, functionally vigorous microbial communities and produce bioactive compounds exerting signals that in turn modulate mammalian metabolism. Intestinal bacterial taxa vary notably regarding their aptitude to use dietary/host-derived carbohydrates (e.g., mucus components) (Sonnenburg et al., 2010).

Bacteroidetes are shown to straightforwardly assimilate dietary carbohydrates as well, since representatives of this bacterial phylum hold the ability to activate numerous carbohydrate utilization pathways. Conversely, in cases of dietary carbohydrate starvation, gut bacteria will typically aggressively catabolize mucins in the GI tract yielding a carbohydrate source, thus possibly compromising the mucus layer adjacent to the epithelium, causing inflammation and likely permeation integrity problems depending on the extent of catabolism. Comparable to Bacteroides, strains of the genus Bifidobacterium encompass genes encoding for glycan-foraging enzymes, which in turn enable those gut bacteria to obtain nutrients from host-derived glycans (Devaraj et al., 2013). Similar to their capacity to hydrolyze starch, gut microbes have evolutionarily developed the capability to degrade several plant- and host-derived glycoconjugates (glycans) and glycosaminoglycans such as cellulose, chondroitin sulfate, hyaluronic acid, mucins and heparin. Catabolic enzymes of microbial origin including endoglycosidases might act on dietary substrates, thereby releasing complex N-glycans from human milk and other dairy sources (Garrido, 2012).

Dietary variations can extend functional consequences on both bacteria and the host alike, leading to the "cannibalization" of indigenous mammalian carbohydrates, which in turn could lead to expansion of beneficial features, prevention of diseases or predisposition to different disease states depending on the specifics and the extent of the phenomena. For instance, human milk oligosaccharide-grown Bifidobacteria contribute to the stabilization of epithelial tight junctions' formation while promoting secretion of interleukin-10 (Chichlowski et al., 2012). The biogeography of the microbiome may be relevant since specific genes/pathways such as simple carbohydrate transport phosphotransferase systems are more prominent in the small intestine as opposed to the colon (Zoetendal et al., 2012), seemingly by design.

## SIMPLE CARBOHYDRATES

High levels of plasma lipopolysaccharides (LPS) with ectopic hepatic lipid accumulation increase gut permeability, and low-grade endotoxemia have all been demonstrated in animals whereby obesity was induced via exposure to high-fat or high-fructose diets. High-fructose diets, in particular, have been strongly related to both hepatic and extra-hepatic insulin resistance as well as obesity-related metabolic disturbances via mechanisms involving gut microbiome and downstream intestinal permeability (Ochoa et al., 2015). While sugars in general constitute a major carbon source modulating growth and virulence in a broad spectrum of gut pathogen and pathobionts, refined/simple carbohydrates support overgrowth for opportunistic bacteria including *Clostridium difficile* and *Clostridium perfringens* by induction of biliary output (Wasielewski et al., 2016; Albenberg and Wu, 2014). Taken together, these observations imply that high-fat/high-refined sugars diets can introduce undesirable ecological alterations in the gut environment while intensifying host response such as inflammation and differentiated glucose metabolism (Albenberg and Wu, 2014). Furthermore, simple carbohydrate overconsumption could produce unfavorable effects at both central and peripheral levels, such as fluctuations in secretion of satiety-regulating peptides as well as neuropeptides. Further negative impact includes increase of gut permeability leading to low-grade inflammation and liver disease as well as induced blood–brain barrier (BBB) permeability, in turn affecting appetite and mood/predisposition toward food, via the reward/dopamine axis related mechanism (Ochoa et al., 2015). While fiber consumption seems to protect against inflammation, the accumulation of simple sugars in the colon induces an increase of the osmotic load, as well as the fermentation rate by the colonic microbiome, subsequently potentially promoting abdominal pain, discomfort and various intestinal dysfunctions.

While enterocytes in the intestine will typically produce fatty acids, utilizing both glucose and fructose as substrates, compared to glucose, fructose may be proven a deprived substrate for *de novo* lipogenesis in enterocytes, while fatty acid accumulation could worsen intestinal function. Consequently, excessive sucrose intake has been recognized as a primary cause of metabolic syndrome, the toxicity resulting from excess fructose rather than sucrose, as fructose extends the induction of glycation phenomena targeting proteins and, physiologically, its metabolic substrate rapidly flows into *de novo* lipogenesis, which in turn strongly promotes liver inflammation (MacDonald, 2016). Additionally, the pro-oxidative and pro-inflammatory effects of fructose can lead to induced gut permeability and endotoxemia both of which conditions do exacerbate chronic inflammation in the gut.

High sugar intake might disturb intestine homeostasis in a variety of mechanisms and ways. The consumption of sugar-rich diets can alter the intestinal mucosa architecture. A high-sugar diet promotes intestinal stem cells differentiation into absorptive enterocytes and secretive enteroendocrine cells in *Drosophila*, which causes the gut to become thinner, and produces high levels of reactive oxygen species (Zhang et al., 2017); specifically, high fructose intake can lead to reduced mucus thickness in the colon and defensin secretion. Recent studies demonstrated that dietary fructose worsens colitis in mice by altering the composition, localization and metabolism of gut microbiota through mechanisms involving GLUT5 (glucose transporter 5) expression (fructose transporter) (García-Montero et al., 2021).

Moreover, high glucose- and high fructose-fed mice have been shown to lose gut microbial diversity (characterized by a reduced proportion of Bacteroidetes and a markedly increased proportion of Proteobacteria) (Do et al., 2018). Dietary sugars that are not absorbed at the intestinal level of the host and reach the colonic environment exposed to the microbiota also regulate gut colonization by beneficial microbes. High-sucrose diets (when comprising 70% of the kilocalories from carbohydrates, mainly in the form of sucrose) have previously been shown to elevate Clostridiales (a class of Firmicutes) while simultaneously reducing Bacteroidales (an order of the phylum Bacteroidetes) abundance in adult rodents, thereby promoting gut dysbiosis (Magnusson et al., 2015). Additionally, dietary fructose intake was negatively associated with the abundance of the bacterial species *Eubacterium eligens*, while it is known that *E. eligens*, along with other members of the phylum Firmicutes, produce fewer polysaccharide-degrading enzymes compared to the members of the phylum Bacteroidetes. Moreover, dietary fructose consumption is negatively associated with microbes belonging to the genus *Streptococcus*, including the species *S. thermophilus*, with this bacterium has been shown to effectively ferment lactose and sucrose in addition to its ability to metabolize fructose (Jones et al., 2019). Recently, a study underlined the importance of intestinal symbiosis to prevent chronic inflammation, as well as the fact that the intestinal microbiota needs to also be studied from an ecosystem perspective instead of merely focusing on select bacterial species whose relative abundance correlates with the inflammatory level (Barnich and Chassaing, 2021).

## COMPLEX CARBOHYDRATES

Oligosaccharides and polysaccharides extend several functions toward the maintenance of colonic health. Raffinose, stachyose, fructooligosaccharides and soluble fiber are shown to be beneficial to gut microflora and overall health of the colon. More specifically, making these carbohydrates available to the gut microbiome, bacteria synthesize specific vitamins (biotin and K), which can be utilized by the host. Furthermore, such feeding conditions support the generation of beneficial fatty acids that are shown to improve colonic health, lower inflammation and reduce risk of colon cancer (Ochoa et al., 2015; Salonen and de Vos, 2014). Two most common oligosaccharides considered prebiotics as they help desirable gut microflora to flourish are raffinose, composed of three monosaccharide units, and stachyose, composed of five monosaccharide units, primarily found in beans and other legumes. Another oligosaccharide group is the fructo-oligosaccharides, comprised of varying numbers of fructose molecules, found in artichokes, onions, garlic, bananas and other plant-based foods (Salonen and de Vos, 2014). Furthermore, in work studying the *in vitro* digestion of the whole blackberry fruit, whereby bioaccessibility, bioactive variation of active ingredients and impacts on human gut microbiota were assessed, results showed that the phenolics were mainly released in gastric phase while carbohydrates in small intestinal phase. The bioaccessibility for phenolics and carbohydrates was 42.80% and 69.30%, respectively, indicating most of phenolics still remain in colon and are available for intestinal flora (Dou et al., 2022).

## NONDIGESTIBLE POLYSACCHARIDES – FIBER

Unrefined grains, starchy and nonstarchy vegetables, legumes, and fruit constitute dietary sources of a broad variety of nondigestible polysaccharides. Fiber, a collective term for nondigestible polysaccharides divided into soluble and insoluble fibers, is not easily digested or absorbed in the small intestine, but rather typically metabolized in the distal colon. Cellulose is degraded by Bacteroides species, primarily associated with plant polysaccharide degradation, or Ruminococcus, and degradation results in the production of SCFAs. Abundance in Bacteroides was observed in population-wide studies with participants on rural (significantly rich plant-based and high fiber foods) versus Western diet. Furthermore, Prevotella populations are typically high in humans with a high intake of plant-based complex carbohydrates. These bacteria utilize xylan, common hemicellulose in human diets, via a variety of metabolic pathways conserved in the Bacteroidetes' phylum. Shifts in diet composition when introducing high plant polysaccharide intake lead to increased production of SCFAs, while by contrast Western diet has been shown to reduce Bacteroides' levels (Salonen and de Vos, 2014; Sandhu et al., 2016). Inulins, plant storage polysaccharides, are extensively studied and well-established prebiotics. Fermentation of inulin and several of its subgroups enhances expansion of Bifidobacterium and Lactobacillus populations, in the gut. Inulins are predominantly found in wheat and a variety of fruits and vegetables including onions, bananas, asparagus and artichokes (Sandhu et al., 2016). The amount of Bifidobacteria in feces of humans on a low-fat Western diet supplemented with inulin is higher than no inulin supplementation. Additionally, inulin-supplemented diets in dextran sulfate sodium-induced colitis murine model produced a significant increase of colonic Lactobacilli and amelioration of colitis symptoms. In studies with infants, where mothers received inulin and galacto-oligosaccharide supplements during pregnancy and breastfeeding, newborns were more protected against allergies, exhibited lower histamine levels and better bowel permeability (Sandhu et al., 2016). A different polysaccharide β-glucan, commonly found in seeds and grains like barley and oats, is shown to reduce hyperglycemia, hyperlipidemia and hypertension (Dawson et al., 2016).

Moreover, in a recent human study conducted in the USA, tree-based analysis of dietary diversity captured associations between fiber intake and gut microbiota composition in a healthy U.S. adult cohort (Kable et al., 2021). More specifically, two to three Automated Self-Administered 24-hour Dietary Recalls (ASA24) were collected over 10–14 d together with a single stool sample from 343 healthy adults in a cross sectional phenotyping study. The study examined a multi-ethnic cohort balanced for age (18y-65y), sex and BMI (18.5–45). Further, the tree structure was annotated with the average total grams of dry weight, fat, protein, carbohydrate or fiber from each food item reported. The alpha and beta diversity measurements, calculated using the tree structure, were analyzed relative to the microbial community diversity determined by QIIME 2 analysis of the bacterial 16S rRNA V4 region, sequenced from stool samples. K-means clustering was used to form groups of individuals consuming similar diets, and gut microbial communities were compared among groups using DESeq2. The authors reported that alpha diversity of diet dry weight was significantly correlated with gut microbial community alpha diversity ($r = 0.171$). The correlation observed was shown improved when diet was characterized using grams of carbohydrates ($r = 0.186$) or fiber ($r = 0.213$). The researchers concluded that consumption of fiber from fruit robustly associated with abundance of pectinolytic bacterial genus, Lachnospira, in the gut of healthy adults, revealing a strong association between the ingested fiber and the gut microbiota profile (Kable et al., 2021).

Interestingly, as mentioned earlier, polysaccharides for intestinal microbiome metabolism are derived from mucus as well as diet. Underlying the ability of intestinal bacteria to switch substrate utilization depends on substrate availability/ source (Albenberg and Wu, 2014). Interestingly, low-fiber diets lead to loss of microbiome diversity which may well extend over three or four generations. Thus, consuming a fiber-rich diet constitutes a critical factor contributing to an individual's overall health and sustained development of a diverse healthy gut microbiome (Dawson et al., 2016; Sandhu et al., 2016).

In both animals and humans, by way of varying the suite and amounts of sugars and sweeteners consumed, we generate a new gut environment that induces in turn the alteration of the demography of our microbial community, changes in microbial metabolism and excreted metabolites, and selects for different microbial strains. Moreover, early-life sugar consumption significantly has been shown to alter the gut microbiome independently of obesity and total caloric intake in a rodent model (Arnone et al., 2021).

## THE GUT MICROBIOME AND FATTY ACID METABOLISM

### GENERAL CONSIDERATIONS

Intestinal bacteria produce a variety of fatty acids which in turn can extend health-promoting effects. Bifidobacteria in the gut generate conjugated linoleic acid, which is shown to influence fatty acid composition in the liver and adipose tissue in mouse models (Devaraj et al., 2013; O'Shea et al., 2012). Additionally, as discussed earlier, intestinal bacteria produce SCFAs such as acetate, butyrate, propionate via dietary carbohydrate fermentation nondigestible by humans. Interestingly, *de novo* gluconeogenesis or lipid synthesis can be derived from certain SCFAs including propionate, hence serving as a means for fuel production and energy yielding for the host (human). Another interesting aspect of SCFAs is that they can extend signaling properties and, in this sense, constitute the mode by which microbes can produce metabolic signals affecting the metabolic regulation at the host level. In fact, SCFAs can modulate carbohydrate metabolism as well as gut physiology via the stimulation of mammalian peptide secretion while serving as fuel for gut epithelial cells. More specifically, SCFAs can stimulate glucagon-like peptide 1 (GLP-1) secretion via the G-protein-coupled receptor FFAR2 (free fatty acid receptor 2) in colon (Devaraj et al., 2013). Through the stimulation of GLP-1 secretion, bacterially produced SCFAs stipulate signals that downregulate glucagon secretion and stimulate glucose-dependent insulin secretion, while promoting glucose homeostasis.

Peptide YY, a hormone released by ileal and colonic epithelial cells in response to feeding seemingly able to suppress appetite, is also shown to be stimulated by SCFAs (Zhou et al., 2006). Interestingly, butyrate-supplemented high-fat diets were demonstrated to partially improve insulin resistance in diet-induced obese mice. Simultaneously, diets low in specific types of carbohydrates are shown to yield reduced butyrate-producing bacteria and fecal butyrate concentrations (Gao et al., 2009), thus lending support to the notion that the type of fuel can determine bacterial metabolite output and by extension ensuing signaling. Propionate promotes G-protein-coupled receptor 41 (GPR41)-mediated activation of sympathetic neurons, in contrast to ketone bodies, thereby affecting energy homeostasis (Kimura et al.,

2011). This documented potential for sympathetic outflow modulation constitutes yet another mechanism outlining the axis of gut microbiome–enteric nervous system–energetics–metabolic homeostasis.

Interestingly, Roux-en-Y gastric bypass (RYGB) surgery, a major bariatric intervention to treat morbid obesity, is shown to have an impact on the gut microbiome. Enhanced populations of Proteobacteria at the expense of those of Bacteroidetes were detected post-RYGB surgery. Such microbial population shifts plausibly result in alterations of metabolite profiles as well as relative preponderance for various fatty acids, including SCFAs. In animal experiments, nonobese rats subjected to RYGB exhibited reduced amounts of both Firmicutes and Bacteroidetes while exhibited significantly increased amounts (52-fold higher concentrations) of Proteobacteria compared to sham-operated counterparts (Bouillot et al., 2010). While obesity can be viewed as a chronic mild inflammatory or at least a pro-inflammatory state, the abundance of butyrate-producing *Faecalibacterium prausnitzii* was demonstrated to be negatively associated with biomarkers of inflammation prior and post-RYGB surgery, indicative of the fact that such bacterial species could be contributors to a healthy gut (Furet et al., 2010). Therefore, GI tract surgeries could extend a significant impact on gut microbial profile ensuing SCFA production and immunological responses.

Antibiotic administration even at the subtherapeutic level constitutes a *de facto* intervention in the GI tract and can alter the microbiome characteristics and by extension metabolic function. In an *in vivo* study, researchers administered subtherapeutic doses of antibiotics to mice observing increase in adiposity and levels of incretin GIP-1. Furthermore, significantly altered taxonomy in the microbiome was seen (increased Lachnospiraceae and Firmicutes at the expense of Bacteroidetes). Moreover, changes in metabolism-related genes (carbohydrates to SCFAs) were observed. More specifically, increased levels of acetate, propionate and butyrate were measured as well as changes in the regulation of hepatic lipid and cholesterol metabolism. Therefore, alteration of gut microbiota by antibiotic administration can result in the modulation of murine metabolic homeostasis. In this context, significant concerns are posed regarding antibiotics in the food chain and how these indirect exposures of consumers to antibiotics, especially chronically, may influence the human gut microbiome and by extension metabolic function and disease predisposition (Cho et al., 2012).

Additional microbial by-products with important relevance in host metabolism and health include secondary bile acids, which affect glucose homeostasis by activating receptors similar to those activated by the parent compounds (e.g., farnesoid X receptor-$\alpha$), and trimethylamine (TMA), derived by choline degradation (Cella et al., 2021). While TMA conversion to trimethylamine N-oxide is involved in CVD and choline deficiency is related to nonalcoholic fatty liver disease and altered glucose metabolism, secondary bile acids have been shown to be carcinogenic, thus significantly increasing risk for colonic tumorigenesis (Ocvirk and O'Keefe, 2021).

## SATURATED FATTY ACIDS

Saturated fatty acids were reported to enhance dysbiosis as well as intestinal inflammation in IL-10-deficient mice by inducing excessive growth of the bile-resistant Gram-negative bacterium *Bilophila wadsworthia*. In separate experiments, feeding C57BL/6J mice high-saturated fat diet significantly promoted the growth of 3 types of sulfidogenic bacteria in the colonic mucosa. These are hydrogen sulfide-producing bacteria as a metabolic by-product that damages intestinal barriers while causing endotoxemia. Providing C57BL/6J mice with a high-saturated fat dietary regime downregulated expression of tight junction proteins, contributing to induced intestinal permeability, endotoxemia as well as elevated levels of LPS-binding protein. Additionally, to higher fecal and plasma endotoxin levels, mice fed the aforementioned diet exhibited lower Bifidobacteria populations but increased Enterobacteriaceae populations in fecal culture. Laugerette et al. (2012) demonstrated a significantly increased intestinal *E. coli* population along with elevated both plasma and adipose inflammation in animals fed palm oil-based diets compared to counterparts fed diets with unsaturated fat. Collectively, these data suggest that diets high in saturated fat may negatively modulate the profile and subsequently the function of gut microbiota, contributing to increased inflammation in animal models (Alcock and Lin, 2015).

Researchers showed that high-fat diets resulted in a significant population reduction of dominant bacteria and groups such as Bifidobacteria, Eubacterium, Bacteroides and rectal *Clostridium coccoides*, constituting gut microflora. Such microflora alterations in turn increase the ratio of Gram-negative to Gram-positive bacteria including an increase in plasma LPS levels. Increased adiposity, body weight, hepatic ectopic lipid accumulation, insulin resistance and type 2 diabetes mellitus were all also associated with the aforementioned intestinal microflora alterations (Estadella, 2013).

LPSs cause endothelial activation by way of receptor complex consisting of Toll-like receptor 4 (TLR4), CD14 and myeloid differentiation factor 2 (MD2). Endothelial activation is characterized as a pro-inflammatory state during which the expression of leukocyte adhesion molecules increases, vascular integrity is lost, cytokine production increases and human leukocyte antigen production is upregulated (Kelleher and Sikalidis, 2021). When the GI is in an inflammatory state, metabolic endotoxemia occurs and bacterial LPS circulation increases by two- to threefold (Bailey and Holscher, 2018). Therefore, a diet high in saturated fat may further encourage a state of inflammation by upregulating LPS transport, while a diet high in fiber may decrease the proportion of Gram-negative bacteria and subsequently prevent endotoxemia, thus contributing to an overall healthier gut environment (Kelleher and Sikalidis, 2021).

## Polyunsaturated Fatty Acids (PUFAs) – Omega-3 and -6 (ω-3 and ω-6) Fatty Acids

The role of omega 3 (ω-3) and omega 6 (ω-6) polyunsaturated fatty acids (PUFAs), particularly omega 3, in regulating microbial metabolism by supporting optimal gut microbial demography more so during early life is of significant interest. The omega-class PUFAs, biosynthetic derivatives of α-linoleic acid and linolenic acid (LA) are found mostly in fatty fish and some plant oils (Sandhu et al., 2016).

The majority of beneficial anaerobic bacteria including Roseburia, Bifidobacteria and Lactobacillus are widely found in the colon, where PUFA metabolism from linoleic acid mainly occurs. Supplementation with omega 3 to an individual's diet during early-life stage supports prevention of gut microbiota changes, thereby reducing the risk for metabolic disorder, as well as chronic inflammation associated with early-life exposure to antibiotics (Sandhu et al., 2016).

Moreover, in adult mice exposed to an omega-3-supplemented diet, in utero and early life consistently increased both Bifidobacterium and Lactobacillus, but also yielded a higher Bifidobacteria-to-Enterobacteriaceae ratio. Omega-3 in particular is an extensively studied PUFA because of its effects on brain function including neuroprotection, restoration of energy metabolism, regulation of neurotransmitter levels and maintenance of membrane structure and composition. Notably, the Western-diet paradigm is typically characterized by high intake of saturated fat alongside with low omega-3 fatty acid intake. High-saturated fat intake at the expense of omega-3, among others, may be yet another reason as to why the "Western" dietary scheme is not generally considered particularly gut microbiome friendly.

According to a number of studies, inclusion of omega-3 PUFAs in the diet could restore inflammatory imbalances and mitigate subsequent harmful effects on cardiovascular diseases and metabolic syndrome (Rousseau G, 2021). A variety of mechanisms may be involved in this regard and include the following: (1) a reduction of bacteria-producing TMA; (2) an increase in bacteria-producing butyrate, which carries anti-inflammatory properties; and (3) a decrease in the production of pro-inflammatory cytokines. Moreover, omega-3 PUFAs could promote maintaining optimal integrity of the intestinal barrier, thereby preventing the translocation of intestinal contents in circulation.

The anti-inflammatory properties of omega-3 PUFA could be related to their incorporation in cell membrane phospholipids, largely at the expense of AA (omega-6 PUFA), with the latter being well established as pro-inflammatory (Simopoulos, 2008). Other possibilities were revealed through the identification of G-protein-coupled receptors (GPCRs) that interact with fatty acids (GPR43, GPR120). More specifically, DHA interacts with GPR120 and could inhibit iKB kinase as well as the production of pro-inflammatory cytokines, for example, tumor necrosis factor-alpha (TNFα). Docosahexaenoic acid and eicosapentaenoic acid may also inhibit NF-κB activity by the interaction with PPARγ or interference with early events prior to NF-κB activation (Rousseau G, 2021).

Moreover, a diet high in omega-3 PUFA is cardioprotective via a mechanism involving Akt activation (Rondeau et al., 2011), which is involved in a critical biochemical pathway component, the reperfusion injury salvage kinase. When activated at the onset of the reperfusion, these kinases confer cardioprotection by mPTP opening inhibition, while DHA can also inhibit the opening of the mPTP and result in a reduction of infarct size although the mechanism of action still remains elusive (Rousseau G, 2021).

Further to the direct effect of omega-3 PUFA, the metabolites involved in the resolution phase of inflammation known as resolvins (Rv) may constitute yet another avenue through which omega-3 PUFAs can exert cardioprotective effects to humans. It has been reported by Tran and colleagues (Tran et al., 2014), that RvD1 administration prior to the onset of reperfusion effectively reduced myocardial infarct size in a porcine model (Tran et al., 2014). Additional observations confirmed that when there is inhibition of the main enzymes involved in DHA transformation to RvD1 (COX-2 and 15-LOX), plasma RvD1 concentrations are significantly reduced and the cardioprotection is abolished (Gilbert et al., 2015). Along similar lines, Keyes et al. demonstrated that RvE1 administration in a rat model of myocardial infarction significantly reduces infarct size while also increases Akt and Erk activity (Keyes et al., 2010). These observations taken together illustrate a potential role for a number of metabolites involved in omega-3 PUFAs-related cardioprotection observed with omega-3 PUFAs-rich diets. Another cardioprotective effect that omega-3 PUFAs and their metabolites could induce may be associated with the impact they may exert on the composition of the microbiota, since omega-3 PUFAs can positively alter gut microbiota demography.

## SHORT-CHAIN FATTY ACIDS

Typically, main metabolic products of colonic fermentation are as follows: SCFAs and varying gaseous volumes of $H_2$ and $CO_2$. SCFAs are generated by plant-derived polysaccharides, whereas they contribute approximately 5%–10% of daily energy requirement in humans. While butyrate is used as fuel, *in situ* by colonocytes, propionate and acetate are largely absorbed and transported to the liver, muscles and other peripheral tissues. Acetate supports resynthesizing of lipids in the liver, whereas propionate constitutes an important substrate for gluconeogenesis (Wasielewski et al., 2016; Thakur et al., 2014; Salonen and de Vos, 2014).

Diets rich in fiber have been shown to increase the production of SCFAs by the intestinal microbiota. SCFAs are very important metabolic products in the maintenance of the intestinal barrier, with physiological concentrations having provable effects on intestinal barrier function. Certain types of bacterial families such as Bacteroides, Bifidobacterium, Propionibacterium, Eubacterium, Lactobacillus, Clostridium, Roseburia and Prevotella produce SCFAs. SCFAs in turn can function as neurohormonal signaling molecules that can cross the BBB transported by monocarboxylate transporters. Imaging studies demonstrated that microbiota-derived acetate can cross the BBB where it subsequently affects hypothalamic gene expression. Butyrate has been demonstrated to influence expression of tight junction proteins (claudin-2, occludin, cingulin, and zonula occludens proteins, ZO-1, ZO-2), while it is shown to be able to reduce bacterial translocation and extend antitumorigenic properties (Kelly et al., 2015).

Furthermore, SCFAs constitute a critical energy source for both colonic and ileal cells while they further affect the intestinal epithelial barrier and defense functions by regulating relevant gene expression and influencing inflammatory status of the gut. Moreover, SCFAs regulate functions of innate immune cells contributing to the immune systematic responses, such as macrophages, neutrophils and dendritic cells. Additionally, SCFAs can extend regulation over the differentiation of T cells and B cells as well as the antigen-specific adaptive immunity mediated by the former. Also, SCFAs constitute potential precursors as in raw materials for glucose and lipid synthesis, which stipulates a theoretical framework for examining the potential role of SCFAs regarding the regulation of energy homeostasis and metabolism. Moreover, there are also studies showing that SCFAs inhibit tumor cell proliferation and promote apoptosis (Yao et al., 2022).

More specifically, Yang and colleagues (2020) demonstrated that microbiota-derived SCFAs promote interleukin 22 (IL-22), a member of the IL-10 family, central to host protection against inflammatory insult in the intestine by inducing antimicrobial peptides and promoting epithelial barrier function. Conducting *in vivo* work, WT B6 mice were administered with or without 200 mM butyrate in drinking water for 3 weeks, and IL-22 was shown to be produced by CD4+ T cells and ILCs through G-protein receptor 41 (GPR41) and inhibit histone deacetylase. The authors reported that SCFAs upregulate IL-22 production by promoting aryl hydrocarbon receptor (AhR) and hypoxia-inducible factor 1α (HIF1α) expression, which are differentially regulated by mTOR and Stat3. Mechanistically, they showed that HIF1α binds directly to the *Il22* promoter, and SCFAs increase HIF1α binding to the *Il22* promoter through histone modification. Hence, SCFA supplementation enhances IL-22 production, which protects intestines from inflammation, and SCFAs promote human CD4+ T-cell IL-22 production. Their reported findings reveal significant roles for SCFAs in inducing IL-22 production in CD4+ T cells and ILCs to maintain intestinal homeostasis and protect against inflammation while optimizing immune responses.

## THE GUT MICROBIOME AND AMINO ACID METABOLISM

Desirable gut bacteria like Bifidobacteria and Lactobacilli produce amino acid–derived bioactive compounds, including several biogenic amines. Amino acids, di-, tri-peptides and a few oligo-peptides from the diet as well as to a lesser degree partially hydrolized proteins reach the colon and ultimately constitute sources yielding substrates for luminal bioconversion via the gut microbiome. Various microbiome-produced enzymes contribute to amino acid metabolism by generating bioactive metabolites in the intestine. A typical class of that type of enzymes is amino acid decarboxylases, widely prevalent in gut microbes. These microbial enzymes, when combined with amino acid transport systems, link dietary compounds with microbial metabolism and signaling with the gut mucosa. Such an example of the gut microbiome is the bacterium *Lactobacillus reuteri*, which can convert dietary L-histidine, to an immunoregulatory signaling molecule, histamine, which in turn suppresses pro-inflammatory TNF production via histamine type 2 receptors in the intestinal epithelium. Another example of microbe-facilitated amino acid metabolism is the generation of γ-amino butyric acid from glutamate, by glutamate decarboxylase (Devaraj et al., 2013), while another is the production of putrescine from ornithine. Such anti-inflammatory amino acid metabolites derived from microbial metabolism utilizing amino acids as substrates may improve pathologies related to obesity, systemic inflammation and type 2 diabetes mellitus status.

In an interesting *in vivo* study involving Sprague–Dawley rats, Li and colleagues investigated the effect of protein feeding to the gut microbiome of rats using soybean protein (Spro), soybean protein-derived peptides (SPre) and casein as feeding regimes (Li et al., 2021). The cecum microflora composition of the rats was determined via 16S rDNA amplicon sequencing, showing that the SPro along with its derived peptides significantly increased the abundance and uniformity of the gut microbiota after 35 days of feeding. The authors reported that Firmicutes/Bacteroidetes (F/B) ratios of the SPep, SPro and casein groups were $2.49 \pm 0.60$, $2.98 \pm 1.12$ and $2.59 \pm 0.74$, respectively. Interestingly, while the rats fed SPro and SPep exhibited similar gut microbiome profiles, SPep significantly promoted Lactobacillus and Phascolarctobacterium growth. Their results indicated that SPep significantly increased the diversity of the gut microbiota and elevated the probiotic portion of the bacterial gut population. The authors concluded that both SPro and SPep were able to modify the demography of gut microbiota in rats, with the effect of SPep being more desirable from a health standpoint as judged by F/B ratio (Li et al., 2021).

In another study, Butteiger et al. demonstrated that soy protein compared to milk protein in a Western-diet regime increases gut microbial diversity and reduces serum lipids in golden Syrian hamsters (Butteiger et al. 2016). More specifically, 32, 6- to 8-week-old male golden Syrian hamsters were fed a Western diet containing 22% (%wt) milk protein isolate (MPI) as the single protein source for 3 week followed by 6 week of one of four diets containing either of the following [22% protein (%wt)]: MPI, soy protein concentrate, partially hydrolyzed soy protein isolate (SPI1) or intact soy protein isolate. Serum lipids, hepatic gene expression and gut microbial populations were evaluated. Sequencing of the 16S ribosomal RNA gene revealed greater microbial diversity in each soy-fed group than in the MPI-fed group ($P < 0.05$). The authors concluded that dietary protein sources in male golden Syrian hamsters fed a Western diet differ in terms of how they affect the gut microbiota with soy protein producing a favorable gut microbiome profile while also potentially promoting the reduction of lipogenesis through alterations of the gut microbial community (Butteiger et al. 2016). These *in vivo* studies lend support to the notion that plant-based/-derived protein may constitute a dietary approach that could extend health benefits, in addition to other shown aspects such as N-balance with lower risk for allergies, also relative to the gut microbiome, while also promoting sustainability and an eco-friendly approach to agriculture and food production.

## THE MICROBIOME AND WEIGHT CHANGE

Overnutrition leading to obesity is associated with a cluster of metabolic and systemic disorders such as insulin resistance, type 2 diabetes mellitus, fatty liver disease, atherosclerosis and hypertension. Alarmingly, obesity rates have more than doubled in the last 2 decades globally. A growing body of evidence suggests that the gut microbiota represents an important factor contributing to energetics and by extension to over-/undernutrition. A pivotal study by Turnbaugh et al. (2006) was among the first studies to demonstrate that gut microbiota contributes to obesity. The microbiome obtained from the colon of genetically obese leptin-deficient mice (*ob/ob*) was compared against that of lean littermates. Researchers reported that *ob/ob* mice microbiota included genes encoding enzymes that hydrolyze indigestible dietary polysaccharides. Higher amounts of fermentation endproducts (i.e., acetate and butyrate) and lower caloric content were identified in the obese mice fecal matter compared to lean counterparts. The results imply that gut microbiota in the obese mice induced extraction of additional calories from the diet by means of metabolic rearrangement, concluding that gut microbiome profile appears important for body weight regulation (Ley et al., 2006). Interestingly, when gut microbiota of either *ob/ob* mice or lean mice was transplanted to lean gnotobiotic mice, in mere 2 weeks, mice that received microbiota from the ob/ob mice extracted more calories from diet, while demonstrating significantly higher adiposity compared to mice receiving the microbiota of lean mice. The results obtained sustenance a critical part of gut microbiome regarding the pathogenesis of obesity and by extension obesity-related disorders. In human experiments, Ley and colleagues (2006) as well as Ravussin and colleagues (2011) successively examined fecal gut microbiota of 12 obese participants who followed an annual weight loss program by engaging in a fat-restricted or a carbohydrate-restricted, but always low-calorie diet. Analogous to similar *in vivo* experiments, abundance of gut bacteria of the Bacteroidetes and Firmicutes phyla was detected, while the microbiome exhibited noteworthy intraindividual consistency over time. Prior to the low-calorie diet initiation, increased populations of Firmicutes at the expense of those of Bacteroidetes were observed in the obese individuals compared to nonobese controls. After weight loss, higher populations of Bacteroidetes (3%–15%) with decreased populations of Firmicutes were seen. More interestingly, the changes observed correlated quantitatively with weight loss rather than dietary caloric content changes in terms of percentages.

In terms of definite dietary schemes, a recent study demonstrated that the Mediterranean diet can positively affect resting metabolic rate as well as salivary microbiota in humans subjects (Daniele et al., 2021). More specifically, salivary microbiota composition and metabolic profile were analyzed in participants with vegan (VEG) or Mediterranean (MED) long-term dietary patterns. The MED participants demonstrated significantly higher percentages of *Subflava* and *Prevotella* bacterial species as compared to VEG participants. Moreover, the authors reported that MED participants showed higher basal metabolic rate (BMR) and lower respiratory quotient (RQ). Furthermore, *Prevotella* abundance was demonstrated to be inversely correlated with RQ and carbohydrate consumption (which was seen to be lower in the MED participants), whereas *Subflava* percentages were demonstrated to be positively correlated to BMR. *Lactobacillus* abundance, which was inversely related to *Subflava* presence in MED participants, was associated with decreased BMR (Harris-Benedict) values. Taken together, these observations demonstrate positive effects of the Mediterranean diet on BMR and on the abundance of microbial species associated with a better macronutrient metabolism (Daniele et al., 2021).

The Mediterranean diet is becoming increasingly more popular due to growing evidence regarding the role it can play in chronic disease prevention and immune response modulation. Characterized by a diet rich in fruits, vegetables, fish, olive oil, red wine and refined cereal products, the foods that are part of Mediterranean diet are typically rich in fiber, omega-3 fatty acids, polyphenols, SCFAs, PUFAs, phytosterols and antioxidants. Together, these bioactive compounds collectively and synergistically extend anti-inflammatory and antioxidative properties, which may be needed in counteracting accumulation of TMA N-oxides and the endotoxin LPS (Kelleher and Sikalidis, 2021).

## FUTURE PERSPECTIVES

Whereas the link between gut microbiome, food and health is becoming increasingly clearer, researchers are struggling to successfully and effectively manipulate the microbiome as a form of treatment. Even though we have gained more knowledge and understanding than ever before as to how the microbiome influences chronic disease, it remains elusive as to how to change a person's microbiome in a particular favorable direction. There appears to be a clear need to assess how delivery and/or interactive systems in the gut's interface can be employed to affect bacterial type and population size in the gut (Kristo et al., 2015) promoting optimal microbiome demography, including but not solely limited to dietary schemes (Sikalidis, 2019). It is clearly important to consider nutrition/diet perspectives as related to implications with clinical nutrition and medical nutrition therapy. Beyond the studied relationship between the microbiome and the obesity, further, there is significant evidence to suggest that there are strong associations between the demographics/quality of the microbiome and risk toward chronic diseases such as T2DM and ensuing CVD, as well as inflammation and related pathologies (Sikalidis and Maykish, 2020), extending through the gut–brain axis to potential roles in Alzheimer's as well as other neurodegenerative diseases (Shukla et al., 2021).

After the successful completion of the human genome project approximately two decades ago, Relman and Falkow urged the scientific community to embark on a "second human genome project", a large-scale genomic survey of our endogenous microflora (Relman and Falkow, 2001). Since then, the field of microbiome research has greatly expanded, leading to large-scale efforts such as the NIH, HMP and the Earth Microbiome Project. Those efforts alongside a significant increase in the interest and ensuing research of the microbiome generated a significant body of literature aiming to shed light on this human–microbiome symbiotic relationship. There is ample evidence that microbiomes are networked and interconnected primarily by means of the flows of mobile genetic elements (MGEs) (Haraoui, 2022). The diversity, demography and profile of those MGEs have significantly expanded over the past decades responsive to continuously growing selective pressures primarily due to several anthropogenic forces applied. A microbial ontology more attuned to these phenomena considering the aforementioned process could potentially provide a more effective theoretical framework toward studying the microbiome and revealing potential ways to utilize its plasticity for the benefit of human health.

## REFERENCES

Albenberg LG, Wu GD. Diet and the intestinal microbiome: associations, functions, and implications for health and disease. *Gastroenterology*. 2014;146(6):1564–1572.

Alcock J, Lin HC. Fatty acids from diet and microbiota regulate energy metabolism. *F1000Research*. 2015;4(F1000 Faculty Rev):738.

Arnone D, Chabot C, Heba AC, Kökten T, Caron B, Hansmannel F, Dreumont N, Ananthakrishnan AN, Quilliot D, Peyrin-Biroulet L. Sugars and gastrointestinal health. *Clin Gastroenterol Hepatol*. 2021. doi: 10.1016/j.cgh.2021.12.011.

Bailey MA, Holscher HD. Microbiome-mediated effects of the Mediterranean diet on inflammation. *Adv Nutr*. 2018;9(3):193–206. doi: 10.1093/advances/nmy013.

Barnich N, Chassaing B. When pathobiont-carbohydrate interaction turns bittersweet! *Cell Mol Gastroenterol Hepatol*. 2021;12(4):1509–1510. doi: 10.1016/j.jcmgh.2021.08.008.

Bashiardes S, Godneva A, Elinav E, Segal E. Towards utilization of the human genome and microbiome for personalized nutrition. *Curr Opin Biotechnol*. 2018;51:57–63.

Bouillot JL, et al. Differential adaptation of human gut microbiota to bariatric surgery-induced weight loss: links with metabolic and low-grade inflammation markers. *Diabetes*. 2010;59:3049–3057.

Butteiger DN, Hibberd AA, McGraw NJ, Napawan N, Hall-Porter JM, Krul ES. Soy protein compared with milk protein in a western diet increases gut microbial diversity and reduces serum lipids in golden Syrian hamsters. *J Nutr*. 2016;146(4):697–705. doi: 10.3945/jn.115.224196.

Cantarel BL, Lombard V, Henrissat B. Complex carbohydrate utilization by the healthy human microbiome. *PLoS One*. 2012;7:e28742.

Cella V, Bimonte VM, Sabato C, Paoli A, Baldari C, Campanella M, Lenzi A, Ferretti E, Migliaccio S. Nutrition and physical activity-induced changes in gut microbiota: possible implications for human health and athletic performance. *Foods*. 2021;10(12):3075. doi: 10.3390/foods10123075.

Chichlowski M, De Lartigue G, German JB, Raybould HE, Mills DA. Bifidobacteria isolated from infants and cultured on human milk oligosaccharides affect intestinal epithelial function. *J Pediatr Gastroenterol Nutr*. 2012;55:321–327.

Cho I, Yamanishi S, Cox L, Methe BA, Zavadil J, Li K, et al. Antibiotics in early life alter the murine colonic microbiome and adiposity. *Nature* 2012;30:621–626.

Daniele S, Scarfò G, Ceccarelli L, Fusi J, Zappelli E, Biagini D, Lomonaco T, Di Francesco F, Franzoni F, Martini C. The Mediterranean Diet Positively Affects Resting Metabolic Rate and Salivary Microbiota in Human Subjects: a Comparison with the Vegan Regimen. *Biology (Basel)*. 2021;10(12):1292. doi: 10.3390/biology10121292.

Dawson SL, Dash SR, Jacka FN. Chapter Fifteen – the importance of diet and gut health to the treatment and prevention of mental disorders. *Int Rev Neurobiol*. 2016;131:325–346.

Devaraj S, Hemarajata P, Versalovic J. The human gut microbiome and body metabolism: implications for obesity and diabetes. *Clin Chem*. 2013;59(4):617–628.

Do MH, Lee E, Oh MJ, Kim Y, Park HY. High-glucose or -fructose diet cause changes of the gut microbiota and metabolic disorders in mice without body weight change. *Nutrients*. 2018;10(6):761. doi: 10.3390/nu10060761.

Dou Z, Chen C, Huang Q, Fu X. In vitro digestion of the whole blackberry fruit: bioaccessibility, bioactive variation of active ingredients and impacts on human gut microbiota. *Food Chem*. 2022;370:131001. doi: 10.1016/j.foodchem.2021.131001.

Estadella D, Da Penha Oller Do Nascimento CM, Oyama LM, Ribeiro EB, Dâmaso AR, De Piano A. Lipotoxicity: effects of dietary saturated and transfatty acids. *Mediators Inflamm*. 2013;2013:137579.

Faming Z, Luo W, Shi Y, et al. Should we standardize the 1700-year-old fecal microbiota transplantation? *Am J Gastroenterol*. 2012;107:1755.

Furet JP, Kong LC, Tap J, Poitou C, Basdevant A, Bouillot JL, et al. Differential adaptation of human gut microbiota to bariatric surgery-induced weight loss: links with metabolic and low-grade inflammation markers. *Diabetes*. 2010;59:3049–3057.

Gao Z, Yin J, Zhang J, Ward RE, Martin RJ, Lefevre M, et al. Butyrate improves insulin sensitivity and increases energy expenditure in mice. *Diabetes*. 2009;58:1509–1517.

García-Montero C, Fraile-Martínez O, Gómez-Lahoz AM, Pekarek L, Castellanos AJ, Noguerales-Fraguas F, Coca S, Guijarro LG, García-Honduvilla N, Asúnsolo A, Sanchez-Trujillo L, Lahera G, Bujan J, Monserrat J, Álvarez-Mon M, Álvarez-Mon MA, Ortega MA. Nutritional components in western diet versus Mediterranean diet at the gut microbiota-immune system interplay. Implications for health and disease. *Nutrients*. 2021;13(2):699. doi: 10.3390/nu13020699.

Garrido D, Nwosu C, Ruiz-Moyano S, Aldredge D, German JB, Lebrilla CB, Mills DA. Endo-beta-N-acetylglucosaminidases from infant-gut associated bifidobacteria release complex N-glycans from human milk glycoproteins. *Mol Cell Proteom.* 2012;11:775–785.

Gilbert K, Malick M, Madingou N, Touchette C, Bourque-Riel V, Tomaro L, Rousseau G. Metabolites derived from omega-3 polyunsaturated fatty acids are important for cardioprotection. *Eur J Pharmacol.* 2015;769:147–153. doi: 10.1016/j.ejphar.2015.11.010.

Gray MW. Lynn Margulis and the endosymbiont hypothesis: 50 years later. *Mol Biol Cell.* 2017;28(10):1285–1287.

Haraoui LP. Networked collective microbiomes and the rise of subcellular 'units of life'. *Trends Microbiol.* 2022;30(2):112–119. doi: 10.1016/j.tim.2021.09.011.

Hemarajata P, Versalovic J. Effects of probiotics on gut microbiota: mechanisms of intestinal immunomodulation and neuromodulation. *Therap Adv Gastroenterol.* 2013;6(1):39–51.

Heras VL, Melgar S, MacSharry J, Gahan CGM. The influence of the western diet on microbiota and gastrointestinal immunity. *Annu Rev Food Sci Technol.* 2022; doi: 10.1146/annurev-food-052720-011032.

Holmes E, Wilson ID, Nicholson JK. Metabolic phenotyping in health and disease. *Cell.* 2008; 134(5):714–717.

Hussein HM, Elyamany MF, Rashed LA, Sallam NA. Vitamin D mitigates diabetes-associated metabolic and cognitive dysfunction by modulating gut microbiota and colonic cannabinoid receptor 1. *Eur J Pharm Sci.* 2022;170:106105. doi: 10.1016/j.ejps.2021.106105.

Institute of Medicine 2013. *The Human–Microbiome, Diet, and Health: Workshop Summary.* Washington, DC: The National Academies Press.

Jones RB, Alderete TL, Kim JS, Millstein J, Gilliland FD, Goran MI. High intake of dietary fructose in overweight/obese teenagers associated with depletion of *Eubacterium* and *Streptococcus* in gut microbiome. *Gut Microbes.* 2019;10(6):712–719. doi: 10.1080/19490976.2019.1592420.

Kable ME, Chin EL, Storms D, Lemay DG, Stephensen CB. Tree-based analysis of dietary diversity captures associations between fiber intake and gut microbiota composition in a healthy U.S. Adult Cohort. *J Nutr.* 2021;nxab430. doi: 10.1093/jn/nxab430.

Kelleher AH, Sikalidis AK. The Effects of Mediterranean Diet on the Human Gut Microbiota; a Brief Discussion of Evidence in Humans. *Gastroenterol Hepatol.* 2021;5(1):16. doi:10.21926/obm.hg.2101056.

Kelly JR, Kennedy PJ, Cryan JF, Dinan TG, Clarke G, Hyland NP. Breaking down the barriers: the gut microbiome, intestinal permeability and stress-related psychiatric disorders. *Front Cell Neurosci.* 2015;9:392.

Keyes KT, Ye Y, Lin Y, Zhang C, Perez-Polo JR, Gjorstrup P, Birnbaum Y. Resolvin E1 protects the rat heart against reperfusion injury. *Am J Physiol Heart Circ Physiol.* 2010;299(1):H153–H164. doi: 10.1152/ajpheart.01057.2009.

Kimura I, Inoue D, Maeda T, Hara T, Ichimura A, Miyauchi S, et al. Short-chain fatty acids and ketones directly regulate sympathetic nervous system via G protein-coupled receptor 41 (GPR41). *Proc Natl Acad Sci U S A.* 2011;108:8030–8035.

Kristo AS, Tzanidaki G, Lygeros A, Sikalidis AK. Bile sequestration potential of an edible mineral (clinoptilolite) under simulated digestion of a high-fat meal; an in vitro investigation. *Food Funct.* 2015;6(12):3818–3827.

Laugerette F, Furet JP, Debard C, Daira P, Loizon E, Géloën A, et al. Oil composition of high-fat diet affects metabolic inflammation differently in connection with endotoxin receptors in mice. *Am J Physiol Endocrinol Metab.* 2012;302(3):E374–E386.

Ley RE, Turnbaugh PJ, Klein S, Gordon IJ. Microbial ecology: human gut microbes associated with obesity. *Nature.* 2006;444(7122):1022–1023.

Li W, Li H, Zhang Y, Zhang C, Zhang J, Liu X. Differences in the gut microbiota composition of rats fed with soybean protein and their derived peptides. *J Food Sci.* 2021;86(12):5452–5465. doi: 10.1111/1750-3841.15948.

MacDonald IA. A review of recent evidence relating to sugars, insulin resistance and diabetes. *Eur J Nutr.* 2016;55(Suppl 2):17–23. doi: 10.1007/s00394-016-1340-8.

Magnusson KR, Hauck L, Jeffrey BM, Elias V, Humphrey A, Nath R, Perrone A, Bermudez LE. Relationships between diet-related changes in the gut microbiome and cognitive flexibility. *Neuroscience.* 2015;300:128–140. doi: 10.1016/j.neuroscience.2015.05.016.

Mondot S, Lepage P. The human gut microbiome and its dysfunctions through the meta-omics prism. *Ann N Y Acad Sci.* 2016;1372(1):9–19.

Moore AM. Nineteenth-century psychiatry of coprophilia and psychosis. *Microbial Ecol Health Dis.* 2019;30:1546267.

Nicholson JK, Holmes E, Wilson ID. Gut microorganisms, mammalian metabolism and personalized health care. *Nat Rev Microbiol.* 2005;3(5):431–438.

Nicholson JK, Elliott P, Holmes E. Metabolome-wide association study identifies multiple biomarkers that discriminate North and South Chinese populations at differing risks of cardiovascular disease: Intermap study. *J Proteome Res.* 2010;9(12):6647–6654.

Ochoa M, Lallès JP, Malbert CH, Val-Laillet D. Dietary sugars: their detection by the gut-brain axis and their peripheral and central effects in health and diseases. *Eur J Nutr.* 2015;54(1):1–24.

Ocvirk S, O'Keefe SJD. Dietary fat, bile acid metabolism and colorectal cancer. *Semin Cancer Biol.* 2021;73:347–355. doi: 10.1016/j.semcancer.2020.10.003.

Opritu R, Bratu M, Opritu B. Fecal transplantation – the new, inexpensive, safe and rapidly effective approach in the treatment of gastrointestinal tract disorders. *J Med Life.* 2016;9(2):160–162.

O'Shea EF, Cotter PD, Stanton C, Ross RP, Hill C. Production of bioactive substances by intestinal bacteria as a basis for explaining probiotic mechanisms: bacteriocins and conjugated linoleic acid. *Int J Food Microbiol.* 2012;152:189–205.

Prescott SL. History of medicine: origin of the term microbiome and why it matters. *Hum Microbiome J.* 2017;4:24–25.

Ravussin Y, Koren O, Spor A, LeDuc C, Gutman R, Stombaugh J, et al. Responses of gut microbiota to diet composition and weight loss in lean and obese mice. *Obesity.* 2011;20:738–747.

Relman DA, Falkow S. The meaning and impact of the human genome sequence for microbiology. *Trends Microbiol.* 2001;9(5):206–208. doi: 10.1016/s0966-842x(01)02041-8.

Rondeau I, Picard S, Bah TM, Roy L, Godbout R, Rousseau G. Effects of different dietary ω-6/3 polyunsaturated fatty acids ratios on infarct size and the limbic system after myocardial infarction. *Can J Physiol Pharmacol.* 2011;89(3):169–176. doi: 10.1139/Y11-007.

Rossella C, Laura F, Grazia MM, Raffaele B, Antonio T, Maria P, Francesco V, Giovanni G. The crosstalk between gut microbiota, intestinal immunological niche and visceral adipose tissue as a new model for the pathogenesis of metabolic and inflammatory diseases: the paradigm of type 2 diabetes mellitus. *Curr Med Chem.* 2022. doi: 10.2174/0929867329666220105121124.

Rousseau G. Microbiota, a new playground for the Omega-3 polyunsaturated fatty acids in cardiovascular diseases. *Marine Drugs.* 2021;19(2):54. doi: 10.3390/md19020054.

Salonen A, de Vos WM. Impact of diet on human intestinal microbiota and health. *Annu Rev Food Sci Technol.* 2014;5(1):239–262.

Sandhu KV, Sherwin E, Schellekens H, Stanton C, Dinan TG, Cryan JF. Feeding the microbiota-gut-brain axis: diet, microbiome and neuropsychiatry. *Transl Res.* 2016;179:223–244.

Sarkar A, Lehto SM, Harty S, Dinan TG, Cryan JF, Burnet PWJ. Psychobiotics and the Manipulation of bacteria–gut–brain signals. *Trends Neurosci.* 2016;39(11):763–781.

Savage D. Microbial ecology of the gastrointestinal tract. *Annu Rev Microbiol.* 1977;31:107–133.

Sender R, Fuchs S, Milo R. Revised estimates for the number of human and bacteria cells in the body. *PLoS Biol.* 2016a;14(8):e1002533.

Sender R, Fuchs S, Milo R. Are we really vastly outnumbered? Revisiting the ratio of bacterial to host cells in humans. *Cell*. 2016b;164:337–340.

Shukla PK, Delotterie DF, Xiao J, Pierre JF, Rao R, McDonald MP, Khan MM. Alterations in the gut-microbial-inflammasome-brain axis in a mouse model of Alzheimer's disease. *Cells*. 2021;10(4):779. doi: 10.3390/cells10040779.

Sikalidis AK. From food for survival to food for personalized optimal health. A historical perspective of how food and nutrition gave rise to nutrigenomics. *J Am Coll Nutr*. 2019;38(1):84–95.

Sikalidis AK, Maykish A. The gut microbiome and type 2 diabetes mellitus; discussing a complex relationship. *Biomedicines*. 2020;8(1):8. doi: 10.3390/biomedicines8010008.

Simopoulos AP. The importance of the omega-6/omega-3 fatty acid ratio in cardiovascular disease and other chronic diseases. *Exp Biol Med (Maywood)*. 2008;233(6):674–688. doi: 10.3181/0711-MR-311.

Sonnenburg ED, Zheng H, Joglekar P, Higginbottom SK, Firbank SJ, Bolam DN, Sonnenburg JL. Specificity of polysaccharide use in intestinal bacteroides species determines diet-induced microbiota alterations. *Cell*. 2010;141:1241–1252.

Speliotes EK, et al. Association analyses of 249,796 individuals reveal 18 new loci associated with body mass index. *Nat Genet*. 2010;42(11):937–948.

Steve LB, Khoruts A. Fecal microbiota transplantation: an interview with Alexander Khoruts. *Global Adv Health Med*. 2014;3(3):73–80.

Thakur AK, Shakya A, Mohammed G, Emerald M, Kumar V. Gut-microbiota and mental health: current and future perspectives. *Pharmacol Clin Toxicol*. 2014;2(1):1–15.

Tran Quang T, Gosselin A-A, Bourque-Riel V, Gilbert K, Charron T, Rousseau G. Effect of Resolvin D1 on experimental myocardial infarction. *Exp Clin Cardiol*. 2014;20:6704–6712.

Turnbaugh PJ, Ley RE, Mahowald MA, Magrini V, Mardis ER, Gordon JI. An obesity-associated gut microbiome with increased capacity for energy harvest. *Nature*. 2006;444(7122):1027–1031.

Wasielewski H, Alcock J, Aktipis A. Resource conflict and cooperation between human host and gut microbiota: implications for nutrition and health. *Ann N Y Acad Sci*. 2016;1372(1):20–28.

Woodruff IO. Organotherapy. *J Adv Ther*. 1910;28:551.

Yang W, Yu T, Huang X, Bilotta AJ, Xu L, Lu Y, Sun J, Pan F, Zhou J, Zhang W, Yao S, Maynard CL, Singh N, Dann SM, Liu Z, Cong Y. Intestinal microbiota-derived short-chain fatty acids regulation of immune cell IL-22 production and gut immunity. *Nat Commun*. 2020;11(1):4457. doi: 10.1038/s41467-020-18262-6.

Yao Y, Cai X, Fei W, Ye Y, Zhao M, Zheng C. The role of short-chain fatty acids in immunity, inflammation and metabolism. *Crit Rev Food Sci Nutr*. 2022;62(1):1–12. doi: 10.1080/10408398.2020.1854675.

Yap IK, Brown IJ, Chan Q, Wijeyesekera A, Garcia-Perez I, Bictash M, et al. Metabolome wide association study identifies multiple biomarkers that discriminate North and South Chinese populations at differing risks of cardiovascular disease: Intermap study. *J Proteome Res*. 2010;9(12):6647–6654.

Zhang X, Jin Q, Jin LH. High sugar diet disrupts gut homeostasis though JNK and STAT pathways in drosophila. *Biochem Biophys Res Commun*. 2017;487(4):910–916. doi: 10.1016/j.bbrc.2017.04.156.

Zhou J, Hegsted M, McCutcheon KL, Keenan MJ, Xi X, Raggio AM, Martin RJ. Peptide YY and proglucagon mRNA expression patterns and regulation in the gut. *Obesity (Silver Spring)*. 2006;14:683–689.

Zoetendal EG, Raes J, van den Bogert B, Arumugam M, Booijink CC, Troost FJ, et al. The human small intestinal microbiota is driven by rapid uptake and conversion of simple carbohydrates. *ISME J*. 2012;6:1415–1426.

# 4 Models for Researching the Gut Microbiome

*Alison Lacombe and Vivian C.H. Wu*
United States Department of Agriculture

*Aleksandra S. Kristo*
California Polytechnic State University

## CONTENTS

## INTRODUCTION

Models are used to study gastrointestinal health to determine the impact of a treatment, critical time points for administration, and potential mechanisms that drive efficacy. For many studies pertaining to probiotics and prebiotics, complex microbiological and metabolomics assays serve as proxy for microbiota function (Mabwi et al., 2021). A "snapshot" of the gut microbiota composition and function can provide valuable insights into what factors alter compositional and metabolic changes subsequent to dietary interventions (Mabwi et al., 2021). However, investigating discreet time points only offers limited information regarding the dynamics of compositional and

DOI: 10.1201/b22970-6

metabolic changes. Therefore, models to investigate alterations in gut function incurred by dietary changes must be placed in the proper context of a defined research question.

Most research on the gut microbiota utilizes clinical studies or animal models. Models attempt to address the intrinsic difficulty in accessing the human intestine to study its microbial composition, metabolite and enzyme production, and inflammatory processes (Mabwi et al., 2021). However, studies with humans and animal models can be limited by the lack of homogeneity with regard to the target population. Due to their technical reproducibility, easy access, and monitoring, *in vitro* and *in silico* models represent a valid alternative to study the microbial behavior of the human gut microbiota. In previous chapters, we have discussed the recent advances in high-throughput sequencing of the gut microbiome and the general impact of nutrition on species profile composition. In this chapter, we will be providing a brief overview of the models utilized to study the interactions between diet and gut microbiota. The intestinal microbiota has been studied in a variety of *in vitro*, *in vivo*, and *ex vivo* models, each presenting distinct benefits and drawbacks, while all models can provide useful insights into the mechanism of human digestion of prebiotics.

## COMPUTATIONAL MODELS

Mathematical models can determine the statistical relationship between dietary interventions and gastrointestinal health; however, these experiments are subject to the assumptions used to build the models (Lamichhane, Sen, Dickens, Orešič, & Bertram, 2018). "Snapshots" of the gut metagenome or metabolome often fail to provide sufficient information on periodic patterns, interdependencies, or temporal variations present within the microbiome (Lamichhane et al., 2018). Longitudinal analysis can elucidate the changes over time and offer better context to the health impacts of dietary interventions; however, this approach presents its own unique set of challenges (Mabwi et al., 2021). Longitudinal studies in human populations are often complicated by limited time points, sample dropout, and uneven sampling frequency (Mabwi et al., 2021). Therefore, other models, such as animals or cell culture, are often employed for complex computational analysis.

Interactions in a microbial community are driven by several mechanisms including competition for nutrients, direct interactions between community members, and interactions with the host and attachment sites in the host environment (Mabwi et al., 2021). This network of bacterial interactions can be altered by the host's age, diet, disease initiation, or other exogenous perturbations (Mabwi et al., 2021). The combinations of the correct models and computational tools are needed to infer ecological relationships of microbiota and its associated metabolic functionality.

Temporal networks that depict how a connected system evolves with time have emerged as useful tools for analyzing the gut microbiome. There are numerous univariate and multivariate analytical methods that can test the significance of dietary intervention at discrete time points or within a time series (Mabwi et al., 2021). These methods have been applied to both metataxonomic and metabolomic temporal data. For longitudinal studies where specific microbial features (e.g., taxa) are differentially abundant, data smoothing, such as spline ANOVA, can discrete time points into a polynomial curve (Mabwi et al., 2021). This analysis can estimate a difference in function in the context of time with differential abundance. With the integration of the difference function over a time interval, a statistical divergence in the data set can be detected. Tools such as MetaDprof and MetaLonDA demonstrated the specificity and sensitivity needed for detecting time periods of differentially abundant features (Mabwi et al., 2021). Most notably, MetaLonDA can handle uneven sample sizes and time intervals, which are common in human subject studies. For example, using inputs from the DIABIMMUNE project, MetaLonDA found significant differences between the Finnish and Russian cohorts in the relative abundances of Bacteroides and Bifidobacterium species during the first year of life (Mabwi et al., 2021). Additionally, MetaLonDA showed that Bacteroides is significantly more abundant from day 96 to day 584 in Finnish infants, while Bifidobacterium is significantly more abundant in Russian infants from day 96 to day 720 (Markowiak & Ślizewska, 2017). This type of computational analysis can inform the treatment of several gut-driven immune disorders often seen in children and provide valuable regional population context.

Compared to taxonomic profiling and metagenomic data, there have been fewer published works on metabolomic data. In dietary studies, the purpose of analyzing metabolomic data is to determine whether two or more metabolite profiles are significantly different. For a comparison of time series data from two experimental groups, Hoteling-T2 statistic can be used as a measure of holistic differences (Chong et al., 2019). When these studies employ multiple groups or levels of treatments, multivariate empirical Bayes analysis of variance may be used to test for significance (Chen et al., 2020). In cases where the specific metabolite might be unknown or is overly complex to analyze, significant discriminatory biomarkers are used in multivariate analysis (Park, Ufondu, Lee, & Jayaraman, 2020a). Linear mixed models offer an attractive option to investigate the longitudinal trend of metabolites and identify metabolites that show significant concentration changes over time (Mabwi et al., 2021). One promising technique is dynamic probabilistic principle coordinate analysis, which models the correlations in multivariate data that occur due to repeated measurements in time (Mabwi et al., 2021).

Integration of complex computation into microbiome studies is important. Even with longitudinal studies, there is often a mismatch between microbial community dynamics and sampling frequency. Most *in vivo* studies collect samples infrequently, because of practical limitations, over days or weeks, whereas microbial community dynamics in the gut microbiota can significantly vary within hours (Park, Ufondu, Lee, & Jayaraman, 2020b). One possible solution is to use studies in parallel with computational models to simulate the microbiome or metabolome dynamics to identify optimal sample collection (Park et al., 2020b). Computational and statistical methods can rigorously address the challenges of microbiome temporal data analysis. For mechanistic studies, a promising collection of software tools has become available to support the analysis of large "omics" data sets from longitudinal studies (Park et al., 2020b). There is no one size fits all regarding a standardized process for reporting and comparing outcomes from different analyses. As a result, the choice of a data analysis tool often relies on trial and error. In this regard, open-source platforms that provide options to conduct multiple analyses on consistently formatted and normalized data sets would be a powerful resource for elucidating diet.

## *IN VITRO* MODELS

*In vitro* models constitute an opportunity to study the gut microbiota in cases that an *in vivo* study would be considered conceptually not feasible or unethical. In essence, *in vitro* gut models function as chemostats, that is, bioreactors inoculated with fecal microbiota and operated under physiological temperature, pH, and anaerobic conditions (Ahmadi et al., 2019). Experimentation within these models is very flexible with regards to studying multiple permutations/combinations of dietary ingredients and their impact on gut microbial populations (Ahmadi et al., 2019). Ultimately, cumulative *in vitro* studies can lead to robust *in vivo* approaches to investigating gut microbiota functionality (Litten-Brown, Corson, & Clarke, 2010; Nguyen, Vieira-Silva, Liston, & Raes, 2015; Ray & Dittel, 2015). In theory, each study yields complementary results that strengthen the overall validity of each individual model and distinguishes between the functionality of gut microbes and human processes.

### FECAL BATCH CULTURES

Many of the microbes that reside within the gut are not cultivable using traditional microbiological techniques such as agar Petri plates (Nagalingam, Kao, & Young, 2011). Preliminary studies of the human microbiome typically start with obtaining donor specimens and culturing the microbes under anaerobic conditions in a bioreactor (Ahmadi et al., 2019). The bioreactor setup can be as simple as an Erlenmeyer flask inside a $CO_2$ incubator on a stir plate or a complex system of pumps and valves meant to closely simulate the physical system of the digestive tract (Ahmadi et al., 2019). The complexity of the bioreactor setup is usually dictated by the question the investigator is attempting to answer. For example, in determining if a potential food ingredient is bifidogenic, investigators can quantify the presence of *Bifidobacteria* using agar and simple biochemical tests. However, such setup cannot reveal the ingredient's effect on other important bacterial species or potential effects in human physiology (Ahmadi et al., 2019; Vrieze et al., 2013a). For a comprehensive *in vitro* or *ex vivo* analysis of microbiome shift with different dietary interventions, metagenomic analysis is still needed. For preliminary studies of the interactions of the gut microbiome and specific nutrients, a video protocol can be found at www.jove.com/v/59524/an-vitro-batch-culture-model-to-estimate-effects-interventional. This protocol details a comprehensive and cost-effective way to use a bioreactor for studying the compositional shift that occurs in a fecal sample following dietary amendments ("An In Vitro Batch-culture Model to Estimate the Effects of Interventional Regimens on Human Fecal Microbiota|Protocol," n.d.).

### CELL CULTURE

*In vitro* human cell models are typically composed of polarized monolayers of single or co-cultured carcinoma cells (Saygili, Dogan-Gurbuz, Yesil-Celiktas, & Draz, 2020). These cell lines are distinguished based on their physiological properties and ability to differentiate (Pearce et al., 2018). The intestinal epithelial consists of several cell types, including enterocytes, goblet cells, stem cells, enteroendocrine cells, Tuft cells, M cells, and Paneth cells, all of which can interact or sense the presence of the gut microbiota and respond accordingly (Pearce et al., 2018). Caco-2 and mucus-secreting HT29-MTX cell lines predominate the literature with regards to the study of probiotics and prebiotics (Pearce et al., 2018). There are important considerations in selecting a cell culture model, and decisions should be guided based on the research question asked.

Caco-2 cell line, derived from colorectal adenocarcinomas, is one of the oldest and most utilized cell cultures in medical research (Pearce et al., 2018). This cell line can function as an undifferentiated large intestinal cell or can spontaneously differentiate into a cell closely resembling a small intestinal enterocyte (Ahmadi et al., 2012). This ability to spontaneously differentiate is difficult to control and presents challenges in the reproduction of scientific studies, despite the fact that these Caco-2 cells are widely used to study the protective effects of probiotics and prebiotics (Pearce et al., 2018). Additionally, Caco-2 cells are commonly used in immunological studies since they can express important pattern recognition receptors, Toll-like receptors, which can provide information about the relative abundance of inflammatory markers known to contribute to the disease process (Payne et al., 2012).

HT-29 is another commonly utilized, polarized, and undifferentiated human colorectal adenocarcinoma cell line (Paul et al., 2018). Recently, several subpopulations have been selected to exhibit more "enterocyte-like" features, but in general, spontaneous differentiation is less common compared to Caco-2 (Payne et al., 2012). HT-29 cell lines have been extensively studied in the field of nutrition and host–microbiome interactions because they produce important inflammatory cytokines, such as interleukins and TNF α (De Simone et al., 2015; Khan Mirzaei et al., 2016) In addition, HT-29 provides an important benefit compared to Caco-2 in that HT-29 cells contain mucus-producing goblet cells. The ability to produce mucus is critical for predicting immune function in the intestinal brush border and studying bacterial–host interactions (Raja et al., 2012; Altamimi et al., 2016).

Prebiotic oligosaccharides have been shown to positively modulate both Caco-2 and HT-29 cells, and exhibit reduced inflammatory activity (Bode, 2009; Kelly, 2008). For example, the HT-29-MTX cell line, treated with methotrexate to produce more mucin, has been a useful tool to show that oligosaccharides and a functional mucin layer can reduce bacterial adhesion to the epithelium (Altamimi et al., 2016). Studies with HT-29-MTX demonstrated that prebiotics can reduce the possibility of an infection by reducing pathogens' adhesion, migration, and internalization, including *Salmonella* and *E. coli*. Co-cultures of Caco-2 and HT-29 render cell culture models more physiologically and functionally relevant, by combing the benefits of mucin secretion and differentiation (Altamimi et al., 2016). In co-cultures of HT-29 Caco-2, anti-adhesive effects of *Streptococcus thermophilus* and *Lactobacillus acidophilus* against enteroinvasive *E. coli* were observed (Resta-Lenert and Barrett, 2003).

## EX VIVO MODELS

*Ex vivo* models are models cultured outside of an organism, while closely mimic functional live tissue systems and the complex cellular environments found *in vivo* (Roeselers et al., 2013). These extended models are used to mimic the intestinal tract in more detail by using advanced tissue engineering approaches. *Ex vivo* model systems can delve deeper into the complexity of the microbiome–host environment and can probe the mechanism by which certain dietary components can improve health outcomes (Roeselers et al., 2013).

## 3D CELL CULTURE

Modern 3D printing techniques allow for the creation of complex biological tissue (Saygili et al., 2020). Bioprinting simultaneously combines living cells and biomaterials through a computer-aided design program to create 3D bioengineered living constructs that mimic natural tissue characteristics, including organs. This microscale fabrication is commonly used for tissue engineering, regenerative medicine, microbiology, and the study of the gut microbiota (Saygili et al., 2020). In 3D bioprinting, there are three major groups of techniques commonly used: layer-by-layer (stereolithographic), line-by-line (extrusion-based), and droplet-based bioprinting (Saygili et al., 2020). Extrusion-based bioprinting is the most common and affordable 3D printing and creates complex, multilayered scaffolds and tissue constructs in biomedical applications. The stereolithography utilizes a photopolymerization process in which UV light creates a pattern over a photopolymerizable liquid polymer, cross-linking the light-sensitive polymers into a hardened layer (Patel, Lee, Park, Kim, & Jeong, 2018). Droplet-based bioprinting utilizes multiple mechanisms to deposit droplets of cell suspension in a high-throughput manner (Saygili et al., 2020). The materials fed through the printer are typically hydrogels that have similar viscoelastic properties to that of biological material (Patel et al., 2018). Hydrogel-based bio-ink materials typically have short-termed stability, the ability to retain nutrients, and controlled cross-linking to facilitate bioprinter deposition (Patel et al., 2018).

The development of 3D tissue systems allowed for the modeling of host–bacterial microbiome interactions in an organoid environment that closely resembles the intestinal tract (Saygili et al., 2020). Organoid models for the gastrointestinal tract were first developed in 2009 and have evolved into two distinct types, adult stem cell (ASC) and pluripotent stem cell (PSC) derivatives (Saygili et al., 2020). ASC- derived intestinal organoids are limited and consist only of basic epithelial cells such as parietal cells, chief cells, and surface pit cells (Saygili et al., 2020). In comparison, PSC has the capacity to differentiate into three germ layers (ectoderm, mesoderm, and endoderm), mesenchymal cells, including smooth muscle cells, fibroblasts, and myofibroblasts. However, to date, the cultivation of environmental cells, such as neural cells, immune cells, and endothelial cells, is extremely difficult (Patel et al., 2018). Without the environmental context of these other systems, organoids are prevented from properly recapitulating the features of the actual organs designed to represent.

## MICROFLUIDICS SYSTEMS AND THE "GUT CHIP"

Recent advances in cell culture 3D printing and microfluidics have facilitated the development of lab-on-a-chip systems that can be used to study the gut microbiota. Gut chip and microfluidic systems typically house channels, chambers, sensors, electrodes, and valves that allow for cellular growth media and air exchange (Ashammakhi et al., 2020). Most microfluidic models of the gut involve an array of microchannels that are separated by a porous and flexible membrane that allows for nutrient exchange and elimination of waste, a design intended to simulate the barrier between the intestinal lumen and the draining vasculature. The target cells are seeded into channels and allowed to adhere, and then media is pumped through the channels to simulate the microenvironment found *in vivo* (Ashammakhi et al., 2020).

Multiple cell types have been used within gut-on-a-chip devices depending on the proposed research question. The most commonly used cell type is Caco-2 cells due to their ease in culturing and capacity to differentiate in 3D cell culture, generating an intestinal structure (von Martels et al., 2017). The presence of fluid flow to provide biomimetic shear stress to cells is critical to this development, with the peristalsis-like strain on cells inducing morphogenesis into 3D intestinal villi. However, the use of Caco-2 if severely is limited by their lack of capacity to produce a significant mucosal layer (von Martels et al., 2017). Therefore, co-culture with HT-29 cells and other types of cells is an attractive option for many studies. In another gut model studying the remodeling of extracellular matrix, Caco-2 cells were co-cultured with subepithelial myofibroblasts to generate a full-thickness model of the intestine (Ashammakhi et al., 2020). Co-cultures in 3D system can go beyond typical cell monolayers through the formation of the villous structures, and the expression of tight junctions, presentation of a brush layer, and production of mucous (von Martels et al., 2017).

The advent of gut chip technologies has allowed for the study of host–microbiota interaction, circumventing the use of costly animal models. A model microfluidic environment consists of two compartments separated, one containing mixed microbiota and the other enterocytes (Marzorati et al., 2014). To recreate physiologically relevant GIT conditions in order to study the gut microbiota, the following are needed: (a) a mucosal area under shear stress for bacterial adherence; (b) transport of low molecular weight metabolites; and (c) microaerophilic conditions. With this model, it is possible to simulate bacterial adhesion and the indirect effect on cells. Compared to traditional cell cultures, the constant nutrient cycling of microfluidics systems allows for observations over longer periods with a lower risk of contamination (Ashammakhi et al., 2020). Recent studies examined the intercellular cross talk between Caco-2BBE cells and peripheral blood mononuclear cells in response to challenges with dextran sulfate sodium (DSS), lipopolysaccharide (LPS) endotoxin, probiotic VSL#3, and non-pathogenic *E. coli* (von Martels et al., 2017). This system facilitated the isolation of each component of the signaling cascade to identify the root cause of the inflammatory response. The gut epithelium disruption with LPS activated the immune component of the model allowing for elucidation of dysfunctional pathways, potentially not revealed by using complex animal models (Ashammakhi et al., 2020).

## SIMULATOR OF THE HUMAN INTESTINAL MICROBIAL ECOSYSTEM (SHIME)

The SHIME was developed in 1993 as a multicompartment dynamic simulator of the human gut (Molly et al., 1993). The development of SHIME® addresses the limitations that *in vivo* studies have capturing colon microbiota in terms of community composition and metabolic activity by adding some of the physical and mechanical aspects of digestion to the study design (Van De Wiele, Van Den Abbeele, Ossieur, Possemiers, & Marzorati, 2015.). Simple fecal batch culture studies only utilize single-stage chemostats to mimic colon conditions. These designs are often limited for diet studies because environmental parameters such as pH, redox potential, available nutrients, and microbial population dynamics constantly change throughout transit. To simulate *in vivo* conditions while still taking advantage of *in vitro* designs, semicontinuous fermenters were developed where the intermittent supplementation of nutritional medium (Van De Wiele et al., 2015). In contrast, fecal batch culture studies that use one single fermenter ignore the heterogeneity in substrate availability, fermentation activity, microbial composition, and other intrinsic characteristics.

The SHIME system is intended to mimic the microbiota, and the initial inoculum originates from a donor's fecal sample. Fecal samples capture a microbial community and metabolic shifts during transit from the proximal colon to the rectum. It is important to consider that the fecal microbiome is significantly different from the *in vivo* colon microbiome, both in terms of composition and metabolic activity (Van De Wiele et al., n.d.). With that in mind, the colon is where the microbiome is the most accessible sample for an individual intestinal community. The purpose of the SHIME system is to adapt the fecal microbiome to the conditions present in the different colon compartments (Van De Wiele et al., n.d.). The SHIME is typically inoculated with fecal material sourced from individual donors, despite research due to pool samples from several people. Pooling samples can partially account for the interindividual variability that exists in microbiome composition and incorporates properties from different enterotypes. Since there is enormous functional redundancy of the gut microbiome, such pooled microbiome and the adaption process of SHIME will shift the fermentation profile, not a strictly necessary step. However, because SHIME models adapt the fecal microbiome to the simulated environment of the colon, it often fails to capture function nuances. For example, the metabolism of polyphenols, such as daidzein, isoxanthohumol, and catechins, is highly dependent on an individual's microbiome (van Duynhoven et al., 2011).

The mucosal microbiome is a crucial part of the gut microbial ecosystem because of its proximity to host epithelial cells. It is thought to have an intrinsically higher impact on human health because of the immunological activity that occurs (Van den Abbeele et al. 2011). The mucosal microbiome is different from the luminal microbiome in composition and, interestingly, the presence of important mucosal colonizers such as *Faecalibacterium prausnitzii* (Willing et al. 2009). Access to the mucosal environment *in vivo* is extremely difficult, and the development of gut simulators that accurately mimic mucosal microbial colonization is needed. The SHIME can mimic some of the mucosal microbial colonization by incorporation of mucin and other compounds in which to establish a biofilm. One result of mucosal SHIME experiments was the higher colonization rate of butyrate-producing *Clostridium* clusters IV and XIVa (Van De Wiele et al., n.d.). This phylogenetic group is considered crucial for delivering butyrate as a primary energy source to colonocytes and improves gut barrier function by strengthening the tight junctions (Van De Wiele et al., n.d.).

This modular nature of SHIME is useful for diet studies and investigating the microbiome's ability to produce a bioactive metabolite (Possemiers et al. 2006). The microbiome behavior in response to dietary inputs can be investigated by comparing upper digestive tract to the colon. The residence times of the different gastric compartments, the composition of the gastric juices, region-specific pH values, feed, feeding regimes, and body temperatures are adapted in the SHIME setup leading to a simulation of the targeted human or animal host. Finally, other features of the SHIME include the gradual emptying of the gastric digest into the intestine compartment. The option of running a dynamic pH profile in the gastric compartment enables the running experiments with real food matrices or food constituents that need to undergo predigestion and removal of sugar monomers or amino acids and peptides before the digest is transferred advancing to the colon compartment (Van De Wiele et al., n.d.).

## ANIMAL MODELS FOR STUDYING GUT MICROBIOTA

As the microbiota of the human gut is gaining increasing research attention, the need for the development of models for non-human microbiota studies is significant. There are several possibilities for *in vivo* models utilized in microbiota research spanning from mice and other rodents such as guinea pigs to primates, zebrafish, pigs, and dogs (Nguyen et al., 2015). Most studies are using rodent models, with murine being the most common, porcine, and zebrafish. In the following section of this chapter, these commonly used models are discussed with particular emphasis on the murine models being the most widely used currently.

### INSECT MODELS

Insects are the most diverse class of animals regarding species numbers and biomass (Muñoz-Benavent, Pérez-Cobas, García-Ferris, Moya, & Latorre, 2021). The microbiota of insects, especially the gut microbiota, is as complex and rich as the phylogeny and ecology of insects. Most insect species have endosymbiotic relationships with a specialized gut microbiota that contributes to health status and important nutritional roles (Muñoz-Benavent et al., 2021). The insect intestine is inhabited by microorganisms from all domains, including bacteria, fungi, archaea, protozoa, and viruses (Muñoz-Benavent et al., 2021). As a result of their co-evolutionary histories with the host, these microorganisms play essential roles in host physiology. Insect symbiotic systems are either ectosymbiotic when the symbiont is on the surface of the host or endosymbiotic when it lives inside specialized host cells (Muñoz-Benavent et al., 2021). For example, termites gut endosymbiotic microbiota enables them to feed on a wood diet due to its unique enzymatic capabilities. Cockroaches possess bacteriocytes, specialized cells in the fat body of the insect, and an abundant and varied intestinal microbiota, whose function is not fully understood (Muñoz-Benavent et al., 2021).

The combination of microorganisms populating the insect gut is driven by several evolutionary and ecological factors, including phylogeny, diet, life stage, and host environment (Muñoz-Benavent et al., 2021). Proteobacteria, Firmicutes, Bacteroidetes, Actinobacteria, and Tenericutes are the most common phyla insect guts, and the distribution of these phyla varies greatly among insect species. Diet is a major driver of the gut microbiota composition in animals. Gene sequencing has revealed the influence of diet on the gut microbiota of insects (Muñoz-Benavent et al., 2021). With termites, there are major distinctions in the gut microbiota between dry-wood, damp-wood, and subterranean environments. A comparative study including 18 species of higher termites identified the diet as a significant factor of bacterial community structure in the termite gut using amplicon libraries of 16S rRNA genes (Muñoz-Benavent et al., 2021). Lower termites have a diet based on lignocellulose that is digested by symbiotic flagellates, which are absent in higher termites and cockroaches (its closest relative) (Muñoz-Benavent et al., 2021). However, in wood feeding, higher termites' bacterial species from *Spirochaetes* and *Fibrobacteres* phyla are responsible for digesting their diet [20]. The analysis of metagenomes from the hindgut microbiota of a wood-feeding higher termite showed a large and diverse set of bacterial genes for cellulose and xylan hydrolysis (Muñoz-Benavent et al., 2021). In addition, $H_2$ metabolism, $CO_2$-reductive acetogenesis, and $N_2$ fixation functions were identified as putative functions of the microbiome (Muñoz-Benavent et al., 2021).

*Drosophila melanogaster*, the common house fly, is a universal model for genetic and genomic studies and is used as a human disease model (Douglas, 2018). The fly genome includes orthologs for many human disease genes. The *Drosophila* research community has developed powerful resources to facilitate translation between the fly and human disease including the Human Disease Model Report in FlyBase (http://flybase.org/) (Douglas, 2018). Programs like FlyBase focus on the genetic mechanisms of drug–microbiome interactions in Drosophila to the treatment of human disease (Douglas, 2018). The *Drosophila* microbiome is dominated by two groups of taxa: gut microorganisms localized to the gut lumen and endosymbionts, which are transmitted with high fidelity from mother to offspring via the oocyte (Douglas, 2018). Endosymbionts, which humans lack, can have substantial effects on the metabolic and immune phenotype of flies (Douglas, 2018). Therefore, the use of endosymbiont-free *Drosophila* strains is recommended for the study of drug–gut microbiome interactions.

The intimate relationship between *Drosophila* and its food adds an important dimension to microbiome interactions. The gut microbiome of laboratory *Drosophila* is generally dominated by bacteria, usually *Acetobacteraceae* (a-proteo-bacteria) and *Lactobacillales* (Firmicutes) (Douglas, 2018). Drosophila diets with high sugar content favor *Acetobacteraceae*, while lactobacilli are favored by *Drosophila* diets dominated by complex carbohydrates like cornmeal-based diets (Douglas, 2018). The capacity of microorganisms to persist and proliferate in the *Drosophila* gut varies among microbial isolates. Many of the bacteria that inhabit *Drosophila* exploit the mobile fly as a vector for transmission among fruits at different stages of decay (Douglas, 2018).

Genomic sequencing analysis demonstrated that diet contributed not only to differential gut microbiota diversity but also to a distinct colonization resistance capacity against pathogens. Another field of interest in medicine is the study of antibiotic resistance genes and their transmission in bacteria through insects. The gut microbiota plays a crucial role in developing and maintaining the insect immune system, so studying these communities is essential to better understand the pathogens they carry and transmit or even find ways to prevent them. For example, the gut microbiota of the mosquitoes can prevent them from becoming infected with *Plasmodium*, the malaria parasite (Muñoz-Benavent et al., 2021).

## AVIAN MODELS

Birds represent a vertebrate class that plays a major role in natural ecosystems and is with diverse gut microbiomes (Hird, Grond, Poulsen, & Jønsson, 2021). As with most vertebrate species, the microbiome of birds is influenced to varying degrees by host physiology and genetics, ecology and behavior, the environment, and diet (Hird et al., 2021). Avian microbiomes are extremely diverse, and there is little similarity between gut microbial community and host phylogeny. Low levels of host specificity and high variability of the gut microbiome may result from the effects of a highly diverse diet. Functional insights into avian gut bacteria stem mainly from poultry studies, where gut microbes aid digestion, synthesize essential molecules for the host (Hird et al., 2021), and interact with the immune system during microbiome establishment and development (Hird et al., 2021). However, poultry are unlikely to be representative of all bird species. Nevertheless, the application of insights and methods developed for poultry may have implications for human diet and disease studies.

Birds represent important reservoirs and carriers of both animal and human pathogens as well as antimicrobial resistance genes (Tellez et al., 2001). Bird microbiomes can reflect active infection status, and noninvasive methods exist to collect fecal samples for migration and population-monitoring programs (Tellez et al., 2001). Avian social behaviors impact the dynamics and assembly of gut bacterial communities (Tellez et al., 2001). Studies on social contact during breeding have yielded some insights into the effects of family interactions on microbiomes. Group living may also increase pathogen transfer among individuals who may select for diverse and stable microbiomes that are more resilient to pathogen invasion, and such advantages may be greater in social than in solitary species (Tellez et al., 2001).

Apart from chickens, few studies have investigated the cross talk between avian immune systems and gut microbes, including gut symbiont responses to microbial infections. In wild ducks, gut microbiome composition is significantly correlated with influenza virus infections (Navarro-gonzalez et al., 2020), and in ostriches, colonization of harmful bacteria can lead to dysbiosis and even death (Navarro-gonzalez et al., 2020). Environmental microbial diversity can also impact both immune functions and cloacal microbiomes of hosts (Zimmer-Faust, Steele, Griffith, & Schiff, 2020). Such pattern-based and experimental manipulation of infections provides an initial foundation to identify defensive microbial symbionts (Zimmer-Faust et al., 2020). These insights can then be used to establish more precisely how microbes combat pathogens.

## MURINE MODELS

Rodents, mice, in particular, have become the most broadly and commonly used model of choice for most studies in this emerging field. While both healthy human and murine gut microbiota are dominated by the same two phyla (i.e., Bacteroidetes and Firmicutes), studies by Ley et al. have demonstrated that approximately 85% of the bacterial genera found in mice are not observed in humans under normal healthy conditions (Ley et al., 2006). While similarities between the murine and human condition have been observed, studies with mice have indicated changes in abundance of bacterial phylotypes. In mice bacteria such as Tenericutes and Enterobacteriaceae

(Nagalingam et al., 2011), explained at least to some extent by differential methodological approaches (16S rRNA vs. stool sample analyses) as per the assessment of the microbiota between humans and (Nguyen et al., 2015). Regardless of the approach, a certain degree of differentiation is always seen.

Another question, as per the suitability of murine models for studying human gut microbiome responses, is the extent to which murine gut microbiota is modified in response to various metabolic conditions and diseases in a similar manner to that reported in the human gut. For example, studies investigating obesity and the gut microbiota have shown a significant overlap in terms of responses between humans and mice. Moreover, genome-wide association studies of obesity in mice have revealed that genes associated with obesity overlap with some genes in human obesity (Nguyen et al., 2015). A plethora of studies have been conducted on mice or humanized mouse models (i.e., germ-free (GF) mice administered human gut microbiota), in which animals were fed diets high in fat or saturated/unsaturated fat to investigate changes in the gut microbiota (Le Chatelier et al., 2013). Furthermore, there is a similar change in the Bacteroidetes/Firmicutes (B/F) ratio in *ob/ob* obese mice and obese humans (Murphy et al., 2010).

The development of inflammatory bowel disease (IBD) has been linked to the composition of gut microbiota, among other factors (Ray & Dittel, 2015). A significant challenge in assessing the alignment and translatability of findings from murine models to human IBD patients is that IBD is essentially a cluster of diseases, further distinguished by stages of activity. Various mouse models have been developed in efforts to mimic the human pathophysiology of IBD by manipulating the murine genome, chemical induction of IBD as well as pathogen-driven models. While genetic models for IBD are a promising practice, targeted genes are often involved in multiple pathways, thus potentially confounding the conclusions derived based on the association between gut microbiota and function in the disease state. For example, none of the approximately 60 colitis murine models mimic accurately the human condition (Peloquin & Nguyen, 2013). Overall, obesity and IBD appear to be quite differently translatable from murine models to humans, illustrating concerns in the accuracy and validity of conclusions.

Interestingly, a noticeable parallel exists between dominant bacterial families of the mouse and human enterotypes. Namely, one mouse enterotype is dominated by *Lachnospiraceae/Ruminococcaceae*, similar to the human *Ruminococcaceae* enterotype (also known as enterotype 3). Additionally, the second mouse enterotype, dominated by *Bacteroidaceae/Enterobacteriaceae*, is similar to the human *Bacteroides* enterotype (enterotype 1) (Arumugam et al., 2011). Interestingly, two enterotypes were also identified in wild mice, dominated by *Bacteroides* and *Robinsoniella*, respectively (Wang et al., 2016). Moreover, the laboratory mouse enterotypes were found to correlate with species richness and inflammation, that is, mice belonging to the low species-richness enterotype (*Bacteroidaceae/Enterobacteriaceae*) demonstrated significantly higher levels of calprotectin, a biomarker of inflammation. This result is consistent with studies of human obesity (Le Chatelier et al., 2013), in which low species-richness individuals were found to have more pronounced inflammation, with microbiota dominated by *Bacteroidetes* and *Proteobacteria*, the same bacterial groups that dominated the high inflammation mouse enterotype.

Overall, these observations underline clear differences at the level of specific genus/species abundances between the murine and human gut microbiota while simultaneously indicating that overall community composition, as well as the driving factors, might be similar (e.g., enterotypes). Although absolute comparisons might be challenging and not straightforward, murine models are likely relevant for studying the processes responsible for microbiota variation and shifts upon perturbations.

Murine models permit interventions for studying the causal role of gut microbiota in health and disease, not otherwise attainable in humans. The use of murine models generates comprehensive knowledge of mouse genetics and thus extends the availability of numerous genetically modified mouse models more than any other model. Other advantages include the relatively low cost of maintenance, high reproductive rate, and short life cycle, all of which increase the efficiency and efficacy of experimental designs using mice. Mice are omnivorous mammals, with gut physiology and anatomy comparable to that of humans. Moreover, murine microbiota models allow for specificity in targeting genes/pathways in the complex gut microbiota–host interactions by employing knockout models. Mouse models are inbred, providing a homogenous genetic background, a cleaner system to dissect signals from gut–bacteria–host interactions and improve the reproducibility of experiments with high power in relatively low numbers of animals per group. Sources of variations such as diets and housing conditions are generally controlled for in experiments, limiting undesired background influence to gut microbiota.

Despite important similarities, with mice being different from humans in anatomy, genetics, and physiology, their use cannot fully recapitulate human systems. In this regard, different mouse models can give rise to diverging shifts in gut microbiota composition. Cross talk between gut microbiota and the host can be largely host-specific; hence, observations in mice may be of limited translatability to humans. Genetic homogeneity while positive in terms of reducing "genetic noise" also implies that the inbred mouse strains cannot capture the inherent genetic variations naturally occurring in the human population. Multiple factors, such as genetic background, birth mode of delivery (caesarean versus vaginal), mode of feeding (breast versus bottle), diet, medical history, and social activities, all contribute to shaping the "actual" gut microbiota in humans. The absence of these factors in mice implies that gut microbiota in murine models cannot closely reflect a "real-life" gut microbiota.

## HUMANIZED GNOTOBIOTIC MICE

Humanized gnotobiotic mice are produced by the inoculation of a human gut microbiota sample in GF mice. This murine model constitutes a powerful tool for gut microbiota studies capturing a large part of the human gut microbiota phylogenetic composition (100% of phyla, 11/12 classes, and ~88% of genus-level taxa) (Nguyen et al., 2015). This approach has been widely employed in a plethora of studies since it allows perturbations in a "human-like system" and is widely regarded as the gold standard for confirming associations and trying to prove causality in gut microbiota research (Faith, McNulty, Rey, & Gordon, 2011; Goodman et al., 2011).

Nevertheless, it must be emphasized that host–microbe relationships in humanized mouse models do not necessarily reflect the entire relationship spectrum seen in humans since the gut microbiota transplanted into a host (mouse) has not co-evolved with the recipient. It has been reported that certain resident bacterial taxa in the human gut microbiota are absent in the humanized mouse gut microbiota (Turnbaugh et al., 2009).

Despite their limitations, humanized mice constitute one of the very few methods to assess causality in microbiota research, and therefore, further development and improvement of this approach is important.

## PORCINE MODELS

The porcine gut microbiota is increasingly and more rigorously studied due to the scale of porcine husbandry industry, but also due to the similarities in anatomy, physiology, and immunology to the human gastrointestinal tract (Litten-Brown et al., 2010). An elegant and in-depth study of swine gut microbiota composition in the Yorkshire pig breed demonstrated that human and pig microbiota shared similar diversity patterns, with the two dominant phyla being Bacteroidetes and Firmicutes (Lamendella, Santo Domingo, Ghosh, Martinson, & Oerther, 2011). However, at the genus level, the swine gut microbiota harbors more Spirochaetes and *Prevotella* than the human gut microbiota (Lamendella et al., 2011).

Another porcine model promising for microbiota research is the miniature pig. Generally, miniature pigs develop obesity when fed *ad libitum* and are thus used as an obesity and metabolic syndrome model. Specifically, the gut microbiota composition of two miniature pig breeds, Gottingen and Ossabaw, was investigated for responses to obesity induction (Meier & Bode, 2013; Pedersen et al., 2013), demonstrating that the major phyla of miniature pig gut microbiota are Firmicutes and Bacteroidetes.

Interestingly, the two miniature pig breeds responded differently to an obesity-inducing diet: Ossabaw gut microbiota displayed more of the characteristics of a "healthy" obese microbiota, while Gottingen gut microbiota demonstrated alterations analogous to metabolic syndromes, such as those found in gut microbiota profiles of type 2 diabetic mice.

## ZEBRAFISH MODEL

Zebrafish is an attractive model used extensively for gut microbiota research due to its small size, high fecundity, and full annotation of its genome. Given that several gut functions and immune genes are conserved between zebrafish and mammals, the zebrafish is an interesting model organism to investigate fundamental processes underlying intestinal inflammation and injury (Brugman, 2016). As revealed by genomic profiling, the zebrafish gut microbiota shares six bacterial divisions with mice and five with humans, although marked differences exist in the relative abundance of these phyla (Zhao et al., 2017). The microbiota of laboratory-reared zebrafish intestine is dominated by *Proteobacteria*, while Firmicutes and Bacteroidetes dominate in mice and humans (Rawls et al., 2004). Despite differences in the composition of their microbiota, the responses of zebrafish and mammals to microbial colonization are similar. As an example, microarray analysis comparing the digestive tracts of GF versus conventionally reared zebrafish revealed differential expression of over 200 genes, of which nearly one-third were conserved in mice (Rawls et al., 2004). The majority of these genes can be linked to epithelial proliferation, nutrient metabolism, and immune responses. In terms of utilization of the zebrafish model, Aryas-Jayo and colleagues investigated the effects of a high-fat diet (HFD) over a period of 25 days on intestinal microbiota and inflammation in zebrafish. The consumption of the HFD resulted in microbial dysbiosis, characterized by an increase in the relative abundance of the phylum Bacteroidetes (Aryas-Jayo et al., 2018).

## FECAL MICROBIOME TRANSLOCATION MODELS

The bidirectional relationships between fecal microbiota and human health have been considered the next frontier for microbiome research and the amelioration of disease (Wu et al., 2019). Recent studies demonstrated an association between intestinal microbiota composition and human disease; however, direct causality remains to be proven. The application of fecal microbiome translocation (FMT) is the closest example of a causal relationship between gut microbiota composition and a resultant cure of several disease states (Chong et al., 2019). Randomized controlled double-blind trials have provided valuable insight into implementing FMT that might be serving as a future diagnostic and therapy in human disease.

In clinical practice, FMT from healthy donors is applied in the treatment of specific dysbiosis-related diseases. The principle of FMT involves restoration of the colonic microflora by introducing healthy bacterial flora through the infusion of stool from a healthy donor. *Clostridioides difficile* is a disorder of the intestinal flora often the result of antibiotics and microorganisms that do not respond to antimicrobial therapy (Vrieze et al., 2013b). Fecal translocation demonstrated efficacy against *C. difficile* infection and performed better than vancomycin. The overall efficacy of FMT is an >90% reduction of *C. difficile*, and it is influenced by various factors depending on the donor, transfer method, and colonic environment (Vrieze et al., 2013a). The overall efficacy of FMT can be increased with multiple infusions, higher initial dosages, and improved delivery, with a higher success rate if FMT is performed by colonoscopy (Ianiro et al., 2018). New scientific studies have reported that in patients suffering from *C. difficile* infection, FMT is followed immediately by a repairing effect and disappearing symptoms of the disease, which relates to normalization of the disturbed microbiota (CDC, 2020). As *C. difficile* infection becomes common, FMT research has increased in prominence and has been used experimentally to treat other gastrointestinal diseases including colitis, constipation, irritable bowel disease, and some neurological conditions such as Parkinson's disease (Vrieze et al., 2013c).

Many authors investigated the potential role of restoring eubiosis with FMT among IBS patients' community to obtain combined effects on intestinal and mental disturbances. Microbiota analysis shows that, after FMT in *C. difficile* patients, there was an increase in the number of the *Bacteroidetes, Clostridium* clusters IV and XIVa, *Faecalibacterium prausnitzii, Butyrivibrio crossotus, Enterococcus, Lactobacillus, Veillonella,* and a decrease in pathogenic bacteria (Antushevich, 2020a). A recent clinical trial demonstrated, in patients administrated FMT for 3 months, lower improvement of clinical symptoms, namely swelling of the liver, disappearance of abdominal pain syndrome, and normalization of the frequency of defecation (Antushevich, 2020a). Fecal translocation may also be a promising therapy for ulcerative colitis, and clinical trials demonstrated a decrease in diarrhea, hematochezia, and improved clinical scores (Antushevich, 2020a). Murine models of dextran sulfate sodium (DSS)-induced colitis found that FMT reduces the levels of TNF-α, IL-1β, and MPO activity and increases the level of IL-10 in the colon (Antushevich, 2020a). Reduction of intestinal inflammation in DSS-induced colitis mice was also observed (Antushevich, 2020a). In FMT group of rats, the authors observed reducing the colonic expression of the pro-inflammatory cytokine genes and bacterial antigens, decreasing weight loss, and increasing length of the colon and antimicrobial peptides and mucins secretion (Vrieze et al., 2013c). Also, an increase of *Lactobacillaceae* and *Bifidobacteriaceae* in the gut was observed (Vrieze et al., 2013c).

It is important to consider the heterogeneity of fecal samples in the human population and the collection of fecal specimen protocols. Fecal collection, transportation condition, storage status, and DNA extraction method all have some impacts on sample quality (Vrieze et al., 2013a). Methodology studies are helpful for investigators to build more reasonable protocols for the fecal sampling and handling process. Although knowledge and evidence were accumulating to contribute to the quality control of fecal sampling of microbiome study, there remain some gaps and challenges (Settanni, Ianiro, Bibbò, Cammarota, & Gasbarrini, 2021a). For example, it might be debated whether the anaerobic condition should be maintained for sample collection since the MetaHIT protocol contains an anaerobic bag in the fecal collection bottle, but the HMP did not (Settanni, Ianiro, Bibbò, Cammarota, & Gasbarrini, 2021b). Another controversy is whether to include the homogenization process before aliquoting since the microbial population from different sampling sites in poop can be quite divergent (Antushevich, 2020b). If homogenization is not performed, how much biomass in a sample is enough to be representative for a complete microbial population in a poop may become a concern. Besides, since most of the comparative methodology studies were currently done at 16S DNA amplicon analysis level, we just begin to learn the optimal condition for shotgun metagenome study (Niederwerder, 2018).

Although it can be relatively simple to perform, cost challenges need to be overcome before this procedure is widely accepted in mainstream clinical practice. Most of the solutions to these challenges already exist, but some need further optimization and testing. Standardized fecal microbiota is being developed as a therapeutic agent, although it clearly challenges some of the existing paradigms of drug development, delivery, and regulation. The dietary record is an important component for gut microbiome study for its potential to provide environmental vectors to explain the compositional results of a relevant gut microbiome analysis (Niederwerder, 2018). Food frequency questionnaire (FFQ) and 24 h dietary record are useful tools for dietary surveillance and have been successfully applied for microbiome studies (Vrieze et al., 2013c). However, it is worth noting that the validity of FFQ and dietary record recalls relying heavily on the completeness of the food composition database that may conventionally only include common macro- and micronutrients.

## CONCLUSION

To elucidate causal relationships between prebiotics, probiotics, and gastrointestinal health, multiple investigative approaches are needed that combine appropriate models with sensitive methods for data analysis. Modern approaches include *in vitro*, *in vivo*, and *ex vivo* models, along with metagenomic and metabolomic analysis of the community composition, its functional repertoire, and the by-products produced. This information is often used to determine the dominant set of taxa that govern the dynamics of multiple metabolic functions at the community level. In addition, information can be revealed about the dynamics of the microbiome and the correlation between specific taxa's abundance with a metabolic function. However, due to the complexity of the human body, it is rare that causation can be unequivocally established using only one model.

## REFERENCES

Ahmadi, S., Wang, S., Nagpal, R., Mainali, R., Soleimanian-Zad, S., Kitzman, D., & Yadav, H. (2019). An In Vitro Batch-culture model to estimate the effects of interventional regimens on human fecal microbiota. *Journal of Visualized Experiments: JoVE, 149,* 59524. https://doi.org/10.3791/59524

Altamimi, M., Abdelhay, O., Rastall, R.A. (2016). Effect of oligosaccharides on the adhesion of gut bacteria to human HT-29 cells, *Anaerobe, 39,* 136–142.

An In Vitro Batch-culture Model to Estimate the Effects of Interventional Regimens on Human Fecal Microbiota | Protocol. (n.d.). Retrieved August 12, 2020, from https://www.jove.com/v/59524/an-vitro-batch-culture-model-to-estimate-effects-interventional

Antushevich, H. (2020a). Fecal microbiota transplantation in disease therapy. *Clinica Chimica Acta, 503,* 90–98. https://doi.org/10.1016/J.CCA.2019.12.010

Antushevich, H. (2020b). Fecal microbiota transplantation in disease therapy. *Clinica Chimica Acta, 503*(October 2019), 90–98. https://doi.org/10.1016/j.cca.2019.12.010

Arumugam, M., Racs, J., Pelletier, E., Le Paslier, D., Yamada, T., Mende, D. R., ... Bork, P. (2011). Enterotypes of the human gut microbiome. *Nature, 473*(7346). https://doi.org/10.1038/nature09944

Ashammakhi, N., Nasiri, R., de Barros, N. R., Tebon, P., Thakor, J., Goudie, M., ... Khademhosseni, A. (2020, October 1). Gut-on-a-chip: Current progress and future opportunities. *Biomaterials, 255.* https://doi.org/10.1016/j.biomaterials.2020.120196

Bode, L. (2009). Human milk oligosaccharides: Prebiotics and beyond. *Nutrition Reviews.* https://doi.org/10.1111/j.1753-4887.2009.00239.x

CDC. (2020). *Coronavirus Disease 2019 (COVID-19) Meat and Poultry Processing Workers and Employers Exposure Risk among Meat and Poultry Processing Workers. 2019,* 1–9.

Chen, T. M., Rui, J., Wang, Q. P., Zhao, Z. Y., Cui, J. A., & Yin, L. (2020). A mathematical model for simulating the phase-based transmissibility of a novel coronavirus. *Infectious Diseases of Poverty, 9*(1), 1–8. https://doi.org/10.1186/s40249-020-00640-3

Chong, P. P., Chin, V. K., Looi, C. Y., Wong, W. F., Madhavan, P., & Yong, V. C. (2019). The microbiome and irritable bowel syndrome – A review on the pathophysiology, current research and future therapy. *Frontiers in Microbiology, 10*(Jun). https://doi.org/10.3389/fmicb.2019.01136

De Simone, V., Franzè, E., Ronchetti, G., Colantoni, A., Fantini, M.C., Di Fusco, D., Sica, G.S., Sileri, P., MacDonald, T.T., Pallone, F., Monteleone, G., & Stolfi, C. (2015). Th17-type cytokines, IL-6 and TNF-α synergistically activate STAT3 and NF kB to promote colorectal cancer cell growth. *Oncogene, 34,* 3493–3503.

Douglas, A. E. (2018). Drosophila and its gut microbes: A model for drug-microbiome interactions. *Drug Discovery Today: Disease Models*, *28*, 43–49. https://doi.org/10.1016/j.ddmod.2019.08.004

Faith, J. J., McNulty, N. P., Rey, F. E., & Gordon, J. I. (2011). Predicting a human gut microbiota's response to diet in gnotobiotic mice. *Science*, *333*(6038). https://doi.org/10.1126/science.1206025

Goodman, A. L., Kallstrom, G., Faith, J. J., Reyes, A., Moore, A., Dantas, G., & Gordon, J. I. (2011). Extensive personal human gut microbiota culture collections characterized and manipulated in gnotobiotic mice. *Proceedings of the National Academy of Sciences of the United States of America*, *108*(15). https://doi.org/10.1073/pnas.1102938108

Hird, S. M., Grond, K., Poulsen, M., & Jønsson, K. A. (2021). *Avian gut microbiomes taking flight*, 1–13. https://doi.org/10.1016/j.tim.2021.07.003

Ianiro, G,. Maida, M., Burisch, J., Simonelli, C., Hold, G., Ventimiglia, M., Gasbarrini, A., & Cammarota, G. (2018). Efficacy of different faecal microbiota transplantation protocols for *Clostridium difficile* infection: A systematic review and meta-analysis. *United European Gastroenterology Journal*, *6*(8), 1232–1244. https://doi.org/10.1177/2050640618780762. PMID: 30288286; PMCID: PMC6169051.

Kelly, G. (2008). Inulin-type prebiotics – A review: Part 1. *Alternative Medicine Review : A Journal of Clinical Therapeutic*, *13*(4), 315–329.

Khan Mirzaei, M., Haileselassie, Y., Navis, M., Cooper, C., Sverremark-Ekström, E., & Nilsson, A.S., (2016). Morphologically distinct *Escherichia coli* bacteriophages differ in their efficacy and ability to stimulate cytokine release *In Vitro*. *Frontiers in Microbiology*, *7*, 437.

Lamendella, R., Santo Domingo, J. W., Ghosh, S., Martinson, J., & Oerther, D. B. (2011). Comparative fecal metagenomics unveils unique functional capacity of the swine gut. *BMC Microbiology*, *11*. https://doi.org/10.1186/1471-2180-11-103

Lamichhane, S., Sen, P., Dickens, A. M., Orešič, M., & Bertram, H. C. (2018). Gut metabolome meets microbiome: A methodological perspective to understand the relationship between host and microbe. *Methods*, *149*(March), 3–12. https://doi.org/10.1016/j.ymeth.2018.04.029

Le Chatelier, E., Nielsen, T., Qin, J., Prifti, E., Hildebrand, F., Falony, G., … Yamada, T. (2013). Richness of human gut microbiome correlates with metabolic markers. *Nature*, *500*(7464). https://doi.org/10.1038/nature12506

Ley, R. E., Turnbaugh, P. J., Klein, S., & Gordon, J. I. (2006). Microbial ecology: Human gut microbes associated with obesity. *Nature*, *444*(7122). https://doi.org/10.1038/4441022a

Litten-Brown, J. C., Corson, A. M., & Clarke, L. (2010). Porcine models for the metabolic syndrome, digestive and bone disorders: A general overview. *Animal*, *4*(6). https://doi.org/10.1017/S1751731110000200

Mabwi, H. A., Kim, E., Song, D. G., Yoon, H. S., Pan, C. H., Komba, E. V. G., … Cha, K. H. (2021). Synthetic gut microbiome: Advances and challenges. *Computational and Structural Biotechnology Journal*, *19*, 363–371. https://doi.org/10.1016/j.csbj.2020.12.029

Markowiak, P., & Ślizewska, K. (2017). Effects of probiotics, prebiotics, and synbiotics on human health. *Nutrients*, *9*(9). https://doi.org/10.3390/NU9091021

Meier, P. P., & Bode, L. (2013). Health, nutrition, and cost outcomes of human milk feedings for very low birthweight infants. *Advances in Nutrition*. https://doi.org/10.3945/an.113.004457

Molly, K., Vande Woestyne, M., & Verstraete, W. (1993). Development of a 5-step multi-chamber reactor as a simulation of the human intestinal microbial ecosystem. *Applied Microbiology and Biotechnology*. May; *39*(2), 254–258. https://doi.org/10.1007/BF00228615. PMID: 7763732

Marzorati, M., Vanhoecke, B., De Ryck, T. *et al.* (2014). The HMI™ module: a new tool to study the Host-Microbiota Interaction in the human gastrointestinal tract *in vitro*. *BMC Microbiology*, *14*, 133. https://doi.org/10.1186/1471-2180-14-133

Muñoz-Benavent, M., Pérez-Cobas, A. E., García-Ferris, C., Moya, A., & Latorre, A. (2021). Insects' potential: Understanding the functional role of their gut microbiome. *Journal of Pharmaceutical and Biomedical Analysis*, *194*. https://doi.org/10.1016/j.jpba.2020.113787

Nagalingam, N. A., Kao, J. Y., & Young, V. B. (2011). Microbial ecology of the murine gut associated with the development of dextran sodium sulfate-induced colitis. *Inflammatory Bowel Diseases*, *17*(4). https://doi.org/10.1002/ibd.21462

Nguyen, T. L. A., Vieira-Silva, S., Liston, A., & Raes, J. (2015). How informative is the mouse for human gut microbiota research? *DMM Disease Models and Mechanisms*, *8*(1). https://doi.org/10.1242/dmm.017400

Niederwerder, M. C. (2018). Fecal microbiota transplantation as a tool to treat and reduce susceptibility to disease in animals. *Veterinary Immunology and Immunopathology*, *206*(October), 65–72. https://doi.org/10.1016/j.vetimm.2018.11.002

Park, S. Y., Ufondu, A., Lee, K., & Jayaraman, A. (2020a). Emerging computational tools and models for studying gut microbiota composition and function. *Current Opinion in Biotechnology*, *66*, 301–311. https://doi.org/10.1016/J.COPBIO.2020.10.005

Park, S. Y., Ufondu, A., Lee, K., & Jayaraman, A. (2020b). Emerging computational tools and models for studying gut microbiota composition and function. *Current Opinion in Biotechnology*, *66*, 301–311. https://doi.org/10.1016/j.copbio.2020.10.005

Patel, M., Lee, H. J., Park, S., Kim, Y., & Jeong, B. (2018). Injectable thermogel for 3D culture of stem cells. *Biomaterials*, *159*, 91–107. https://doi.org/10.1016/j.biomaterials.2018.01.001

Paul, W., Marta, C., & Van De Wiele, T. (2018, August 1). Resolving host–microbe interactions in the gut: The promise of in vitro models to complement in vivo research. *Current Opinion in Microbiology*, *44*, 28–33. https://doi.org/10.1016/j.mib.2018.07.001

Payne, A. N., Zihler, A., Chassard, C., & Lacroix, C. (2012, January). Advances and perspectives in in vitro human gut fermentation modeling. *Trends in Biotechnology*, *30*, 17–25. https://doi.org/10.1016/j.tibtech.2011.06.011

Pearce, S. C., Coia, H. G., Karl, J. P., Pantoja-Feliciano, I. G., Zachos, N. C., & Racicot, K. (2018, November 12). Intestinal in vitro and ex vivo models to study host-microbiome interactions and acute stressors. *Frontiers in Physiology*, *9*. https://doi.org/10.3389/fphys.2018.01584

Pedersen, A. N., Kondrup, J., & Børsheim, E. (2013). Health effects of protein intake in healthy adults: a systematic literature review. *Food & Nutrition Research*, *30*, 57. https://doi.org/10.3402/fnr.v57i0.21245. PMID: 23908602; PMCID: PMC3730112.

Peloquin, J. M., & Nguyen, D. D. (2013). The microbiota and inflammatory bowel disease: Insights from animal models. *Anaerobe*, *24*. https://doi.org/10.1016/j.anaerobe.2013.04.006

Possemiers, S., Bolca, S., Grootaert, C., Heyerick, A., Decroos, K., Dhooge, W., De Keukeleire D., Rabot, S., Verstraete, W., Van de Wiele, T. (2006). The prenylflavonoid isoxanthohumol from hops (Humulus lupulus L.) is activated into the potent phytoestrogen 8-prenylnaringenin in vitro and in the human intestine. *Journal of Nutrition*, Jul; *136*(7), 1862–1867. https://doi.org/10.1093/jn/136.7.1862. PMID: 16772450.

Raja, M., Puntheeranurak, T,. Hinterdorfer, P., Kinne, R. (2012). Chapter Two - SLC5 and SLC2 Transporters in epithelia—cellular role and molecular mechanisms. *Current Topic in Membrane*, *70*, 29–76.

Rawls, J.F., Samuel, B.S., & Gordon, J.I. (2004). Gnotobiotic zebrafish reveal evolutionarily conserved responses to the gut microbiota. *PNAS*, *101*(13), 4596–4601.

Ray, A., & Dittel, B. N. (2015). Interrelatedness between dysbiosis in the gut microbiota due to immunodeficiency and disease penetrance of colitis. *Immunology, 146*(3). https://doi.org/10.1111/imm.12511

Resta-Lenert, S., & Barrett, K.E. (2003). Live probiotics protect intestinal epithelial cells from the effects of infection with enteroinvasive Escherichia coli (EIEC). Gut, *52*(7), 988–997. https://doi.org/10.1136/gut.52.7.988. PMID: 12801956; PMCID: PMC1773702.

Roeselers, G., Ponomarenko, M., Lukovac, S., & Wortelboer, H. M. (2013). Ex vivo systems to study host-microbiota interactions in the gastrointestinal tract. *Best Practice and Research: Clinical Gastroenterology, 27*, 101–113. https://doi.org/10.1016/j.bpg.2013.03.018

Saygili, E., Dogan-Gurbuz, A. A., Yesil-Celiktas, O., & Draz, M. S. (2020, June 1). 3D bioprinting: A powerful tool to leverage tissue engineering and microbial systems. *Bioprinting, 18*. https://doi.org/10.1016/j.bprint.2019.e00071

Settanni, C. R., Ianiro, G., Bibbò, S., Cammarota, G., & Gasbarrini, A. (2021a). Gut microbiota alteration and modulation in psychiatric disorders: Current evidence on fecal microbiota transplantation. *Progress in Neuro-Psychopharmacology and Biological Psychiatry, 109*, 110258. https://doi.org/10.1016/J.PNPBP.2021.110258

Settanni, C. R., Ianiro, G., Bibbò, S., Cammarota, G., & Gasbarrini, A. (2021b). Gut microbiota alteration and modulation in psychiatric disorders: Current evidence on fecal microbiota transplantation. *Progress in Neuro-Psychopharmacology and Biological Psychiatry, 109*(August 2020). https://doi.org/10.1016/j.pnpbp.2021.110258

Tellez, G., Petrone, V. M., Escorcia, M., Morishita, T. Y., Cobb, C. W., & Villasenõr, L. (2001). Evaluation of avian-specific probiotic and Salmonella enteritidis-, Salmonella typhimurium-, and Salmonella Heidelberg-specific antibodies on cecal colonization and organ invasion of Salmonella enteritidis in broilers. *Journal of Food Protection, 64*(3), 287–291. https://doi.org/10.4315/0362-028X-64.3.287

Turnbaugh, P. J., Ridaura, V. K., Faith, J. J., Rey, F. E., Knight, R., & Gordon, J. I. (2009). The effect of diet on the human gut microbiome: A metagenomic analysis in humanized gnotobiotic mice. *Science Translational Medicine, 1*(6). https://doi.org/10.1126/scitranslmed.3000322

Van de Wiele, T., Van den Abbeele, P., Ossieur, W., Possemiers, S., Marzorati, M. (2015). The Simulator of the Human Intestinal Microbial Ecosystem (SHIME®). In *The Impact of Food Bioactives on Health, Verhoeckx, K., Cotter, P., López-Expósito, I., Kleiveland, C., Lea, T., Mackie, A., Requena, T., Swiatecka, D., & Wichers, H. (Eds.)*. Springer, Cham. https://doi.org/10.1007/978-3-319-16104-4_27

Van den Abbeele, P., Roos, S., Eeckhaut, V., MacKenzie, D.A., Derde, M., Verstraete, W., Marzorati, M., Possemiers, S., Vanhoecke, B., Van Immerseel, F., Van de Wiele, T. (2012). Incorporating a mucosal environment in a dynamic gut model results in a more representative colonization by lactobacilli. *Microbial Biotechnology*, 106–115. https://doi.org/10.1111/j.1751-7915.2011.00308.x. PMID: 21989255; PMCID: PMC3815277.

van Duynhoven, J., Vaughan, E.E., Jacobs, D.M., Kemperman, R.A., van Velzen, E.J., Gross, G., Roger, L.C., Possemiers, S., Smilde, A.K., Doré, J., Westerhuis, J.A., Van de Wiele, T. (2011). Metabolic fate of polyphenols in the human superorganism. *Proceedings of the National Academy of Sciences of the United States of America, 108* Suppl, 4531–4538. https://doi.org/10.1073/pnas.1000098107. Epub 2010 Jun 25. PMID: 20615997; PMCID: PMC3063601.

von Martels, J. Z. H., Sadaghian Sadabad, M., Bourgonje, A. R., Blokzijl, T., Dijkstra, G., Faber, K. N., & Harmsen, H. J. M. (2017, April 1). The role of gut microbiota in health and disease: In vitro modeling of host-microbe interactions at the aerobe-anaerobe interphase of the human gut. *Anaerobe, 44*, 3–12. https://doi.org/10.1016/j.anaerobe.2017.01.001

Vrieze, A., De Groot, P. F., Kootte, R. S., Knaapen, M., Van Nood, E., & Nieuwdorp, M. (2013a). Fecal transplant: A safe and sustainable clinical therapy for restoring intestinal microbial balance in human disease? *Best Practice and Research: Clinical Gastroenterology*, 27, 127–137. https://doi.org/10.1016/j.bpg.2013.03.003

Vrieze, A., De Groot, P. F., Kootte, R. S., Knaapen, M., Van Nood, E., & Nieuwdorp, M. (2013b). Fecal transplant: A safe and sustainable clinical therapy for restoring intestinal microbial balance in human disease? *Best Practice and Research: Clinical Gastroenterology*, 27(1), 127–137. https://doi.org/10.1016/j.bpg.2013.03.003

Vrieze, A., De Groot, P. F., Kootte, R. S., Knaapen, M., Van Nood, E., & Nieuwdorp, M. (2013c). Fecal transplant: A safe and sustainable clinical therapy for restoring intestinal microbial balance in human disease? *Best Practice and Research: Clinical Gastroenterology*, 27(1), 127–137. https://doi.org/10.1016/j.bpg.2013.03.003

Wang, T., Wu, J., Qi, J., Hao, L., Yi, Y., & Zhang, Z. (2016). Kinetics of inactivation of Bacillus subtilis subsp. niger spores and Staphylococcus albus on paper by chlorine dioxide gas in an enclosed space. *Applied and Environmental Microbiology*. https://doi.org/10.1128/AEM.03940-15

Willing, B., Halfvarson, J., Dicksved, J., Rosenquist, M., Järnerot, G., Engstrand, L., Tysk, C., Jansson, J.K. (2009). Twin studies reveal specific imbalances in the mucosa-associated microbiota of patients with ileal Crohn's disease. *Inflammatory Bowel Disease*, 15(5), 653–660. https://doi.org/10.1002/ibd.20783. PMID: 19023901.

Wu, W. K., Chen, C. C., Panyod, S., Chen, R. A., Wu, M. S., Sheen, L. Y., & Chang, S. C. (2019). Optimization of fecal sample processing for microbiome study—The journey from bathroom to bench. *Journal of the Formosan Medical Association*, 118(2), 545–555. https://doi.org/10.1016/J.JFMA.2018.02.005

Zhao, Y., Czilwik, G., Klein, V., Mitsakakis, K., Zengerleabc, R., & Paust, N. (2017). C-reactive protein and interleukin 6 microfluidic immunoassays with on-chip pre-stored reagents and centrifugo-pneumatic liquid control. *Lab on a Chip*, 17, 166.

Zimmer-Faust, A. G., Steele, J. A., Griffith, J. F., & Schiff, K. (2020). The challenges of microbial source tracking at urban beaches for quantitative microbial risk assessment (QMRA). *Marine Pollution Bulletin*, 160. https://doi.org/10.1016/J.MARPOLBUL.2020.111546

# 5 Dietary Modulation of Gut Microbiota by Cultured Products

*Salam A. Ibrahim and Rabin Gyawali*
North Carolina A&T State University

*Raphael D. Ayivi*
North Carolina A&T State University
University of North Carolina Greensboro

*Hafize Fidan*
University of Food Technologies

*Saeed Paidari*
Islamic Azad University

*Reza V. Bakhshayesh*
Agricultural Biotechnology Research Institute of Iran
University of Tabriz

## CONTENTS

DOI: 10.1201/b22970-7

## INTRODUCTION

Proper diet and nutrition are fundamentally important for human health and metabolic development and have been advocated by various stakeholders in the quest to decrease the surging rate of health and metabolic diseases. More specifically, the human gut microbiota has been associated with the proper regulation and functionality of the human metabolic and immune system (Gentile & Weir, 2018). As a result of the important role of the gut microbiota in combatting diseases and promoting health and wellness, it is critical for the modulatory functionality of the gut microbiota to be adequately supported in its functionality. Cultured food products, probiotics, and fermented functional foods have all been proposed as conventional approaches to naturally boosting the modulatory effect of the gut microbiota. Cultured food products allude to all fermented dairy or milk products or fermented food beverages with lactic acid bacteria as a key culturing agent (Ayivi et al., 2020). Moreover, the growing demand by consumers and dietary health experts to adopt cleaner and greener strategies in enhancing the human immune system warrants rapid attention and a paradigm shift away from chemical supplements that could pose a human health risk coupled with long-term side effects. The interplay between diet, nutrition, and probiotic consumption results in a synergistic effect on the gut microbiota that boosts the immune system in its fight against attacks from foreign bodies, pathogens, and disease-causing organisms (Yang et al., 2020). Probiotics have been shown to possess a high therapeutic effect on human health. Moreover, studies have confirmed the immunomodulatory properties of probiotics and diet on the gut microbiota through the promotion of beneficial bacteria and the suppression of deleterious microorganisms (Ibrahim et al., 2021). However, there is little available research that has addressed the role of cultured products and diet together and their contingent effect on the modulation of the gut microbiota.

This chapter thus embraces a nutraceutical concept and elucidates the promising and potential role of diet, probiotics, and nutrition in the modulatory action of the gut microbiota. We will also discuss the role of various factors such as cultured products, probiotics, and fermented functional foods in gastrointestinal (GI) disease prevention, cholesterol regulation, lactose intolerance (LI) mediation, and some cardiovascular disease (CVD) prevention strategies. In addition, we wish to promote a comprehensive background of pertinent information regarding the ways in which diet, nutrition, and cultured probiotic food products could immensely enhance human health by promoting the modulatory action of the gut microbiota.

## BIOTHERAPEUTIC PROPERTIES OF CHOLESTEROL-LOWERING PROBIOTICS

### CONCEPT OF PROBIOTICS

The commensal gut microbiome is fundamentally salient in immunological and metabolic activities, inhibiting the development of unwanted microbes through antimicrobial agent production or direct competition for binding sites and resources. Probiotics, as defined by the World Health Organization (WHO), are living and nonpathogenic microbial supplements that, when administered in sufficient amounts to the host organism, confer health benefits by increasing gut health and intestinal mucosal integrity (FAO & WHO, 2002). 'Probiotic' is a Greek term meaning 'for life'; however, the definition has evolved over the years. The evolution of the probiotic term over the years has significantly been associated with the increasing interest in the use of viable bacterial supplements and the progress made in understanding their mechanisms of action. Originally, the phrase referred to secretory compounds from specific bacteria that were beneficial in the development of other species. Later, the probiotic term was associated with extracts of tissue that increased microbial development, as well as animal feed additives that improved intestinal microbiota (Fuller, 1999).

Probiotics improve gut health, improve intestinal mucosal integrity, and suppress potentially pathogenic microorganisms through competition for nutrients and space for gut adherence, antihypertensive effects, reduction in allergic symptoms, cancer prevention, mineral absorption facilitation, cholesterol-lowering effects, arthritis amelioration, and dermis symptoms. In 2013, the global market for probiotics was USD 32.06 billion. In 2015, the value of the probiotics market was estimated at USD 33.19 billion. By 2020, it was expected to reach USD 46.55 billion, USD 64.02 billion by 2022 (Byakika, Mukisa, Byaruhanga, & Muyanja, 2019). The probiotic market thus has promising growth potential. This market is projected to further develop due to rising global consumer health awareness, fueled by the usefulness of probiotics in preventing and treating a variety of health issues, in addition to the soaring global demand for functional food products (El-Saadony et al., 2021). These developments in recent years have influenced the rising demand and consumption of functional foods, as many individuals are now more interested in disease prevention than cure. The positive impact of a probiotic on its host is proportional to its concentration in the intestinal lumen, which must be at least $10^7$ CFU/g of fecal material. For the host organism to adequately experience the efficiency of the probiotic, the product should have a minimum of $10^6$ CFU/g or mL, and a total of $10^8$ to $10^9$ probiotic bacteria should be taken daily (Kechagia et al., 2013).

## Probiotic Microorganism

*Lactobacillus* and *Bifidobacterium* are considered as the most widely and commonly used probiotic microorganisms nowadays (Nami et al., 2018). In addition, other probiotic strains that have gained prominence and consumer acceptance include *Lactococcus* (Shehata, El-Sahn, El Sohaimy, & Youssef, 2019), *Streptococcus* (Shastri et al., 2020), *Enterococcus* (Nami et al., 2019), *Bacillus* (Lim, Oh, Yu, & Kim, 2021), *Saccharomyces* (Rodríguez-Nogales et al., 2018), *Propionibacterium* (Nair & Kollanoor Johny, 2018), *Leuconostoc* (Le & Yang, 2019), *Weissella* (Yadav, Yadav, Singh, Singh, & Mani, 2019), or *Escherichia coli* originating from the GIT (Behrouzi et al., 2020) or *clostridia* (Liu, Xie, Wan, & Deng, 2020) (Table 5.1). Although pathogenic strains such as *Bacillus anthracis* and *Bacillus cereus* are notable in the *Bacillus* family, their toxicity is strain-dependent, and some strains do not create enterotoxins, thus making them suitable for use as probiotics.

## Important Criteria in Selecting Probiotics

Probiotic applications in animal food and feed are also on the rise, but this must be done with caution because the strain can spread from animal to human. Consequently, stringent standards for probiotic safety and quality must be implemented and

**TABLE 5.1**

**Some Known Lactic Acid and Probiotic Bacteria**

| | | Probiotic Microorganisms | |
|---|---|---|---|
| **Lactobacillus spp.** | **Bifidobacterium spp.** | **Other Lactic Acid Bacteria** | **Nonlactic Acid Bacteria** |
| L. acidophilus | B. adolescentis | Enterococcus faecalis | Bacillus cereus var. to yoi<br>B. coagulans GBI-30 |
| L. casei | B. animalis | E. faecium | E. coli strain nissle |
| L. crispatus | B. bifidum | Lactococcus lactis | Propionibacterium freudenreichii |
| L. acidophilus | B. breve | Leuconostoc mesenteroides | Saccharomyces cerevisiae |
| L. gallinarum | B. infantis | Pediococcus acidilactici | S. boulardii |
| L. gasseri | B. adolescentis | Sporolactobacillus inulinus | |
| L. johnsonii | B. animalis | Streptococcus thermophilus | |
| L. paracasei | B. bifidum | Weissella paramesenteroides | |
| L. plantarum | B. breve | | |
| L. reuteri | B. lactis | | |
| L. rhamnosus | B. longum | | |
| L. brevis | | | |
| L. fermentum | | | |
| L. salivarius | | | |
| L. helveticus | | | |

adhere to global requirements commencing with strain selection, manufacturing and labeling, and ending with postmarket surveillance of adverse effects (Byakika et al., 2019). According to several reports, some probiotics can change into opportunistic pathogens, causing illnesses including sepsis and pneumonia (Antoun, Hattab, Akhrass, & Hamilton, 2020). Before a probiotic strain is approved for entry into the consumer market, extra attention should be paid to many adverse qualities such as gene transfer, translocation, the creation of toxic metabolites, and immunomodulation. Even though probiotics (fermented foods) have long been consumed by humans, their safety requires special care, as novel strains from unusual sources and genetically engineered probiotic strains are currently in various phases of commercialization.

The introduction of new probiotic strains generally consists of the isolation and selection of appropriate strains from a diverse microbial population. This is done by searching a set of cell banks, separating traditional dairy products, or isolating healthy humans and animals. First, the isolates are isolated by culturing them in vitro, after which the best probiotic strains are identified by simple in vitro methods by creating conditions such as GI tract and intestinal epithelium (Vasiljevic & Shah, 2008). The features of probiotics are always strain-specific and cannot be generalized to other strains. The criteria of probiotic selection and validation should satisfy key requirements and possess certain qualities that have been integral in probiotic experiment investigations. The choice of probiotics requires well-established and important criteria as follows (FAO & WHO, 2002):

i. Tolerance to acid and bile, which appears to be important for oral administration,
ii. Adherence to epithelial and mucosal surfaces, which is recognized as an important feature for immune modulation, pathogen competitive exclusion, and the adhesion and colonization of pathogens,
iii. Antibacterial action against microorganisms that cause disease, and
iv. The activity of bile salt hydrolase (BSH).

Apart from adhesion to mucus and/or human epithelial cells and cell lines, the principal tests described above are identical to the Indian Council of Medical Research and Department of Biotechnology (ICMR-DBT) criteria for probiotic strain in vitro characterization (Ganguly et al., 2011). The Joint FAO/WHO Working Group advises at a minimum the following screening tests in terms of organism safety (FAO & WHO, 2002):

1. Antibiotic resistance patterns,
2. Metabolic activities such as bile salt deconjugation and D-lactate synthesis,
3. Assessing side effects in humans,
4. Surveillance of epidemiological adverse issues in consumers,
5. Toxin production (for strains belonging to a species known for toxin production), and
6. Hemolytic activity for strains belonging to a species known for hemolysis.

The following assays for microbiological safety evaluation are recommended by the ICMR-DBT guidelines (Ganguly et al., 2011):

1. Antibiotic resistance testing,
2. Checking for unwanted side effects,
3. Testing for toxin production and hemolytic activity, particularly for strains belonging to a species known to produce a toxin or have hemolytic potential, and
4. Ensuring that the candidate strain does not cause infections in immunocompromised individuals.

Nonetheless, the significance of these metrics is still debatable due to issues of relevance, in vivo and in vitro inconsistencies, and a lack of uniformity of operating protocols. Because no single criterion is required for all probiotic uses, the best way to determine a strain's qualities is to conduct studies on a specific population and physiologic function. Evidence supporting a strain's probiotic efficacy should thus be disseminated in medical journals or as peer-reviewed scientific work, according to the Joint FAO/WHO Working Group. Negative results also add to the overall body of evidence supporting probiotic efficacy and should likewise be published.

## Synthesis and Metabolism of Plasma Lipoprotein

Two important organs in the body, the stomach and the liver, are responsible for lipoprotein production. The liver synthesizes bile which is then transported to the gallbladder and utilized there prior to being transported to the intestine via a cystic duct. When a fatty meal reaches the small intestine, bile salts assist in the emulsification of the fats. This allows the fatty meal to be digested and absorbed in the intestines. Next, in the epithelial cells of the gut, fatty acids, triglycerides, and cholesterol mix and are covered by a layer of protein, called chylomicrons (Kaplan, Pesce, & Kazmierczak, 2003). A system of lymphatic cells then absorbs the chylomicrons after which they are released into the bloodstream. Chylomicrons are thus converted to cholesterol and triglycerides upon reaching the liver. It is noteworthy that lipids are immiscible with the bile salts in the intestines. Lipids descend to the ileum, where absorption of a greater proportion of the bile salts occurs and then reabsorbed into the bloodstream. The liver, therefore, is responsible for the recirculation of returned bile salts that stay in the gallbladder, together with bile, to be employed in the aforementioned process once again. The small intestine, however, does not absorb all of the bile salts, and some of them move into the colon, where they are discarded along with feces. By manufacturing bile salts from its cholesterol store, the liver compensates for the loss of bile salts. In addition to dietary sources of cholesterol, liver cells produce cholesterol and are thus another important source of the body's cholesterol pool. A variety of factors, including heredity and food, influence the liver's ability to generate cholesterol.

## CHOLESTEROL-LOWERING OF PROBIOTICS

Hypercholesterolemia is closely linked to the occurrence of ischemic heart disease in both men and women. A slight reduction in serum cholesterol of 1% can lead to a 2%–3% reduction in heart attacks. In previous years, the only treatment was the use of lipid-lowering drugs such as statins, which prevent the synthesis of cholesterol. However, not only is the cost of these drugs very high, but their use in pregnant women and people with liver failure or kidney disease is very dangerous. Moreover, even in otherwise healthy individuals, the use of lipid-lowering drugs can cause abdominal pain, allergic reactions, unusual emotions, hair loss, changes in vision, headaches, muscle cell breakdown, and decreased sexual potency. This has naturally prompted patients to look for other safe options such as weight loss, dietary supplements, lean diets, and exercise. Less than 300 mg of cholesterol per day is recommended according to FDA guidelines published in 2010. However, in 2015, in the absence of scientific evidence, the DGAC Advisory Committee retracted the claim that there was a significant link between dietary cholesterol intake and serum cholesterol. Because diet and lifestyle changes alone would not decrease the risks associated with coronary heart disease (DGA, 2015), despite this claim, lowering cholesterol intake seems to play a significant role in managing blood lipids. It is more expensive to lower one's blood fat than to modify their diet. The growing need to lower blood cholesterol levels has thus provided an opportunity to explore new alternative approaches to doing so including the use of plant sterols, soluble fiber, and, most importantly, probiotics. For example, recent studies conducted on laboratory animals as well as humans suggest that foods containing probiotic lactic acid bacteria may be effective in lowering blood lipids (Kharc & Gaur, 2020; Thumu & Halami, 2020). As a result, finding probiotics that have a hypocholesterolemic impact is of considerable interest as probiotics are of Generally Recognized as Safe status and are thus free of hazardous compounds. Moreover, probiotics are less expensive than traditional cholesterol-lowering medications. A meta-analysis of 30 randomized controlled studies found that probiotics reduced TC and LDLc by 7.8 mg/dL and 7.3 mg/dL, respectively, in 1624 patients compared to control subjects. High-density lipoprotein (HDL) and TG values were unchanged (Galie et al., 2009). According to meta-analysis research, the particular probiotic strains that lowered TC in patients included *L. plantarum* (MD of 1.56 mg/dL), VSL #3 (MD of 11.04 mg/dL), and *B. lactis* and *L. acidophilus* (MD of 8.30 mg/dL) (Wang et al., 2018). In another study, the *L. acidophilus* strain decreased high levels of TC and LDLc (MD 0.35 mmol/L) in those who had normal-to-moderate hypercholesterolemia (Esmaeili, Zamindar, Paidari, Ibrahim, & Mohammadi Nafchi, 2021; Shimizu, Hashiguchi, Shiga, Tamura, & Mochizuki, 2015; Tarrah et al., 2021).

Although the ability of probiotic bacteria to lower cholesterol has been reported in several different strains of these microorganisms, the primary mechanisms by which they can lower cholesterol have remained largely unknown. Most of the hypotheses proposed to date have been based on laboratory experiments, and little attempt has been made to evaluate the possible mechanisms of hypercholesterolemia based on in vivo examination.

## CHOLESTEROL-LOWERING EFFECT MECHANISMS

Biological molecules such as lipids have insoluble qualities in aquatic conditions because they have a nonpolar, hydrophobic area that prevents their dissolving in water (Croft et al., 1988). Phospholipids and glycolipids are present in eukaryotic and bacterial cells. The arrangement of lipid and protein units in variable concentrations forms HDLs, very-low-density lipoproteins, chylomicrons, and low-density lipoproteins (LDLs), and from chylomicrons to HDL, the number of proteins increases. HDL eliminates excess cholesterol from the tissues and is re-transported in the liver, whereas chylomicrons distribute ingested fat to the body tissues (Croft et al., 1988). The rate and levels of synthesized cholesterol are regulated by the daily consumption levels of cholesterol. De novo synthesis regulates cholesterol levels in the body, keeping them between 150 and 200 mg/dL. In healthy adults, just 0.3 g of cholesterol is excreted out of approximately 1 g produced each day. Cholesterol is an important component of the production of bile acids (BAs), steroid hormones, and membrane formation. Because bile salts with conjugated systems are extremely soluble, the majority enter the enterohepatic circulation following absorption, resulting in blood buildup (McAuliffe, Cano, & Klaenhammer, 2005). It has been reported that the hypocholesterolemic function of proteins is related to cholesterol assimilation during cell growth, which reduces the quantity of cholesterol accessible for absorption in the intestine (Huey-Shi Lye, Rahmat-Ali, & Liong, 2010).

The hypothetical concept of cholesterol-lowering probiotic effects includes the following: activity of BSH for the deconjugation of bile (Huey-Shi Lye et al., 2010; H-S Lye, Rusul, & Liong, 2010), probiotic cell binding of cholesterol and cholesterol molecules incorporation into the probiotic cellular membrane (De Preter et al., 2007), production of short-chain fatty acids (SCFAs) from oligosaccharides (De Preter et al., 2007), deconjugated bile coprecipitates with cholesterol (Kumar et al., 2012), and coprostanol formation from converted cholesterol (Kumar et al., 2012) are all part of the hypothesis of probiotics. Although numerous hypocholesterolemic probiotic mechanisms exist, the activity of BSH has been attributed to the most significant probiotic cholesterol-lowering mechanism. Although the hypocholesterolemic mechanism of probiotics is not entirely understood, cholesterol and bile salt metabolism are known to be intertwined. For example, bile salts are produced by the liver hepatocytes, which aid in the transport of fat and dietary cholesterol across the intestinal epithelium.

## DECONGESTING BILE SALTS USING BILE SALT HYDROLYZING ENZYME

The enzyme BSH (choloylglycine hydrolase; EC 3.5.1.24) produces free BAs and amino acid residues upon hydrolyzing glycine- and/or taurine-conjugated bile salts (Figure 5.1), with a preference for glycol-conjugated bile salts over tauro-conjugated bile salts. Bile salt conjugation significantly depends on the characteristics of the host, and in mammals, the site of conjugation depends on the type of host. For example, the microbial flora of *Lactobacillus* in the small intestine of mice are present at the site where bile salt degeneration occurs, whereas, in humans, substantial flora begin only at the end of the ileum and develop fully in the large intestine. Several

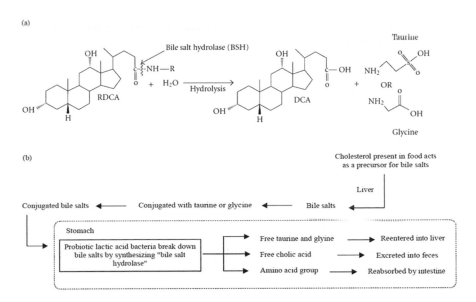

**FIGURE 5.1 (A)** The enzyme BSH hydrolyzes conjugated bile salts. (b) The involvement of BSH in hypocholesterolemia and cholesterol as a mediator in the synthesis of new BAs. R: Amino acid glycine or taurine. RDCA: Glyco- or tauro-deoxycholic acid, DCA: Deoxycholic acid. Adapted from: Jones, Chen, Ouyang, Metz, and Prakash (2004) and Anandharaj, Sivasankari, and Parveen Rani (2014).

researchers have proposed that the activity of BSH activity should be considered in the probiotic selection criteria as they possess the ability to lower cholesterol. This is because some probiotic microorganisms lacking this enzyme are not able to significantly reduce cholesterol. Therefore, if bile secretion is an essential mechanism for lowering cholesterol levels, the cultures used in in vivo tests should be selected from the appropriate source. Numerous studies have demonstrated the distribution of BSH activity in *Bifidobacterium* and *Lactobacillus* is genus, species, or even strain-dependent. Most probiotic lactic acid bacteria originating from the human intestines and feces have shown BSH activity. However, it is important to note that strains with BSH activity isolated from the intestine or feces can also survive without this enzyme and grow under bile salt conditions. BAs also stimulate cholesterol assimilation through anaerobic development. The microbial metabolism of intestinal BAs and the enterohepatic cycle defines the makeup of the pool of human BAs. Bile, which is held in the gallbladder, is comprised primarily of conjugated BAs. Only 5% of the BAs released in bile are reabsorbed in the terminal ileum and are recirculated in the liver via the enterohepatic circulation to the large intestines, whereby 95% of BAs are expelled in feces. While an array of colonic bacteria perform deconjugation activities, 7a-dehydroxylation appears to be limited to a small number of intestinal bacteria. Consequently, the BAs profile expelled in feces and consisting primarily of secondary BAs is highly dependent on gut microbial metabolism. The pool measure, metabolite anatomy, and compartment fixations are important aspects of the BA results because they relate to the normal gut microbiota composition and how it metabolizes BAs and influences host metabolic processes and obesity (Joyce et al., 2014). The organisms use BAs to change the expression of genes controlled by the farnesoid X receptor, resulting in a unique activation by the acids and their metabolites (Sayin et al., 2013). Consequently, the more bile salts are secreted, the more cholesterol will be removed from the bloodstream. Recently, the use of LAB degenerated bile salts to reduce serum cholesterol levels in patients with hypertension and prevent hypertension in normal people has been receiving more attention. The induction of such physiological effects was strongly connected to probiotic consumption, prompting a further investigation to determine whether the effects were due to native microbiota regulation or specific metabolic action of the consumed probiotic strains (Hassan et al., 2019). Until recently, only one probiotic product associated with claims of cardiovascular health has been approved in the market by Health Canada. Cardioviva, which is also available in the United States and Europe, contains two billion encapsulated *Lactobacillus reuteri* NCIMB 30242 and has been clinically proven to lower LDL cholesterol levels by 11.6% in people with high cholesterol levels (Jones, Martoni, & Prakash, 2012).

## CHOLESTEROL DEPOSITION WITH CONJUGATED BILE SALT

Simultaneous removal of deconjugated bile salts associated with cholesterol, in vitro, has been described by several researchers. Cholesterol may be deposited with bile salts degraded at pH below 5.5 at the same time as bacterial fermentation and the formation of SCFAs. At acidic pH, degraded bile salts protonate and precipitate, while glycine-conjugated bile salts remain unreacted without heterolysis and precipitate to some extent leaving taurine-conjugated bile salts ionized in solution (Dashkevicz & Feighner, 1989). Scientific reports have confirmed that the removal of cholesterol from an environment by disruption of unstable cholesterol micelles occurs as a result of the loss of bile salts, followed by a decrease in pH and the deposition of cholesterol with free bile salts (Jones et al., 2004; Molinero, Ruiz, Sánchez, Margolles, & Delgado, 2019). In vitro culture of *L. casei* significantly reduced cholesterol levels by destabilizing cholesterol micelles and coprecipitating them with decongested bile salts at pH less than six (Brashears, Gilliland, & Buck, 1998). Conjugated bile salts associated with the simultaneous deposition of cholesterol are ambient and pH-dependent. Simultaneous deposition of cholesterol occurs at pH around 3.78–6.69 (Liong & Shah, 2005). The highest deposition of cholesterol with colic acid occurs at a pH of less than five, and the lowest simultaneous deposition of cholesterol occurs in the presence of sodium glycocholate regardless of the pH level. Thus, it can be inferred that cholesterol deposition is not solely only pH-dependent (Bhat & Bajaj, 2020).

### Cholesterol Integration into Bacterial Cell Walls

Cholesterol incorporation into bacterial cellular membranes reduces cholesterol absorption from the intestine into the blood, resulting in a decrease in total serum cholesterol. The amino acids that make up the peptidoglycan of probiotic bacteria's cell walls, and the exopolysaccharides released by these microbes, are principally responsible for the close interaction between cholesterol in the medium and the probiotic bacteria's cell surface. The lipids of probiotic lactic acid bacteria are primarily concentrated in the membrane, suggesting that cholesterol incorporated into membrane cells altered the fatty acid composition of the cells (Esmaeili, Paidari, et al., 2021). Moreover, membrane cells with incorporated cholesterol had increased concentrations of unsaturated and saturated fatty acids, thereby improving membrane strength. The cholesterol is then incorporated into the cell membrane of the bacteria which would reduce cholesterol absorption from the intestine into the blood. Interestingly, the content and peptidoglycan structure in bacterial cell walls could also have an impact on each strain's ability to accumulate cholesterol. In a study consisting of 34 *Bifidobacterium* strains (*Bifidobacterium animalis*, *Bifidobacterium bifidum*, *Bifidobacterium longum*, *Bifidobacterium adolescentis*, and *Bifidobacterium pseudocatenulatum*), it was discovered that these bacteria were capable of assimilating 4–81 mg cholesterol/g of dry biomass. Among the different strains investigated, *B. bifidum* MB 109 and *B. bifidum* MB 107 were able to digest the maximum quantities (Bordoni et al., 2013). Shehata et al. (2019) examined the bacterium *Lactococcus lactis* subspecies in terms of cholesterol-lowering in vitro. The results showed that 43.70% of cholesterol was absorbed by growing cells, 12.93% by resting cells, and 6.35% by dead cells. Electron imaging also confirmed cholesterol attachment to bacterial cell walls (Shehata et al., 2019). This process is attributed to the relationship between cholesterol incorporation and the pH of the growth medium. When compared to cultures produced at a pH of 6.0, cell membranes from cultures grown without pH control had considerably higher cholesterol. Moreover, cholesterol levels were found to be greater in cell membranes from cultures that did not have pH control. Cell membranes produced without pH control had greater cholesterol concentrations than whole cells grown under the same circumstances, but there was no significant difference in cholesterol content between cell membranes and entire cells grown at pH 6.0. It has been confirmed that *L. brevis* strains in Iran can assimilate cholesterol up to 80% after 9 hours of incubation compared to other isolated species of lactic acid bacteria originating from traditional dairy products (ewe milk, traditional yogurt, and sour buttermilk). However, the quantity of cholesterol eliminated in the *L. acidophilus* membrane fraction did not account for the overall amount removed by the culture. According to scientists, some cholesterol may loosely interact with the cells and fail to be integrated into the membrane, resulting in loss during the isolation process. Probiotics also reduced cholesterol levels by incorporating cholesterol into cellular membranes during development. By using a fluorescent probe, the probable locations of the cholesterol-binding process inside the phospholipid bilayer membrane of probiotic cells were investigated. Although the absorption of cholesterol by this pathway is strain- and growth-dependent, these findings are, however, yet to be confirmed in vivo (Hassan et al., 2019).

## Lowering Serum Cholesterol by Probiotics

Another mechanistic health characteristic of some lactic acid bacteria and bifidobacteria for decreasing cholesterol levels is cholesterol assimilation. Cholesterol is largely assimilated during bacterial development, where it is attached to the cellular surface without transformation and integrated into the membrane phospholipid layer. In a high-cholesterol mouse model, Park et al. investigated the hypocholesterolemic characteristic of *L. acidophilus ATCC 43121*. The consumption of probiotics by the mice reduced total serum cholesterol levels by up to 25% and confirmed a significant ($P < 0.05$) reduction in LDL, intermediate-density lipoprotein, and LDL cholesterol levels. Probiotics must exhibit viability and growth in order to be able to absorb cholesterol. In one study, *L. plantarum 49* and *L. plantarum 201* were shown to lower TC serum levels after 14 days of bacterium consumption (da Costa et al., 2019). In another study, *L. mesenteroides* subsp. *mesenteroides KDK411* and *L. curvatus KFP419* were found to have potential hypercholesterolemia action in rats through the absorption and excreting of cholesterol per evidence in the feces (Park, Kim, Shin, Kim, & Whang, 2007).

Despite these results, some in vivo investigations have yielded contradictory results. Since the cholesterol content of the feces of rats fed with *L. acidophilus ATCC 43121* ($3 \times 10^7$ CFU/d) did not change from that of the control group, Park et al. did not ascribe this mechanism to the hypocholesterolemic effect of the probiotics. Moreover, adult individuals' serum TC, LDL cholesterol, HDL cholesterol, and TAG concentrations were not affected by treatment with *L. rhamnosus LC705* (two capsules/d containing $2 \times 10^{10}$ CFU, for 4 weeks), even with a small rise in serum cholesterol. As a result, we can conclude that the ability of bacteria to assimilate cholesterol in the medium appears to be strain-specific and reliant on the strain's growth. The occurrence of the hypocholesterolemic effect can be hindered if the strain can remove cholesterol but does not survive during passage through the GI tract.

## Binding of Cholesterol

Growing bacterial cells maintained a considerable quantity of cholesterol, and sonication from cells of *Bifidobacterium* breve ATCC 15700 exuded more than 40% of cholesterol. Even after several washes, detachment of the absorbed cholesterol was impossible, indicating a strong binding potential between cholesterol and the growing cells. Additionally, nongrowing *Lactococcus* cells have been confirmed to have the capability of absorbing cholesterol in vitro; thus, the mechanism of cholesterol removal has been studied from different perspectives. Probiotics endowed with cholesterol-lowering properties possess the attribute of cholesterol-binding potential in the small intestine. Nami et al (2019) reported that probiotic *L. plantarum YS5* exhibited an elevated cholesterol-removal capacity by growing cells (84%) and moderate cholesterol-removal capacity by resting (41.14%) cells and dead (32.71%) cells. Moreover, *L. fermentum* lowered cholesterol levels in vitro, according to Pereira and Gibson (2002). It has been suggested that cholesterol assimilation by gut cells may lower the quantity of cholesterol available for intestinal absorption (Miremadi, Ayyash, Sherkat, & Stojanovska, 2014; Pigeon, Cuesta, & Gilliland, 2002). Viable as well as heat-killed cells were capable of cholesterol removal from growing media by *L. lactis* subsp. *lactis N7*. Viable cells were also able to substantially eliminate more cholesterol than dead cells (Kimoto-Nira et al., 2007). *L. gasseri* strains have been confirmed to eliminate cholesterol in vitro by adhering to the cellular surface, although this capacity seemed to be growth- and strain-specific. The capacity of probiotics to eliminate cholesterol throughout various growth conditions, notwithstanding, bolstered the aforementioned result (Kimoto, Ohmomo, & Okamoto, 2002).

## Other Mechanisms

Metabolic products such as SCFAs synthesized by probiotics have a pivotal role in cholesterol removal. SCFAs serve as ligands to activate peroxisome proliferator-activated receptors (PPARs). Angiopoietin-like protein 4 (ANGPTL4), a lipoprotein lipase (LPL) inhibitor, is produced by brown and white fat in the liver and intestines and is regulated by PPARγ (Hoda, 2011). According to Sheril et al. (2013), butyrates activate PPARs predominantly, followed by propionate, and finally acetate. As a result of PPAR activation and the upregulation of ANGPTL4 levels, SCFAs decrease LPL activities. This action suppresses fat storage by regulating fatty acid oxidation in muscle and adipocytes. Therefore, to have a hypocholesterolemic impact, the probiotic microorganisms must create enough propionate to counteract the effects of acetate on cholesterogenesis. For example, *L. plantarum MA2* (1011 cells/d) incorporated into a cholesterol-enriched diet and fed to Sprague–Dawley rats for 5 weeks exhibited a higher fecal propionate concentration than that of the control group.

Cholesterol can be converted to coprostanol (5-cholestan-3-ol) and coprostanone in small concentrations. These metabolites have a poor intestinal absorption rate and are excreted in the feces with a decrease in cholesterol absorption. The cholesterol reductase enzyme must be present in the cholesterol-lowering probiotics in order to convert cholesterol. This enzyme is present in probiotic bacteria such as *Lactobacillus bulgaricus FTCC 0411, L. acidophilus FTCC 0291, L. acidophilus ATCC 314, L. casei 1311 FTDC ATCC 393, B. bifidum PRL2010,* and *Eubacterium coprostanoligenes ATCC 51222* (Gérard, 2014; H-S Lye et al., 2010; Zanotti et al., 2015). There is limited information in the literature regarding the strains that are positive for this enzyme; however, the activity of this enzyme is strain-specific.

The Niemann-Pick C1-Like 1 (NPC1L1) protein is found in the small intestines on the brush surface membrane of enterocytes and plays an integral role in cholesterol absorption (Jia, Betters, & Yu, 2011). In a study by Huang et al., hypercholesterolemic rats were treated with *L. acidophilus ATCC 4356* for 28 days, and it was found that NPC1L1 levels in segments of the jejunum and the duodenum were considerably decreased ($P < 0.05$) (Huang et al., 2013). This was corroborated and confirmed by Duval et al. that activators of the liver X receptor (LXR) suppressed the expression of the NPC1L1 gene in the gut. Interestingly, in mammals, cholesterol metabolism is primarily regulated by LXRs. LXRα- and LXRβ- are the two kinds of LXR that have been identified so far and regulate the metabolism of lipids and carbohydrates. These LXRs are nuclear receptors and constitute members of a superfamily that functions as ligand-activated transcription factors. Huang and Zheng (2010) found that the expression of LXR-α and LXR-β was upregulated by the *L. acidophilus ATCC 4356* strain, whereas the expression of NPC1L1 was downregulated in a dose- and time-dependent manner in Caco-2. In addition, *L plantarum* LRCC 5273 effectively decreased hypercholesterolemia in mice by activating hepatic and intestinal LXR-, leading to BA excretion and increased fecal cholesterol in the small intestine (Heo et al., 2018).

Choline, phosphatidylcholine, L-carnitine, and betaine were metabolized by the intestinal microbiota to trimethylamine (TMA), which is then oxidized to trimethylamine N-oxide (TMAO) by hepatic flavin monooxygenases (FMO3) (Zhou et al., 2020).

TMAO levels in the blood have been linked to negative outcomes in CVD patients such as chronic heart failure and coronary heart disease. Consequently, attention to TMAO levels could be a potentially useful predictive indicator for unfavorable cardiac events in patients with chronic heart failure following myocardial infarction. In addition, the formation of gut microbiota-dependent TMAO is inhibited and has proven to be a viable method for atherosclerosis therapy (Z. Wang et al., 2015). However, it is yet unclear which gut microorganisms play the most important role in CVD, and the precise processes involved need to be investigated further (Molinero et al., 2019).

### Relationship between Nutrition and Gut Microbiota

The GI tract is one of the most significant and important systems in the human body. For example, the small intestine itself is responsible for two important processes, notably digestion and resorption. The lining of the small intestine is rich in glands that secrete intestinal juice, which contains enzymes that catalyze polypeptides, fats, and disaccharides. The small intestine is associated with the digestion of food due to secreted secretions of the pancreas, liver, and mucous membranes. In addition, the small intestine secretes hormones that participate in the body's immune defenses. The undigested, unabsorbed food that reaches the end of the small intestine passes into the large intestine, which forms the last section of the digestive tract and has no practical significance for digestion. The large intestine is thus simply a reservoir of fecal masses periodically excreted from the body. However, the cavity that comprises the large intestine is inhabited by the normal intestinal microflora, the presence and standard composition of which are very important for overall human health. The intestinal microflora is characterized by diverse species composition including microorganisms such as fungi, bacteria, protozoa, and viruses that colonize the GI tract (Valdes, Walter, Segal, & Spector, 2018). The large intestine microbiota breaks down complex carbohydrates and sugars through the metabolism of SCFAs, acetate, butyric acid, and propionate. Protein fermentation ends with a more diverse metabolic profile. Some nitrogen products, especially N-nitroso compounds, are carcinogenic and can cause mutations in DNA. These compounds occur endogenously due to microbial fermentation of proteins in the colon or can be obtained as a result of nutrition (Duncan et al., 2007).

Intestinal bacteria partially break down dietary fiber and other undigested food residues. The bacterial breakdown of food residues results in end products that include SCFAs and gases. Intestinal bacteria can also synthesize some vitamins (from group B (biotin, pyridoxine, cobalamin, riboflavin, folate, nicotinic acid, thiamine) and vitamin K). Some representatives of the intestinal microflora are antagonists of food pathogens and inhibit their development, growth, and metabolic activity (Holscher, 2017).

The digestion and resorption of nutrients occur in the intestinal tract, particularly the small intestine. Chronic inflammation of the small intestine causes digestion problems and impedes nutrient absorption. Dysfunction of the small intestine significantly hampers the rate of digestion and resorption. In general, factors such as the presence of vitamins, minerals, and other nutritional deficiencies, food intolerance, and food allergies are all hindered when the functionality of the small intestine is impaired (Gentile & Weir, 2018).

With regard to intestinal disorders, it is essential to exclude, from the diet, foods that impair the motor function of the intestine. In other words, the food must be mechanically, chemically, and thermally sparing. It is thus necessary to reduce fat consumption as the quantity and quality of fats impact their degree of digestion by the body. Therapeutic diets are also required to provide the necessary amount of energy and protein. In addition, to address intestinal disorders, therapeutic diets should include a substantial amount of vitamins and minerals (Cardona, Andrés-Lacueva, Tulipani, Tinahones, & Queipo-Ortuño, 2013).

The primary bacterial groups that make up the intestinal microflora of the human body are *Firmicutes, Bacteroidetes, Proteobacteria, Verrucomicrobia*, and *Actinobacteria*. The amount and species composition of the intestinal microflora of a healthy person varies with age and the composition of the food, and most of these bacteria are commensal (they coexist with the human body without causing disease). Children are born with a sterile digestive tract, which begins to colonize with micro-organisms after a few hours. *Enterobacteria* and *Bifidobacteria* are the first settlers. However, a healthy stomach and the proximal part of the small intestine contain very few organisms, which is due to the bactericidal action of hydrochloric acid in gas-tric juice. The colon, on the other hand, is dominated by anaerobic microorganisms, while the small intestine is predominantly aerobic and anaerobic. Bacteria in the intestinal lumen break down different types of sterols and steroids. The bacteria also convert the cholic acid of bile salts into deoxycholate, break down toxins, produce biotin and pantothenic acid, stimulate the immune system, and cause the fermenta-tion of cellulose (Schmidt, Raes, & Bork, 2018).

Many factors affect the degree of microbial presence in the gut. Factors that influence the ecosystem of the intestinal microbiota include the mode of birth, the mother's microbiota, breastfeeding, exposure to environmental bacteria, intake of antibiotics/probiotics, and diet (Figure 5.2). It was found that in terms of com-position, variety, and functional competencies, the microbiota of 2- to 3-year-old

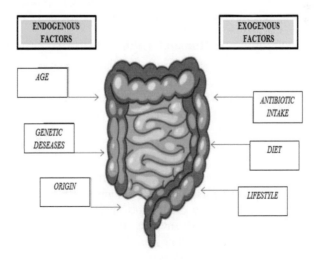

**FIGURE 5.2**    Factors influencing the gut microflora.

children is close to that of adults (Yang, Ye, Yan, He, & Xing, 2019). It is believed that the composition of the microbiota after three years of age is complete and functional. Moreover, eating habits and overall healthy lifestyles could generally promote a healthy intestinal microbiota (Yang et al., 2019).

There is a strong link between nutrient intake and the composition of intestinal microbiota. It is known that intestinal microorganisms can affect the synthesis of specific vitamins or the breakdown of certain nutrients, that is, the effects of micro-biota on nutrition. Moreover, the intestinal microbiota also differs among people from different latitudes and is also buttressed by environmental and genetic factors, as well as the use and administration of antibiotics (Goodrich et al., 2016). Nutrition, however, is suggested as the main reason for the differences in the composition of the gut microbiota between people.

Studies have shown that different food components are used by different bacterial communities and ensure the colonization of this community; in this way, the domi-nant bacterial species can be formed depending on the diet. Among the nutrients, carbohydrates, fiber, protein, fat, phytochemicals, and vitamins play a significant role in creating the intestinal microbiota (Duncan et al., 2007). Studies examining the effects of a high-fat diet on the intestinal fat microbiota have shown that such a diet reduces microbial diversity and increases the number of Bacteroides, Alistipe, and Bilophila. High-fat diets increase the concentration of SCFAs in the feces com-pared to low-fat diets and significantly reduce the levels of *bifidobacteria* (Heiman & Greenway, 2016). Phytochemicals are biologically active substances derived from plants that give plants their color, odor, and natural stability. It is known that a diet rich in fruits, vegetables, grains, and legumes reduces the risk of various diseases. The prophylactic effects, therefore, of these foods are partly due to antioxidants in their composition. The beneficial health effects of foods with probiotics such as dairy products have been well studied. For example, in recent years, we have seen increas-ing evidence that probiotics may play an essential role in the proper functioning of gut health and digestion, urogenital tract, immune system, respiratory features, and allergies, and can significantly combat various infectious diseases (Yang et al., 2019).

## Role of the Gut Microbiota in Human Health and Disease Prevention

The microflora in the digestive system plays a significant role in human health. Prebiotics, probiotics, and symbiotics are used to protect this microflora from patho-gens. For example, probiotic bacteria inhibit pathogenic microorganisms, increase the digestibility of food, strengthen the immune system, lower blood cholesterol lev-els, and increase the absorption of prebiotics. On the other hand, prebiotics are indi-gestible carbohydrates that increase the number and activity of bacteria in the colon and enhance the effect of probiotics. While prebiotics is used selectively by the ben-eficial microflora in the colon, they prevent the proliferation of potential pathogens. Probiotics and prebiotics can be used in combination with foods called symbiotics. With this application, the life span of probiotic bacteria is extended, resulting in enhanced colonization in the colon. Meanwhile, studies on the clinical use of probiotic microorganisms continue to increase. The use of probiotics is particularly associated with the treatment and enhanced outcomes of the following: diseases of the intestinal system, liver, *H. pylori*, oral and dental health, diseases of the genitourinary system,

LI, symptoms of constipation, stimulating the immune system, allergies, cancer, prevention of various types of diarrhea, and regulation of cholesterol levels (Liu, Tran, & Rhoads, 2018). There are many studies on probiotic use in diarrhea due to the use of antibiotics, and inflammatory bowel diseases (IBDs) such as ulcerative colitis (UC), chronic illness, spastic irritable bowel syndrome, and necrotizing enterocolitis (Ryma, Samer, Soufli, Rafa, & Touil-Boukoffa, 2021). Oligosaccharides cannot be hydrolyzed or absorbed in the small intestine. However, they can be fermented by *Lactobacillus* spp. and *Bifidobacterium* spp. and have prebiotic properties. In the food industry, the most widely used oligosaccharides are the following: fructooligosaccharides, galactooligosaccharides (GOS), transgalactooligosaccharides, xylooligosaccharides, gentio, lactulose, lactosaccharose, inulin, isomaltooligosaccharides, preharisaccharides, and salt. Inulin has also been widely used in food in recent years and can be fermented by *Lactobacillus* spp. and *Bifidobacterium* spp., and has prebiotic characteristics (Liu et al., 2018).

## Cardiovascular Disease

Globally, CVD is extensive, and the death toll attributed to this disease is increasing. Estimates by the WHO confirm that approximately 23 million people worldwide will have CVD by 2023, affecting up to 22% of the global economy. As human societies progress, lifestyle changes, and mobility declines, anomalies such as impaired insulin production or insulin resistance have led to increased levels of triglycerides, total cholesterol, low-density lipoprotein (LDL-C), and decreased LPL-C lipoprotein. High (HDL-C) cholesterol rises in the blood, thus posing an elevated CVD health risk in susceptible individuals. In addition, cholesterol oxidized by the formation of arterial plaques is a major cause of coronary heart disease. These factors, in combination with widespread smoking, contribute to the bulk of critical modifiable risk factors, which are responsible for approximately half of all deaths globally. Aortic and other peripheral vascular blood vessel inflammation is also a less prevalent health concern linked to atherosclerosis. According to Lee et al. (2012), CVD is attributed as one of the major precursors of death and sickness in the world, accounting for 29% of overall worldwide mortality (Lee et al., 2013). In addition to these variable basic factors, ACD mortality is influenced by extremely widespread physiologic and metabolic changes. Dyslipidemias, obesity, high blood sugar, hypertension, and insulin resistance are the most common diseases (Ramos, Esteves, Prates, Moreno, & Santos, 2022). For example, people with hypercholesterolemia are three times more susceptible to having a heart attack than those with a normal lipid profile.

### Liver Disease

During the first years of use of lactulose in hepatic encephalopathy, the colon pH decreases as a result of the bacterial metabolism of lactulose, which facilitates the proliferation of *Lactobacillus* and other acidophilic bacteria that can tolerate acid while preventing the formation of ammonia. *Lactobacillus* is thought to avoid the proliferation of the responsible acidophobic, proteolytic bacteria. Some researchers contend that bacterial proliferation in the colon increases with lactulose, that the increased bacterial population uses ammonia as a source of nitrogen or that there is metabolic inhibition in bacteria due to lower pH in the colon ammonia-producing bacteria not producing ammonia (Aller et al., 2011).

As is well known, probiotics can inhibit bacteria (especially gram-negative ones) with fecal enzyme activity by various mechanisms. In addition, the administration of lactulose alone or in combination with probiotics (especially *Bifidobacteria*) is one of the most recommended treatment methods. At low pH, most ammonia is in the form of ammonium ions (NH4 +), which the gut cannot absorb, and this reduces the passage of ammonia into the blood. The use of lactulose in combination with *Bifidobacteria* may support this protective effect (Xu, Wan, Fang, Lu, & Cai, 2011).

The second important mechanism associated with probiotics in treating encephalopathy is that probiotics help to more effectively clear ammonia and other toxins from the liver by reducing inflammation and oxidative stress in liver cells. Probiotics can play a protective role against inflammation and cell damage in the liver.

Details on the inhibition of the absorption of toxins other than ammonia, the last possible mechanism for the positive effects of probiotics, are not fully defined. However, the potential mechanism is advanced kidney disease undergoing hemodialysis (Aller et al., 2011).

Gut microbiota may cause nonalcoholic fatty liver disease by luminal ethanol production. Probiotics are used in order to treat changes in microbiota that have been reported in nonalcoholic fatty liver disease. A mixture of three genera of bacteria (a multistrain formulation composed of *Streptococcus*, *Thermophilus,* and several species of *Bifidobacterium* and *Lactobacillus*) administered to Lepob/ob mice over 4 weeks improved insulin sensitivity, total fatty acid content, serum alanine aminotransferase levels, and the histological spectrum of liver damage (Meroni, Longo, & Dongiovanni, 2019).

## Dental Diseases

The activity of probiotics on the health of the oral cavity and teeth is related to the ability of probiotics to produce an antimicrobial agent against oral pathogens. Probiotic bacteria can release various antimicrobial substances such as organic acid, hydrogen peroxide, carbon dioxide, diacetyl, bacteriocin, and adhesion inhibitors, which have high antimicrobial potential. Probiotics can also adhere to the surface of the teeth as well as the mouth surface. This is an essential point with regard to the long-term probiotic effects of bacteria. *Lactobacilli* can adhere to hydroxyapatite on teeth. Most adhesion experiments for probiotic purposes were based on the daily consumption of cheese and yogurt. Another vital ability of probiotics is their effect on the immune system. Probiotics are thought to have mechanisms that can alter the host's immune system. Dendritic cells scattered on the mucosa surface play a crucial role in the pre-identification of bacteria and activation of T-cell responses. Depending on the signal, either immune tolerance or an active immune response against a particular antigen is established in the dendritic cells. Due to the ability of probiotic bacteria to produce various antimicrobial substances and adhesion inhibitors that affect the oral flora, probiotics can significantly affect the environmental conditions necessary for the survival of bacteria by altering the pH of the environment and the redox potential (Haukioja, 2010).

## Gastrointestinal Diseases

### Inflammatory bowel Disease

Inflammatory bowel disease is an inflammatory, intermittent, chronic GI tract disease that recurs spontaneously. IBD is a term used to describe a group of complex disorders of the GI tract. IBDs include two main forms: Crohn's disease (CD) and UC, which share similar clinical symptoms. Symptoms and signs of the disease include stool changes in CD; however, recurrence is observed when stool change disappears. Inflammation of the mucosa is reduced when broad-spectrum enteric-coated antibiotics are used for UC. Triggering environmental conditions, genetic predisposition, and intestinal bacteria plays a role in the occurrence of IBD. Studies in humans and animals have shown that the percentage of beneficial microorganisms such as probiotics decreases the incidence of IBD (Lakatos, 2006).

Manipulation of the intestinal flora has become an interesting approach to preventing and treating IBD. Different results were obtained with other probiotic strains and their combined use in experimental models of colitis (Ryma et al., 2021).

**Ulcerative colitis:** Another well-known chronic IBD is UC whereby inflammation occurs as a result of abnormal reactions of the immune system. Many studies have shown that probiotics effectively maintain remission in UC. When fecal suspensions of healthy individuals are given to patients with UC by enema, the symptoms can be relieved and remission achieved.

In placebo-controlled studies, the incidence of relapse was found to be significantly reduced in probiotic users. With the establishment of remission, NF-κB, IL-1β, TNF-α decreased, and IL-10 increased (Baumgart & Carding, 2007; Ryma et al., 2021).

**Crohn's disease:** This is another IBD that leads to inflammation of the digestive tract. The distribution of bacteria in the gut of individuals with CD is very different from that of normal individuals. For this reason, although it was thought possible to approximate the flora of normal individuals through the use of probiotics, it was not possible to make a definite assessment of the results obtained (Nagao-Kitamoto, Kitamoto, Kuffa, & Kamada, 2016). CD is characterized by a discontinuous pattern, affecting the entire GI tract. In CD patients, the inflammation is transmural with large ulcerations and granulomas.

Several clinical trials and experimental studies displayed the role of *Saccharomyces boulardii* as a good biotherapeutic agent for preventing and treating several GI diseases including CD. *S. boulardii* stimulates effects that resemble the protective effects of the normal healthy gut flora (Kelesidis & Pothoulakis, 2012).

*Pouchitis* is inflammation occurring in the ileal region after ileal-anal anastomosis, in which the irregularities in the intestinal flora act as a triggering factor. In a study investigating the efficacy of a probiotic preparation (VSL#3) containing $5 \times 10(11)$ per gram of viable lyophilized bacteria of four strains of *Lactobacilli*, three strains of *Bifidobacteria*, and one strain of *Streptococcus salivarius* subsp. *thermophilus*, it was confirmed that this probiotic preparation was as efficient as compared to a placebo in the maintenance of remission of chronic pouchitis. The results showed that fecal concentration of *Lactobacilli*, *Bifidobacteria*, and *S. thermophilus* increased significantly from baseline levels only in the VSL#3-treated group. Thus, oral administration of the new probiotic preparation was effective in preventing flare-ups of chronic pouchitis (Gionchetti et al., 2000). While 85% of study subjects had a decrease in disease effects after 9 months, there was evidence of disease recurrence in all individuals in the placebo group.

## Complications after Surgery

The incidence of complications is high in patients who have undergone surgery and are kept in the intensive care unit. Among the complications, infections occupy a vital place. Early probiotic therapy and appropriate nutritional support have been valuable and effective options compared to the prophylactic use of antibiotics to control these complications. For example, perioperative care for patients with colorectal cancer includes antibiotics that are used in postoperative care and provide some protection against infections. Antibiotics carry risks of microbial resistance and disruption of the microbiome. Probiotics, on the other hand, can help to maintain the balance of the microbiome after surgery by preserving the integrity of the intestinal mucosa and reducing bacterial translocation. The authors demonstrated that probiotics were successful in postoperative infectious and noninfectious complications, analysis of bacterial translocation rate, and assessment of intestinal permeability. There was a tendency for lower levels of postoperative contagious and noninfectious complications with probiotics compared to placebo. Probiotics reduced bacterial translocation, maintained the permeability of the intestinal mucosa, and provided a better balance of beneficial pathogens (Pitsillides, Pellino, Tekkis, & Kontovounisios, 2021).

## Cancer Treatment

Diet plays a role in the development of colorectal cancer. A diet rich in meat and animal fats, and low in fiber, changes the distribution of colon flora. As *Clostridium* and *Bacteroides* strains increase, *Bifidobacterium* strains decrease. Because flora and the immune system play a role in tumor development, it is thought that, theoretically, prebiotics and probiotics that regulate flora can also be used to prevent tumor development. For example, lactulose causes a decrease in 7-$\alpha$ dehydroxylase activity through changes in the bacterial flora of the colon. 7-$\alpha$ dehydroxylase is the enzyme that causes the formation of secondary BAs. Secondary BAs are considered cocarcinogens. In addition, secondary BAs enter the enterohepatic circulation and form a continuous cycle, affecting BAs and cholesterol synthesis. The production of 7-$\alpha$ dehydroxylase and other potentially toxic enzymes of bacterial origin is reduced after administration of lactulose. Thus, lactulose administration helps in the reduction of toxic substances such as ammonia, which is also a known potential carcinogen. One hypothesis is that butyrate formed in the colon using lactulose has a DNA-protective impact. In addition to the many positive effects on health, probiotics also have anticancer, tumor-suppressant, and therapeutic effects (Pitsillides et al., 2021). Studies investigating probiotic–cancer interactions have demonstrated the capabilities of probiotics, such as the cancer-preventing effects. Probiotics enhance the host's immune response, deteriorate the structure of potentially carcinogenic compounds, create qualitative and quantitative changes in the intestinal flora, and have antimutagenic effects on the colon. Among the positive effects of probiotic action could be the ability of probiotics to produce anticancer compounds, alteration of metabolic activities, such as inhibition of the conversion of precancers into carcinogens in the intestinal microflora, prevention or retardation of toxin absorption, and modification of physicochemical conditions as enhanced intestinal barrier mechanisms.

Mohammed et al. (2010) reported that *Alexandrium minutum* possesses advantageous, anticancerous activity with mild apoptotic effects (Altonsy, Andrews, & Tuohy, 2010). Prebiotics are also efficient in the treatment of colon cancer due to their ability to ferment dietary fibers and enhance the level of metabolites. For example, wheat aleurone fermentation was reported to be enhanced by the addition of LGG/Bb12, resulting in an increased concentration of butyrate (Altonsy et al., 2010). The beneficial effects of the probiotic lactic acid bacteria *Lactobacillus plantarum* A7 and a commercial strain of *Lactobacillus rhamnosus* GG on human colon cancer cell lines (Caco-2 and HT-29) and normal cells (L-929) have been reported. It was determined that lactobacilli can exert antiproliferative effects on the various cancer cell lines including colon cancer (Sadeghi-Aliabadi, Mohammadi, Fazeli, & Mirlohi, 2014). A wealth of data implicates that ErbB receptors have essential roles in tumor development. *Bacillus polyfermenticus* has been clinically used in the growth of tumors by suppressing ErbB2 and ErbB3 protein. Generally, probiotic bacteria are known to exert anticancer activity in animal studies (Ma et al., 2010).

### Lactose Intolerance

Lactose intolerance is one of the most common forms of food intolerance and occurs when lactase activity is reduced in the small intestine lining. LI is characterized by GI symptoms, including vomiting, diarrhea, flatulence, and abdominal pain, which are caused by the fermentation of unabsorbed lactose in the colon. The severity of LI and the symptoms mentioned above can vary considerably from individual to individual. Lactase deficiency can be primary, secondary, or congenital. The most common form is primary lactase deficiency, a consequence of lactase deficiency characterized by a progressive decrease in lactase activity (Leis, de Castro, de Lamas, Picáns, & Couce, 2020).

If there is no or low lactase activity in the gut, undegraded lactose disturbs the osmotic balance and causes the accumulation of fluids and electrolytes in the gut. In enlarged intestines, motility increases, and diarrhea occurs.

Lactose, which reaches the colon without being broken down, is fermented by bacteria, resulting in hydrogen, methane, and carbon dioxide. Yogurt is the most superior probiotic product due to its beneficial effects on LI (Gyawali et al., 2020; Ibrahim et al., 2021). Because some microorganisms in yogurt contain the enzyme lactase, they break down lactose before it reaches the colon and prevents LI symptoms and signs.

People who have digestive problems with lactose can tolerate yogurt because there is beta-galactosidase activity in the bacteria found in yogurt. *S. thermophilus* and *Lactobacillus delbrueckii* subsp. *bulgaricus* contain the enzyme beta-galactosidase (lactase), which improves the digestion of lactose. Bacteria in yogurt metabolize lactose by releasing bacterial lactase due to lysis through the effect of bile salts in the small intestine after digestion. In addition, because fermented dairy products are darker than milk, their passage time through the GI tract is longer which allows for better digestion.

## Cultured Food Products

Cultured foods (fermented foods) are defined as 'foods or beverages produced through controlled microbial growth, and the conversion of food components through enzymatic action' (Marco et al., 2017). Specifically, lactic acid bacteria such as *Streptococcus, Lactobacillus,* and *Leuconostoc* are predominant in cultured foods. In addition, other microorganisms such as fungi and yeast also have several applications in food fermentation. Cultured foods are consumed worldwide, and the presence of beneficial microorganisms and their metabolites is considered to be an alternative to alleviate conditions associated with gut problems (Marco et al., 2017). These microorganisms known as probiotics are known to provide beneficial effects on gut microflora. According to Fuller (1989), cultured food products that have beneficial effects on host health by improving intestinal microbial balance are generally known to have a probiotic effect (Fuller, 1999). Some health benefits of cultured foods include boosting the immune system, improving intestinal health, alleviating the condition of LI, decreasing the prevalence of allergic reactions, preventing CVD, and minimizing the potential risk of certain cancers (Tamang, Shin, Jung, & Chae, 2016).

Daily consumption of cultured food products helps deliver commensal microbes through the GI tract for modulation of the gut microbiota. Foods such as yogurt, kefir, kimchi, cheese, and Kombucha contain microbial cells ranging between 6 and 9 log CFU/g or mL, and these cells are known to survive passage through the human GI tract (Derrien & van Hylckama Vlieg, 2015). These microbes could help alter the gut microbiota composition. Production of SCFAs, direct inhibition or stimulation of competitors, and other indirect effects are responsible for such changes in the microbial composition of the intestine (Derrien & van Hylckama Vlieg, 2015).

## ROLE OF CULTURED PRODUCTS IN GUT MICROBIOTA MODULATION

Recently, there has been significant interest in cultured foods due to their health benefits and as carriers of beneficial microorganisms such as probiotics and health-promoting metabolites. As a result of these foods, the diversity of the gut microbiota is potentially influenced. Table 5.2 lists selected cultured food products shown to influence gut microbiota.

### Yogurt

Yogurt and other fermented products of dairy origin are generally considered by consumers to be good sources of health-promoting organisms (Tremblay & Panahi, 2017). Yogurt by definition is a fermented cultured milk product containing two strains of live bacteria, namely *Lactobacillus delbrueckii* subsp. *bulgaricus* and *Streptococcus thermophilus*. These microbes should be at least $10^7$cfu/g and live at the time of consumption (Savaiano & Hutkins, 2021). Often other genera of probiotic *Lactobacillus* and *Bifidobacterium* strains are also added into yogurt for additional health benefits. For instance, yogurt-based diets have been linked to a decreased risk of bladder cancer, reduced weight gain, and a reduced risk of metabolic syndrome

## TABLE 5.2
## Intervention Studies and Impact of Cultured Food Products on Gut Microbiota

| Foods | Study Population | Intervention | Findings | References |
|---|---|---|---|---|
| Yogurt | Thirty-eight children with *H. pylori* infection | Four-week ingestion of probiotics-containing yogurt | Reduced *E. coli:Bifidobacterium* spp. ratio in children infected in *H. pylori* | Yang and Sheu (2012) |
| Yogurt drink | Twenty-three healthy preschool children | Six months of daily ingestion of a probiotic (*Lactobacillus casei* strain Shirota) containing drink | *Bifidobacterium* and total *Lactobacillus* increased, and *Enterobacteriaceae*, *Staphylococcus*, and *Clostridium perfringens* decreased | C. Wang et al. (2015) |
| Yogurt | Fifty-eight volunteers: healthy women and men aged between 18 and 55 years | Four-week commercial yogurt consumption supplemented with *Bifidobacterium animalis* subsp. *lactis* and *Lactobacillus acidophilus* | Viable counts of fecal lactobacilli were significantly higher, and those of enterococci were significantly lower | Savard et al. (2011) |
| Kefir | Forty-five (23 male and 22 female) patients completed the study | 400 mL/day kefir was administered twice a day to the patients for 4 weeks, which contains *Lactobacillus* bacteria (treatment group, 25 patients) | Lactobacillus bacterial load of feces of all subjects in the treatment group was between $10^4$ and $10^9$ CFU/g, and the first and last measurements were statistically significant | Yılmaz, Dolar, and Özpınar (2019) |
| Kefir | Eighty-two patients with symptoms of dyspepsia and *H. pylori* infection | Patients were given 250 mL of kefir twice daily (triple therapy + kefir, $n=46$) or 250 mL of milk containing placebo (triple therapy + placebo, $n=36$) for 14 days | Results showed a 14-day regimen of triple therapy with kefir is more effective in achieving *H. pylori* eradication than triple therapy alone | Bekar et al. (2011) |
| Probiotic milk | Six healthy female volunteers, 20–24 years of age | The volunteers consumed two servings of drink daily for 3 weeks, and then stopped consuming for an additional 3 weeks of the study period | Bacteroidetes increased during ingestion and decreased again after the end of ingestion. Firmicutes changed in the opposite way | Unno et al. (2015) |
| Probiotic milk | Thirty-two women (aged 20–69 years) | Thirty-two subjects consumed (125 g/serving) twice a day either the probiotic milk ($n=17$) or an acidified milk product ($n=15$) for 4 weeks | Probiotic milk product containing dairy starters and *Bifidobacterium animalis* potentiates colonic SCFA production and decreases abundance of a pathobiont *Bilophila wadsworthia* compared to a milk product | Veiga et al. (2014) |

*(Continued)*

**TABLE 5.2 (*Continued*)**
**Intervention Studies and Impact of Cultured Food Products on Gut Microbiota**

| Foods | Study Population | Intervention | Findings | References |
|---|---|---|---|---|
| Soy milk | Twenty-eight healthy adults | The drink consisted of 250 mL, twice a day between meals, of either fermented soy milk or regular soy milk first for 2 weeks, then switched to the other drink after 2 weeks | Bifidobacterium spp. and Lactobacillus spp. increased. The population of coliform organisms decreased when subjects consumed fermented soymilk | Cheng et al. (2005) |
| Soy milk | Ten healthy volunteers (six male, four female, 21–25 years old) | Subjects consumed fermented soy milk (100 g/day) and nonfermented soy milk (100 g/day) for 2 weeks | During the administration of fermented soy milk, the number of bifidobacteria and lactobacilli in the feces increased and clostridia decreased | Inoguchi et al. (2012) |
| Kimchi | Twenty-four obese women aged 30–60 years | Consuming 180 g of fresh or fermented kimchi per day (60 g/pkg × 3 meals) for 8 weeks | Abundance of *Bacteroides* and *Prevotella* increased while that of *Blautia* was decreased after intake of fermented kimchi | Han et al. (2015) |
| Kimchi | Six participants (age range 34–57) were assessed for *H. pylori* infection | Subjects consumed 300 g of kimchi with their normal diet. For control subjects consumed 60 g of kimchi | Did not show any therapeutic effect on *H. pylori* in the stomach. However, kimchi increased the population of *Lactobacillus* spp. | Kil et al. (2004) |

(Tremblay & Panahi, 2017). Over a century ago, Elie Metchnikoff proposed that by modifying the intestinal microbiome with bacteria present in yogurt, one's health could be improved (Mackowiak, 2013). Odamaki et al. (2012) assessed 420 healthy people and found that frequent yogurt consumption containing probiotic *Bifidobacterium longum* BB536 reduced the amount of enterotoxigenic *Bacteroides fragilis* in the gut. These results also corroborated the conclusion that endotoxin-producing bacteria are significantly suppressed by the habitual consumption of yogurt (Odamaki et al., 2012). A four-week intervention study with yogurt containing probiotic bacteria reduced the intestinal *Escherichia coli: Bifidobacterium* spp. ratio in children infected with *Helicobacter pylori* when compared with the control. This study showed reduced *H. pylori* loads and elevated serum IgA concentrations in infected children (Yang & Sheu, 2012). Donovan and Shamir (2014) confirmed the enormous health benefits associated with yogurt consumption including the prevention of GI diseases, as well as the maintenance of healthy gut microbiota (Donovan & Shamir, 2014). For example, consumption of probiotic yogurt drink fermented with the strain, *L. casei* Shirota, showed an increase in the total fecal *Lactobacillus* count and decreased *Enterobacteriaceae* and *Staphylococcus* counts

(Tsuji et al., 2014; C. Wang et al., 2015). The consumption of fermented yogurt containing *Bifidobacterium lactis* and *Lactobacillus fermentum* strains was also shown to elevate fecal *Bifidobacterium* and *Lactobacillus* counts (Ahmed, Prasad, Gill, Stevenson, & Gopal, 2007; Ibrahim et al., 2021; Savard et al., 2011; West et al., 2011). It has been reported that consumption of yogurt is associated with an increase in *Lactobacillus gasseri* and a decrease in *Enterobacteriaceae* and *Staphylococcus* levels. Another important health benefit associated with yogurt is the alleviation of LI symptoms due to the expression and release of β-galactosidase by the yogurt cultures (Gyawali et al., 2020; Ibrahim et al., 2021).

## Milk Kefir

Kefir is a cultured dairy product produced by the action of yeasts, lactic acid bacteria, and acetic acid bacteria fermentation of lactose in milk (Guzel-Seydim, Kok-Tas, Greene, & Seydim, 2011). Recently, kefir drink has raised increased interest among health-conscious consumers due to its superior health benefits. The impact of kefir on gut microbiota was investigated by Santos et al. (2003), where isolated kefir strains exhibited adhesion properties to the human enterocyte-like Cco-2 cells indicating a potential ability to colonize the human gut (Santos, San Mauro, Sanchez, Torres, & Marquina, 2003). Some studies on kefir strains have shown an increase in *Lactobacillus, Bifidobacterium,* and *Lactococcus* populations, and a decrease in *Proteobacteria* and *Enterobacteriaceae* counts in the gut microbiota (Kim et al., 2015). In another human study ($n=45$), *Lactobacillus kefiri* was identified in fecal samples after 800 mL/day of kefir was consumed for 4 weeks. The total *Lactobacillus* count in stool samples was significantly higher than as compared to the control samples in patients with CD (Bekar, Yilmaz, & Gulten, 2011). Likewise, a double-blind randomized controlled trial investigated the impact of consumption of 500 mL/day kefir on the eradication of *Helicobacter pylori* in patients with dyspepsia. The results showed that the control group (250 mL/day milk) had a lower eradication rate of *H. pylori* compared to the kefir group which had significantly higher levels of *H. pylori* (Bekar et al., 2011). Kefir also helped to improve LI symptoms, improve the immune system, lower cholesterol, and was shown to have anticarcinogenic and antimutagenic properties (Guzel-Seydim et al., 2011).

## Probiotic Fermented Milk

Probiotic milk is an important functional food that is consumed globally. It is obtained by milk fermentation which results in pH reduction. The common microbes involved in this process are *Lactobacillus delbrueckii* subsp. *bulgaricus, Streptococcus thermophilus, Lactobacillus acidophilus,* and *Lactobacillus kefiri* (Ebringer, Ferenčík, & Krajčovič, 2008). Probiotic fermented milk confers several health benefits. For example, fermented milk consumption was associated with microbial changes in the gut in a crossover intervention study of six healthy women. The study showed an increase in the *Firmicutes: Bacteroidetes* ratio after 3 weeks of fermented milk consumption (Unno et al., 2015). Similarly, Veiga et al. (2014) observed a decrease in *Bilophila wadsworthia* (a pathobiont) and higher counts in butyrate-producing bacteria, SCFA (butyrate) in women with irritable bowel syndrome after fermented milk consumption for 4 weeks (Veiga et al., 2014). Joseph et al. (2019) studied intestinal microbial changes in school children (n = 42, normal and overweight) after consumption of a probiotic drink containing *Lactobacillus casei* Shirota (Joseph et al., 2019). The results suggested that frequent consumption of probiotic drinks helped to significantly alter the composition of *Bifidobacterium* spp. and *Lactobacillus* spp. in the gut microbiota. Elevated fecal SCFAs (butyric and propionic acid) were observed in overweight children compared to normal-weight children which correspond to the presence of a higher number of gut microbiota. Sidira et al. (2010) assessed the effect of probiotic milk containing *Lactobacillus casei* ATCC 393 on modulation of intestinal microbiota in a rat model (Sidira et al., 2010). Daily administration (9 days) of milk led to significant reduction in staphylococci, enterobacteria, coliforms, and streptococci counts indicating protection against pathogens.

In a double-blind, placebo-controlled trial, Miyazaki et al. (2015) confirmed that frequent daily consumption of fermented milk products containing the prebiotic GOS and *Bifidobacterium breve* strain Yakult prevented dry skin in adult women in good health (Miyazaki et al., 2015). The results showed that the probiotic strain and GOS improved skin by limiting the production of phenols by the gut microbiota. A similar study examined the effects of the consumption of a fermented milk product containing the probiotic *L. casei* strain Shirota on the stress response of healthy medical students. The study confirmed that the frequent consumption of *L. casei* significantly lowered the percentage of *Bacteroidaceae* compared to the placebo group (Kato-Kataoka et al., 2016).

## ROLE OF CULTURED BEVERAGES IN GUT MICROBIOTA MODULATION

Kombucha is the most popular nonalcoholic fermented drink obtained by sugared tea fermentation with a cocktail of bacterial cultures (lactic acid and acetic acid bacteria) and symbiotic culture of bacteria and yeast. During fermentation, ethanol is produced from sucrose conversion by yeast and carbon dioxide, plus organic acids, while acetic acid and acetaldehyde are produced by acetic acid bacteria (Dufresne & Farnworth, 2000).

An evaluation was performed on the effect of Kombucha tea and its association with the gut microbiota on a progressive nonalcoholic fatty liver disease. The study confirmed a reduction in *Allobaculum*, *Turicibacter*, and *Clostridum* genera, whereas *Lactobacillus* was abundant in kombucha tea-fed mice (Jung et al., 2019). Even though kombucha is rich in microbial culture, limited available studies have explored the link between the composition of the gut microbiota and the effect of kombucha consumption in mammals (Coton et al., 2017).

Fermented soymilk is a soy-based functional drink with known health benefits. Increased counts of *Lactobacillus* and *bifidobacteria* spp. and decreased counts of *coliform* and *Clostridium perfringens* were linked to the consumption of 250 mL soybean milk twice daily for 2 weeks (Cheng et al., 2005). These results were in agreement with the findings of Inoguchi et al. (2012) in which consumption of 100 g of fermented soy milk (once/daily for 2 weeks) was associated with a decrease in *Clostridia* spp and an increased number of *Lactobacillus* spp. (Inoguchi et al., 2012) in ten healthy adults. Similarly, consumption of extracts of fermented plants for 8 weeks by 22 hypercholesterolemic patients was found to increase *bifidobacteria* and *Lactobacillus* spp. and decrease *E. coli* and *C. perfringens* counts (Chiu et al., 2017).

## ROLE OF FERMENTED VEGETABLES IN GUT MICROBIOTA MODULATION

Kimchi is a traditionally fermented vegetable product of Korean origin and contains various lactic acid bacteria such as *Lactobacillus, Leuconostoc, Pediococcus*, and *Weissella* (Choi, Lee, & Paik, 2015). Kimchi also possesses several health-promoting properties including antiaging, antihypertension, anticancer, anti-obesity, and anticonstipation effects (Das et al., 2020). An et al. (2019) investigated the effect of kimchi on the intestinal microbiota of rats (An et al., 2019). The microbiota's diversity was higher in the diet supplemented with kimchi as compared to the control. It was reported that obesity-associated *Firmicutes* decreased while leanness-associated *Bacteroidetes* increased. These results thus indicate that fermented kimchi can help reduce obesity and improve the host's health by modulating gut microbiota. Han et al. (2015) were interested in understanding the anti-obesity impact of kimchi by evaluating the relationship between gut microbiota and kimchi after its consumption (Han et al., 2015). The results showed an increase in *Prevotella* and *Bacteroides* and a decrease in the genus *Blautia* in the gut microbial population. This indicated that participants of the kimchi intervention group aligned with a 'lean enterotype' pattern as *Prevotella* and *Bacteroides* were associated with anti-obesity effects. In a randomized study with human subjects, consumption of 300 g/day kimchi for 4 weeks increased counts of *Lactobacillus* and *Leuconostoc* and decreased stool pH compared to 60 g/day of kimchi (Kil et al., 2004). Based on these results, kimchi was found to be an excellent source for colon health as it increased the population of beneficial bacteria and was also found to decrease toxic enzyme activity (Anusha Siddiqui, Redha, Esmaeili, & Mehdizadeh, 2022).

## EFFECTS OF PHENOLIC COMPOUNDS ON GUT MICROBIOTA

During the last few decades, scientists have conducted numerous research projects on the effects of nutritional diet on gut microbiota. Their results have revealed the direct impacts of nutritional habits on the microbial load, and survival, of essential bacteria in the GI tract (Suganya, Son, Kim, & Koo, 2021). Therefore, the evaluation of different structural food materials seems to be essential for a precise determination of their effects on gut microbiota and human health. In recent years, among diverse foodstuffs, cultured probiotics have played a major role in transferring essential nutritional compounds to the human body. This transfer has occurred via the development of the intestinal microflora and continuous modulation of the load and species of the distal gut as well as manipulation of the human gut microbiome (Shabbir et al., 2021). The term cultured probiotics, as mentioned before, is designated to a wide range of foodstuffs, and can be modified via the addition of various essential nutritional compounds, for example, polyphenols and antioxidants. Polyphenols, for example, have been the subject of a great deal of research due to their ability to prevent the formation of bioactive oxygen as well as their potential for synergism with numerous body compounds.

Polyphenols are considered to be a secondary plant metabolite containing a minimum of two hydroxyl groups linked to a carious number of aromatic structures, mostly found in plant residues, stems, leaves, and flowers. Polyphenols are mostly classified into flavonoids such as anthocyanins and nonflavonoids, for example, phenolic acids (Pandey & Rizvi, 2009).

The human body gains its essential polyphenolic compounds by consumption of various common agricultural products, namely tomatoes, onions, apple, berry, hazelnuts, plums, and black olive. Since polyphenol compounds consist of a large number of nutritional chemicals, there is not a prepared dietary reference intake value for determining the daily or even monthly intake of their source foodstuff. According to an investigation, Eastern countries consume an average of 2 g (per day) of polyphenolic compounds in comparison with 800 mg per day for Western countries due to the Western countries' typically lower consumption of natural food materials such as vegetables and fruits. Additionally, according to a report based on investigations in 2020, an average of 0.9 g/person/day was consumed by the total global population, primarily from coffee, tea, and fruits. Regarding various scientific reports, a deficiency of flavonoids and anthocyanins as the most important phenolics compounds can intensify the risk of various illnesses and diseases such as cancer, pancreatitis, and GI problems. On the contrary, excessive intake of polyphenols is reported to be hazardous due to their high affinity to interact with drugs and body enzymes (Rong et al., 2017).

Phenolic compounds are poorly absorbed (lower than 10%) due to their structure which inhibits their application and in functionalized food material same as in probiotics cultured foods. In this regard, modulated gut microbiota can help the body to biotransform polyphenolic compounds to smaller flavonoids or anthocyanins via different reactions in the GI tract same as is the case with oxidation, methylation, and isomerization. According to the results of Tao et al., gut microbiota can effectively transform bundle side flavonoids to aglycone acacetin and then into other various forms (Tao, Duan, Jiang, Qian, & Qian, 2016). Thus, it could be concluded that the biotransformation of flavonoids can not only increase their absorbance but also positively increase their stability in the GI tract. In this regard, there are various reported microorganisms and probiotics that have the ability to biotransform these phenolic compounds. Additionally, according to the results conducted on *Lactobacillus acidophilus,* these bacteria can remarkably transform glycosides into aglycones and aglycones that can then be beneficially used by host microorganisms. There are numerous reports on the application of *Gordonibacter, Urolithinfacients, Lactobacillus plantarum, Streptococcus intermedious*, etc., as probiotics that serve to increase the bioavailability of polyphenols in the human intestine tract (Kasprzak-Drozd, Oniszczuk, Stasiak, & Oniszczuk, 2021).

In conclusion, a healthy body is derived from the accurate and proper functioning of the GI tract which, in turn, is related to modulated dietary nutrition. The consumption of various cultured probiotics-containing polyphenolic compounds can thus beneficially increase the bioavailability and absorption of flavonoids and anthocyanins resulting in the preparation of proper chemicals for the consumption of gut microbiota. Proper functioning of the gut microbiota via proper nutrition such as the daily intake of cultured probiotics can be considered to be the easiest way not only to increase body health but also to prevent various cancers, diabetes, and GI diseases.

## CONCLUSION

In the last few decades, probiotic consumption has gained much attention due to its association with health benefits. Additionally, there has been increasingly widespread knowledge regarding the role of nutrition and diet in supporting a healthy gut microbiota. In vitro, experimental, and clinical researches have all demonstrated the synergistic effect of diet and probiotic use on enhancing the modulatory mechanism of the gut microbiota in specifically addressing human health and disease challenges. Consequently, it has also been established from the literature that cultured and fermented functional food products exert a positive impact on the overall metabolic functionality of the human system. The mechanism of probiotic action against disease-causing organisms helps to enhance the performance of the gut microbiota by the production of metabolites that support proper coordination and hormonal imbalance. Diet and nutrition are thus important key factors that influence the composition of the gut microbiota and serve as a driving force in promoting human health and wellness. As presented in this chapter, the importance of diet and cultured food products in the modulation of the gut microbiome cannot be overemphasized. Thus, the blending of diet, nutrition, and probiotic consumption as a part of an individual's lifestyle will result in a natural and therapeutic approach to disease prevention via the resultant modulatory effect on the gut microbiota without compromising the immune system.

## REFERENCES

Ahmed, M., Prasad, J., Gill, H., Stevenson, L., & Gopal, P. (2007). Impact of consumption of different levels of bifidobacterium lactis HN019 on the intestinal microflora of elderly human subjects. *Journal of Nutrition Health and Aging, 11*(1), 26.

Aller, R., De Luis, D., Izaola, O., Conde, R., Gonzalez Sagrado, M., Primo, D., . . . Gonzalez, J. (2011). Effect of a probiotic on liver aminotransferases in nonalcoholic fatty liver disease patients: a double blind randomized clinical trial. *European Review for Medical Pharmacological Sciences, 15*(9), 1090–1095.

Altonsy, M. O., Andrews, S. C., & Tuohy, K. M. (2010). Differential induction of apoptosis in human colonic carcinoma cells (Caco-2) by atopobium, and commensal, probiotic and enteropathogenic bacteria: mediation by the mitochondrial pathway. *International Journal of Food Microbiology, 137*(2–3), 190–203.

An, S. J., Kim, J. Y., Kim, I. S., Adhikari, B., Yu, D. Y., Kim, J. A., . . . Cho, K. K. (2019). Modulation of intestinal microbiota by supplementation of fermented kimchi in rats. *Journal of Life Science, 29*(9), 986–995.

Anandharaj, M., Sivasankari, B., & Parveen Rani, R. (2014). Effects of probiotics, prebiotics, and synbiotics on hypercholesterolemia: a review. *Chinese Journal of Biology, 2014*, 1-7.

Antoun, M., Hattab, Y., Akhrass, F.-A., & Hamilton, L. D. (2020). Uncommon pathogen, lactobacillus, causing infective endocarditis: case report and review. *Case Reports in Infectious Diseases, 2020*, 1–4.

Anusha Siddiqui, S., Redha, A. A., Esmaeili, Y., & Mehdizadeh, M. (2022). Novel insights on extraction and encapsulation techniques of elderberry bioactive compounds. *Critical Reviews in Food Science and Nutrition*, 1–16.

Ayivi, R. D., Gyawali, R., Krastanov, A., Aljaloud, S. O., Worku, M., Tahergorabi, R., . . . & Ibrahim, S. A. (2020). Lactic acid bacteria: food safety and human health applications. *Dairy, 1*(3), 202–232.

Baumgart, D. C., & Carding, S. R. (2007). Inflammatory bowel disease: cause and immuno-biology. *The Lancet, 369*(9573), 1627–1640.

Behrouzi, A., Mazaheri, H., Falsafi, S., Tavassol, Z. H., Moshiri, A., & Siadat, S. D. (2020). Intestinal effect of the probiotic Escherichia coli strain Nissle 1917 and its OMV. *Journal of Diabetes & Metabolic Disorders, 19*(1), 597–604.

Bekar, O., Yilmaz, Y., & Gulten, M. (2011). Kefir improves the efficacy and tolerability of triple therapy in eradicating Helicobacter pylori. *Journal of Medicinal Food, 14*(4), 344–347.

Bhat, B., & Bajaj, B. K. (2020). Multifarious cholesterol lowering potential of lactic acid bacteria equipped with desired probiotic functional attributes. *3 Biotech, 10*(5), 1–16.

Bordoni, A., Amaretti, A., Leonardi, A., Boschetti, E., Danesi, F., Matteuzzi, D., . . . Rossi, M. (2013). Cholesterol-lowering probiotics: in vitro selection and in vivo testing of bifido-bacteria. *Applied Microbiology and Biotechnology, 97*(18), 8273–8281.

Brashears, M., Gilliland, S., & Buck, L. (1998). Bile salt deconjugation and cholesterol removal from media by Lactobacillus casei. *Journal of Dairy Science, 81*(8), 2103–2110.

Byakika, S., Mukisa, I. M., Byaruhanga, Y. B., & Muyanja, C. (2019). A review of criteria and methods for evaluating the probiotic potential of microorganisms. *Food Reviews International, 35*(5), 427–466.

Cardona, F., Andrés-Lacueva, C., Tulipani, S., Tinahones, F. J., & Queipo-Ortuño, M. I. (2013). Benefits of polyphenols on gut microbiota and implications in human health. *The Journal of Nutritional Biochemistry, 24*(8), 1415–1422.

Cheng, I.-C., Shang, H.-F., Lin, T.-F., Wang, T.-H., Lin, H.-S., & Lin, S.-H. (2005). Effect of fermented soy milk on the intestinal bacterial ecosystem. *World Journal of Gastroenterology: WJG, 11*(8), 1225.

Chiu, H.-F., Chen, Y.-J., Lu, Y.-Y., Han, Y.-C., Shen, Y.-C., Venkatakrishnan, K., & Wang, C.-K. (2017). Regulatory efficacy of fermented plant extract on the intestinal microflora and lipid profile in mildly hypercholesterolemic individuals. *Journal of Food and Drug Analysis, 25*(4), 819–827.

Choi, H.-J., Lee, N.-K., & Paik, H.-D. (2015). Health benefits of lactic acid bacteria iso-lated from kimchi, with respect to immunomodulatory effects. *Food Science and Biotechnology, 24*(3), 783–789.

Coton, M., Pawtowski, A., Taminiau, B., Burgaud, G., Deniel, F., Coulloumme-Labarthe, L., . . . Coton, E. (2017). Unraveling microbial ecology of industrial-scale Kombucha fermen-tations by metabarcoding and culture-based methods. *FEMS Microbiology Ecology, 93*(5), 1–16.

Croft, J., Cresanta, J., Webber, L., Srinivasan, S., Freedman, D., Burke, G., & Berenson, G. (1988). Cardiovascular risk in parents of children with extreme lipoprotein cholesterol levels: the Bogalusa Heart Study. *Southern Medical Journal, 81*(3), 341–349, 353.

da Costa, W. K. A., Brandão, L. R., Martino, M. E., Garcia, E. F., Alves, A. F., de Souza, E. L., . . . Vidal, H. (2019). Qualification of tropical fruit-derived Lactobacillus plantarum strains as potential probiotics acting on blood glucose and total cholesterol levels in Wistar rats. *Food Research International, 124*, 109–117.

Das, G., Paramithiotis, S., Sivamaruthi, B. S., Wijaya, C. H., Suharta, S., Sanlier, N., . . . Patra, J. K. (2020). Traditional fermented foods with anti-aging effect: a concentric review. *Food Research International, 134*, 109269.

Dashkevicz, M. P., & Feighner, S. D. (1989). Development of a differential medium for bile salt hydrolase-active Lactobacillus spp. *Applied and Environmental Microbiology, 55*(1), 11–16.

De Preter, V., Vanhoutte, T., Huys, G., Swings, J., De Vuyst, L., Rutgeerts, P., & Verbeke, K. (2007). Effects of Lactobacillus casei Shirota, Bifidobacterium breve, and oligo-fructose-enriched inulin on colonic nitrogen-protein metabolism in healthy humans. *American Journal of Physiology-Gastrointestinal and Liver Physiology, 292*(1), G358–G368.

Derrien, M., & van Hylckama Vlieg, J. E. (2015). Fate, activity, and impact of ingested bacteria within the human gut microbiota. *Trends in microbiology, 23*(6), 354–366.

Donovan, S. M., & Shamir, R. (2014). Introduction to the yogurt in nutrition initiative and the First Global Summit on the health effects of yogurt. *The American Journal of Clinical Nutrition, 99*(5), 1209S–1211S.

Dufresne, C., & Farnworth, E. (2000). Tea, Kombucha, and health: a review. *Food Research International, 33*(6), 409–421.

Duncan, S. H., Belenguer, A., Holtrop, G., Johnstone, A. M., Flint, H. J., & Lobley, G. E. (2007). Reduced dietary intake of carbohydrates by obese subjects results in decreased concentrations of butyrate and butyrate-producing bacteria in feces. *Applied and Environmental Microbiology, 73*(4), 1073–1078.

Ebringer, L., Ferenčík, M., & Krajčovič, J. (2008). Beneficial health effects of milk and fermented dairy products. *Folia Microbiologica, 53*(5), 378–394.

Esmaeili, Y., Paidari, S., Baghbaderani, S. A., Nateghi, L., Al-Hassan, A., & Ariffin, F. (2021). Essential oils as natural antimicrobial agents in postharvest treatments of fruits and vegetables: a review. *Journal of Food Measurement and Characterization, 16,* 507–522.

El-Saadony, M. T., Alagawany, M., Patra, A. K., Kar, I., Tiwari, R., Dawood, M. A., Dhama, K., Abdel-Latif, H. M. (2021). The functionality of probiotics in aquaculture: an overview. *Fish & Shellfish Immunology, 1*(117), 36–52.

Esmaeili, Y., Zamindar, N., Paidari, S., Ibrahim, S. A., & Mohammadi Nafchi, A. (2021). The synergistic effects of aloe vera gel and modified atmosphere packaging on the quality of strawberry fruit. *Journal of Food Processing and Preservation, 45*(12), e16003.

FAO & WHO. (2002). *Joint FAO/WHO working group report on drafting guidelines for the evaluation of probiotics in food.* Geneva: World Health Organization.

Fuller, R. (1989). Probiotics in man and animals. *Journal of Applied Bacteriology, 66,* 365–378.

Fuller, R. (1999). Probiotics for farm animals. *Probiotics: A Critical Review,* 15–22.

Galie, N., Manes, A., Negro, L., Palazzini, M., Bacchi-Reggiani, M. L., & Branzi, A. (2009). A meta-analysis of randomized controlled trials in pulmonary arterial hypertension. *European Heart Journal, 30*(4), 394–403.

Ganguly, N., Bhattacharya, S., Sesikeran, B., Nair, G., Ramakrishna, B., Sachdev, H., . . . Kathuria, S. (2011). ICMR-DBT guidelines for evaluation of probiotics in food. *The Indian Journal of Medical Research, 134*(1), 22.

Gentile, C. L., & Weir, T. L. (2018). The gut microbiota at the intersection of diet and human health. *Science, 362*(6416), 776–780.

Gérard, P. (2014). Metabolism of cholesterol and bile acids by the gut microbiota. *Pathogens, 3*(1), 14–24.

Gionchetti, P., Rizzello, F., Venturi, A., Brigidi, P., Matteuzzi, D., Bazzocchi, G., . . . Campieri, M. (2000). Oral bacteriotherapy as maintenance treatment in patients with chronic pouchitis: a double-blind, placebo-controlled trial. *Gastroenterology, 119*(2), 305–309.

Goodrich, J. K., Davenport, E. R., Beaumont, M., Jackson, M. A., Knight, R., Ober, C., . . . Ley, R. E. (2016). Genetic determinants of the gut microbiome in UK twins. *Cell Host & Microbe, 19*(5), 731–743.

Guzel-Seydim, Z. B., Kok-Tas, T., Greene, A. K., & Seydim, A. C. (2011). Functional properties of kefir. *Critical Reviews in Food Science and Nutrition, 51*(3), 261–268.

Gyawali, R., Oyeniran, A., Zimmerman, T., Aljaloud, S. O., Krastanov, A., & Ibrahim, S. A. (2020). A comparative study of extraction techniques for maximum recovery of β-galactosidase from the yogurt bacterium Lactobacillus delbrueckii ssp. bulgaricus. *Journal of Dairy Research, 87*(1), 123–126.

Han, K., Bose, S., Wang, J., Kim, B. S., Kim, M. J., Kim, E. J., & Kim, H. (2015). Contrasting effects of fresh and fermented kimchi consumption on gut microbiota composition and gene expression related to metabolic syndrome in obese Korean women. *Molecular Nutrition & Food Research, 59*(5), 1004–1008.

Hassan, A., Din, A. U., Zhu, Y., Zhang, K., Li, T., Wang, Y., . . . Wang, G. (2019). Updates in understanding the hypocholesterolemia effect of probiotics on atherosclerosis. *Applied Microbiology and Biotechnology, 103*(15), 5993–6006.

Haukioja, A. (2010). Probiotics and oral health. *European Journal of Dentistry, 4*(3), 348–355.

Heiman, M. L., & Greenway, F. L. (2016). A healthy gastrointestinal microbiome is dependent on dietary diversity. *Molecular Metabolism, 5*(5), 317–320.

Heo, W., Lee, E. S., Cho, H. T., Kim, J. H., Lee, J. H., Yoon, S. M., . . . Kim, Y.-J. (2018). Lactobacillus plantarum LRCC 5273 isolated from Kimchi ameliorates diet-induced hypercholesterolemia in C57BL/6 mice. *Bioscience, Biotechnology, and Biochemistry, 82*(11), 1964–1972.

Hoda, M. (2011). Probiotics bacteria from Egyptian infants cause cholesterol removal in media and survive in yoghurt. *Food and Nutrition Sciences, 2*, 150–155.

Holscher, H. D. (2017). Dietary fiber and prebiotics and the gastrointestinal microbiota. *Gut microbes, 8*(2), 172–184.

Huang, Y., & Zheng, Y. (2010). The probiotic Lactobacillus acidophilus reduces cholesterol absorption through the down-regulation of Niemann-Pick C1-like 1 in Caco-2 cells. *British Journal of Nutrition, 103*(4), 473–478.

Huang, Y., Wang, X., Wang, J., Wu, F., Sui, Y., Yang, L., & Wang, Z. (2013). Lactobacillus plantarum strains as potential probiotic cultures with cholesterol-lowering activity. *Journal of Dairy Science, 96*(5), 2746–2753.

Ibrahim, S. A., Gyawali, R., Awaisheh, S. S., Ayivi, R. D., Silva, R. C., Subedi, K., . . . Krastanov, A. (2021). Fermented foods and probiotics: an approach to lactose intolerance. *Journal of Dairy Research, 88*(3), 357–365.

Inoguchi, S., Ohashi, Y., Narai-Kanayama, A., Aso, K., Nakagaki, T., & Fujisawa, T. (2012). Effects of non-fermented and fermented soybean milk intake on faecal microbiota and faecal metabolites in humans. *International Journal of Food Sciences and Nutrition, 63*(4), 402–410.

Jia, L., Betters, J. L., & Yu, L. (2011). Niemann-pick C1-like 1 (NPC1L1) protein in intestinal and hepatic cholesterol transport. *Annual Review of Physiology, 73*, 239–259.

Jones, M., Martoni, C., & Prakash, S. (2012). Cholesterol lowering and inhibition of sterol absorption by Lactobacillus reuteri NCIMB 30242: a randomized controlled trial. *European Journal of Clinical Nutrition, 66*(11), 1234–1241.

Jones, M. L., Chen, H., Ouyang, W., Metz, T., & Prakash, S. (2004). Microencapsulated genetically engineered Lactobacillus plantarum 80 (pCBH1) for bile acid deconjugation and its implication in lowering cholesterol. *Journal of Biomedicine and Biotechnology, 2004*(1), 61–69.

Joseph, N., Vasodavan, K., Saipudin, N. A., Yusof, B. N. M., Kumar, S., & Nordin, S. A. (2019). Gut microbiota and short-chain fatty acids (SCFAs) profiles of normal and overweight school children in Selangor after probiotics administration. *Journal of Functional Foods, 57*, 103–111.

Joyce, S. A., MacSharry, J., Casey, P. G., Kinsella, M., Murphy, E. F., Shanahan, F., . . . Gahan, C. G. (2014). Regulation of host weight gain and lipid metabolism by bacterial bile acid modification in the gut. *Proceedings of the National Academy of Sciences, 111*(20), 7421–7426.

Jung, Y., Kim, I., Mannaa, M., Kim, J., Wang, S., Park, I., . . . Seo, Y.-S. (2019). Effect of Kombucha on gut-microbiota in mouse having non-alcoholic fatty liver disease. *Food science and biotechnology, 28*(1), 261–267.

Kaplan, L. A., Pesce, A. J., & Kazmierczak, S. C. (2003). *Clinical chemistry: theory, analysis, correlation* (Vol. 1): Mosby Incorporated, St. Louis, MO.

Kasprzak-Drozd, K., Oniszczuk, T., Stasiak, M., & Oniszczuk, A. (2021). Beneficial effects of phenolic compounds on gut microbiota and metabolic syndrome. *International Journal of Molecular Sciences, 22*(7), 3715.

Kato-Kataoka, A., Nishida, K., Takada, M., Kawai, M., Kikuchi-Hayakawa, H., Suda, K., . . . Matsuki, T. (2016). Fermented milk containing Lactobacillus casei strain Shirota preserves the diversity of the gut microbiota and relieves abdominal dysfunction in healthy medical students exposed to academic stress. *Applied and Environmental Microbiology, 82*(12), 3649–3658.

Kechagia, M., Basoulis, D., Konstantopoulou, S., Dimitriadi, D., Gyftopoulou, K., Skarmoutsou, N., & Fakiri, E. M. (2013). Health benefits of probiotics: a review. *ISRN Nutrition, 2013*, 481651. https://doi.org/10.5402/2013/481651

Kelesidis, T., & Pothoulakis, C. (2012). Efficacy and safety of the probiotic Saccharomyces boulardii for the prevention and therapy of gastrointestinal disorders. *Therapeutic Advances in Gastroenterology, 5*(2), 111–125.

Khare, A., & Gaur, S. (2020). Cholesterol-lowering effects of Lactobacillus species. *Current Microbiology, 77*(4), 638–644.

Kil, J.-H., Jung, K.-O., Lee, H.-S., Hwang, I.-K., Kim, Y.-J., & Park, K.-Y. (2004). Effects of kimchi on stomach and colon health of Helicobacter pylori-infected volunteers. *Preventive Nutrition and Food Science, 9*(2), 161–166.

Kim, D.-H., Chon, J.-W., Kim, H.-S., Yim, J.-H., Kim, H., & Seo, K.-H. (2015). Rapid detection of Lactobacillus kefiranofaciens in kefir grain and kefir milk using newly developed real-time PCR. *Journal of Food Protection, 78*(4), 855–858.

Kimoto-Nira, H., Mizumachi, K., Nomura, M., Kobayashi, M., Fujita, Y., Okamoto, T., . . . Ohmomo, S. (2007). Lactococcus sp. as potential probiotic lactic acid bacteria. *Japan Agricultural Research Quarterly: JARQ, 41*(3), 181–189.

Kimoto, H., Ohmomo, S., & Okamoto, T. (2002). Cholesterol removal from media by lactococci. *Journal of Dairy Science, 85*(12), 3182–3188.

Kumar, M., Nagpal, R., Kumar, R., Hemalatha, R., Verma, V., Kumar, A., . . . Jain, S. (2012). Cholesterol-lowering probiotics as potential biotherapeutics for metabolic diseases. *Experimental Diabetes Research, 2012*, 1-14.

Lakatos, P. L. (2006). Recent trends in the epidemiology of inflammatory bowel diseases: up or down? *World Journal of Gastroenterology: WJG, 12*(38), 6102.

Le, B., & Yang, S.-H. (2019). Effect of potential probiotic Leuconostoc mesenteroides FB111 in prevention of cholesterol absorption by modulating NPC1L1/PPARα/SREBP-2 pathways in epithelial Caco-2 cells. *International Microbiology, 22*(2), 279–287.

Lee, H., Lee, S., Hwang, I., Park, Y., Yoon, S., Han, K., . . . Yim, H. (2013). Prevalence, awareness, treatment and control of hypertension in adults with diagnosed diabetes: the Fourth Korea National Health and Nutrition Examination Survey (KNHANES IV). *Journal of Human Hypertension, 27*(6), 381–387.

Leis, R., de Castro, M.-J., de Lamas, C., Picáns, R., & Couce, M. L. (2020). Effects of prebiotic and probiotic supplementation on lactase deficiency and lactose intolerance: a systematic review of controlled trials. *Nutrients, 12*(5), 1487.

Lim, H., Oh, S., Yu, S., & Kim, M. (2021). Isolation and characterization of probiotic Bacillus subtilis MKHJ 1-1 possessing L-asparaginase activity. *Applied Sciences, 11*(10), 4466.

Liong, M., & Shah, N. (2005). Acid and bile tolerance and cholesterol removal ability of lactobacilli strains. *Journal of Dairy Science, 88*(1), 55–66.

Liu, M., Xie, W., Wan, X., & Deng, T. (2020). Clostridium butyricum modulates gut microbiota and reduces colitis associated colon cancer in mice. *International Immunopharmacology, 88*, 106862.

Liu, Y., Tran, D. Q., & Rhoads, J. M. (2018). Probiotics in disease prevention and treatment. *The Journal of Clinical Pharmacology, 58*, S164–S179.

Lye, H.-S., Rahmat-Ali, G. R., & Liong, M.-T. (2010). Mechanisms of cholesterol removal by lactobacilli under conditions that mimic the human gastrointestinal tract. *International Dairy Journal, 20*(3), 169–175.

Lye, H.-S., Rusul, G., & Liong, M.-T. (2010). Removal of cholesterol by lactobacilli via incorporation and conversion to coprostanol. *Journal of Dairy Science, 93*(4), 1383–1392.

Ma, E. L., Choi, Y. J., Choi, J., Pothoulakis, C., Rhee, S. H., & Im, E. (2010). The anticancer effect of probiotic Bacillus polyfermenticus on human colon cancer cells is mediated through ErbB2 and ErbB3 inhibition. *International Journal of Cancer, 127*(4), 780–790.

Mackowiak, P. A. (2013). Recycling Metchnikoff: probiotics, the intestinal microbiome and the quest for long life. *Frontiers in Public Health, 1*, 52.

Marco, M. L., Heeney, D., Binda, S., Cifelli, C. J., Cotter, P. D., Foligné, B., . . . Pihlanto, A. (2017). Health benefits of fermented foods: microbiota and beyond. *Current Opinion in Biotechnology, 44*, 94–102.

McAuliffe, O., Cano, R. J., & Klaenhammer, T. R. (2005). Genetic analysis of two bile salt hydrolase activities in Lactobacillus acidophilus NCFM. *Applied and Environmental Microbiology, 71*(8), 4925–4929.

Meroni, M., Longo, M., & Dongiovanni, P. (2019). The role of probiotics in nonalcoholic fatty liver disease: a new insight into therapeutic strategies. *Nutrients, 11*(11), 2642.

Miremadi, F., Ayyash, M., Sherkat, F., & Stojanovska, L. (2014). Cholesterol reduction mechanisms and fatty acid composition of cellular membranes of probiotic Lactobacilli and Bifidobacteria. *Journal of Functional Foods, 9*, 295–305.

Miyazaki, M., Yoshitomi, H., Miyakawa, S., Uesaka, K., Unno, M., Endo, I., . . . Shimada, K. (2015). Clinical practice guidelines for the management of biliary tract cancers 2015: the 2nd English edition. *Journal of Hepato-Biliary-Pancreatic Sciences, 22*(4), 249–273.

Mohammed, O. A., Simon, C. A, Kieran, M. T. (2010). Differential induction of apoptosis in human colonic carcinoma cells (Caco-2) by Atopobium, and commensal, probiotic and enteropathogenic bacteria: Mediation by the mitochondrial pathway. *International Journal of Food Microbiology, 137*(2–3), 190–203.

Molinero, N., Ruiz, L., Sánchez, B., Margolles, A., & Delgado, S. (2019). Intestinal bacteria interplay with bile and cholesterol metabolism: implications on host physiology. *Frontiers in Physiology, 10*, 185.

Nagao-Kitamoto, H., Kitamoto, S., Kuffa, P., & Kamada, N. (2016). Pathogenic role of the gut microbiota in gastrointestinal diseases. *Intestinal research, 14*(2), 127.

Nair, D. V., & Kollanoor Johny, A. (2018). Characterizing the antimicrobial function of a dairy-originated probiotic, Propionibacterium freudenreichii, against multidrug-resistant Salmonella enterica serovar Heidelberg in turkey poults. *Frontiers in Microbiology, 9*, 1475.

Nami, Y., Haghshenas, B., Bakhshayesh, R. V., Jalaly, H. M., Lotfi, H., Eslami, S., & Hejazi, M. A. (2018). Novel autochthonous lactobacilli with probiotic aptitudes as a main starter culture for probiotic fermented milk. *LWT, 98*, 85–93. https://doi.org/10.1016/j.lwt.2018.08.035

Nami, Y., Vaseghi Bakhshayesh, R., Mohammadzadeh Jalaly, H., Lotfi, H., Eslami, S., & Hejazi, M. A. (2019). Probiotic properties of Enterococcus isolated from artisanal dairy products. *Frontiers in Microbiology, 10*, 300.

Odamaki, T., Sugahara, H., Yonezawa, S., Yaeshima, T., Iwatsuki, K., Tanabe, S., . . . Xiao, J.-z. (2012). Effect of the oral intake of yogurt containing Bifidobacterium longum BB536 on the cell numbers of enterotoxigenic Bacteroides fragilis in microbiota. *Anaerobe, 18*(1), 14–18.

Pandey, K. B., & Rizvi, S. I. (2009). Plant polyphenols as dietary antioxidants in human health and disease. *Oxidative medicine and cellular longevity, 2*(5), 270–278.

Park, Y.-H., Kim, J.-G., Shin, Y.-W., Kim, S.-H., & Whang, K.-Y. (2007). Effect of dietary inclusion of Lactobacillus acidophilus ATCC 43121 on cholesterol metabolism in rats. *Journal of Microbiology and Biotechnology, 17*(4), 655–662.

Pereira, D. I., & Gibson, G. R. (2002). Cholesterol assimilation by lactic acid bacteria and bifidobacteria isolated from the human gut. *Applied and Environmental Microbiology, 68*(9), 4689–4693.

Pigeon, R., Cuesta, E., & Gilliland, S. (2002). Binding of free bile acids by cells of yogurt starter culture bacteria. *Journal of Dairy Science, 85*(11), 2705–2710.

Pitsillides, L., Pellino, G., Tekkis, P., & Kontovounisios, C. (2021). The effect of perioperative administration of probiotics on colorectal cancer surgery outcomes. *Nutrients, 13*(5), 1451.

Ramos, C. L., Esteves, E. A., Prates, R. P., Moreno, L. G., & Santos, C. S. (2022). Probiotics in the prevention and management of cardiovascular diseases with focus on dyslipidemia. In Dwivedi, M. K., Amaresan, N., Sankaranarayanan, A., Kemp, H. E., (Eds.), *Probiotics in the prevention and management of human diseases* (pp. 337–351): Elsevier, Academic Press, USA.

Rodríguez-Nogales, A., Algieri, F., Garrido-Mesa, J., Vezza, T., Utrilla, M. P., Chueca, N., . . . . Gálvez, J. (2018). Intestinal anti-inflammatory effect of the probiotic Saccharomyces boulardii in DSS-induced colitis in mice: impact on microRNAs expression and gut microbiota composition. *The Journal of Nutritional Biochemistry, 61*, 129–139.

Rong, S., Hu, X., Zhao, S., Zhao, Y., Xiao, X., Bao, W., & Liu, L. (2017). Procyanidins extracted from the litchi pericarp ameliorate atherosclerosis in ApoE knockout mice: their effects on nitric oxide bioavailability and oxidative stress. *Food & Function, 8*(11), 4210–4216.

Ryma, T., Samer, A., Soufli, I., Rafa, H., & Touil-Boukoffa, C. (2021). Role of probiotics and their metabolites in inflammatory bowel diseases (IBDs). *Gastroenterology Insights, 12*(1), 56–66.

Sadeghi-Aliabadi, H., Mohammadi, F., Fazeli, H., & Mirlohi, M. (2014). Effects of Lactobacillus plantarum A7 with probiotic potential on colon cancer and normal cells proliferation in comparison with a commercial strain. *Iranian Journal of Basic Medical Sciences, 17*(10), 815.

Santos, A., San Mauro, M., Sanchez, A., Torres, J., & Marquina, D. (2003). The antimicrobial properties of different strains of Lactobacillus spp. isolated from kefir. *Systematic and applied Microbiology, 26*(3), 434–437.

Savaiano, D. A., & Hutkins, R. W. (2021). Yogurt, cultured fermented milk, and health: a systematic review. *Nutrition Reviews, 79*(5), 599–614.

Savard, P., Lamarche, B., Paradis, M.-E., Thiboutot, H., Laurin, É., & Roy, D. (2011). Impact of Bifidobacterium animalis subsp. lactis BB-12 and, Lactobacillus acidophilus LA-5-containing yoghurt, on fecal bacterial counts of healthy adults. *International Journal of Food Microbiology, 149*(1), 50–57.

Sayin, S. I., Wahlström, A., Felin, J., Jäntti, S., Marschall, H.-U., Bamberg, K., . . . Bäckhed, F. (2013). Gut microbiota regulates bile acid metabolism by reducing the levels of tauro-beta-muricholic acid, a naturally occurring FXR antagonist. *Cell Metabolism, 17*(2), 225–235.

Schmidt, T. S., Raes, J., & Bork, P. (2018). The human gut microbiome: from association to modulation. *Cell, 172*(6), 1198–1215.

Shabbir, U., Rubab, M., Daliri, E. B.-M., Chelliah, R., Javed, A., & Oh, D.-H. (2021). Curcumin, quercetin, catechins and metabolic diseases: the role of gut microbiota. *Nutrients, 13*(1), 206.

Shastri, M. D., Chong, W. C., Vemuri, R., Martoni, C. J., Adhikari, S., Bhullar, H., . . . Eri, R. D. (2020). Streptococcus thermophilus UASt-09 upregulates goblet cell activity in colonic epithelial cells to a greater degree than other probiotic strains. *Microorganisms, 8*(11), 1758.

Shehata, M. G., El-Sahn, M. A., El Sohaimy, S. A., & Youssef, M. M. (2019). In vitro assessment of hypocholesterolemic activity of Lactococcus lactis subsp. lactis. *Bulletin of the National Research Centre, 43*(1), 1–10.

Sheril, A., Lange, K., Amolo, T., Grinstead, J. S., Haakonsson, A. K., Szalowska, E., ... & Kersten, S. (2013). Short-chain fatty acids stimulate angiopoietin-like 4 synthesis in human colon adenocarcinoma cells by activating peroxisome proliferator-activated receptor γ. *Molecular and Cellular Biology, 33*(7), 1303–1316.

Shimizu, M., Hashiguchi, M., Shiga, T., Tamura, H.-o., & Mochizuki, M. (2015). Meta-analysis: effects of probiotic supplementation on lipid profiles in normal to mildly hypercholesterolemic individuals. *PloS One, 10*(10), e0139795.

Sidira, M., Galanis, A., Ypsilantis, P., Karapetsas, A., Progaki, Z., Simopoulos, C., & Kourkoutas, Y. (2010). Effect of probiotic-fermented milk administration on gastrointestinal survival of Lactobacillus casei ATCC 393 and modulation of intestinal microbial flora. *Microbial Physiology, 19*(4), 224–230.

Suganya, K., Son, T., Kim, K.-W., & Koo, B.-S. (2021). Impact of gut microbiota: how it could play roles beyond the digestive system on development of cardiovascular and renal diseases. *Microbial Pathogenesis, 152*, 104583.

Tamang, J. P., Shin, D.-H., Jung, S.-J., & Chae, S.-W. (2016). Functional properties of microorganisms in fermented foods. *Frontiers in Microbiology, 7*, 578.

Tao, J.-h., Duan, J.-a., Jiang, S., Qian, Y.-y., & Qian, D.-w. (2016). Biotransformation and metabolic profile of buddleoside with human intestinal microflora by ultrahigh-performance liquid chromatography coupled to hybrid linear ion trap/orbitrap mass spectrometer. *Journal of Chromatography B, 1025*, 7–15.

Tarrah, A., dos Santos Cruz, B. C., Sousa Dias, R., da Silva Duarte, V., Pakroo, S., Licursi de Oliveira, L., . . . Oliveira de Paula, S. (2021). Lactobacillus paracasei DTA81, a cholesterol-lowering strain having immunomodulatory activity, reveals gut microbiota regulation capability in BALB/c mice receiving high-fat diet. *Journal of Applied Microbiology, 131*(4), 1942–1957.

Thumu, S. C. R., & Halami, P. M. (2020). In vivo safety assessment of Lactobacillus fermentum strains, evaluation of their cholesterol-lowering ability and intestinal microbial modulation. *Journal of the Science of Food and Agriculture, 100*(2), 705–713.

Tremblay, A., & Panahi, S. (2017). Yogurt consumption as a signature of a healthy diet and lifestyle. *The Journal of Nutrition, 147*(7), 1476S–1480S.

Tsuji, H., Chonan, O., Suyama, Y., Kado, Y., Nomoto, K., Nanno, M., & Ishikawa, F. (2014). Maintenance of healthy intestinal microbiota in women who regularly consume probiotics. *International Journal of Probiotics & Prebiotics, 9*(1/2), 31.

Unno, T., Choi, J.-H., Hur, H.-G., Sadowsky, M. J., Ahn, Y.-T., Huh, C.-S., . . . Cha, C.-J. (2015). Changes in human gut microbiota influenced by probiotic fermented milk ingestion. *Journal of Dairy Science, 98*(6), 3568–3576.

Valdes, A. M., Walter, J., Segal, E., & Spector, T. D. (2018). Role of the gut microbiota in nutrition and health. *BMJ, 361*, 36–44

Vasiljevic, T., & Shah, N. P. (2008). Probiotics—from Metchnikoff to bioactives. *International Dairy Journal, 18*(7), 714–728.

Veiga, P., Pons, N., Agrawal, A., Oozeer, R., Guyonnet, D., Brazeilles, R., . . . Whorwell, P. J. (2014). Changes of the human gut microbiome induced by a fermented milk product. *Scientific Reports, 4*(1), 1–9.

Wang, C., Nagata, S., Asahara, T., Yuki, N., Matsuda, K., Tsuji, H., . . . Yamashiro, Y. (2015). Intestinal microbiota profiles of healthy pre-school and school-age children and effects of probiotic supplementation. *Annals of Nutrition and Metabolism, 67*(4), 257–266.

Wang, L., Guo, M.-J., Gao, Q., Yang, J.-F., Yang, L., Pang, X.-L., & Jiang, X.-J. (2018). The effects of probiotics on total cholesterol: a meta-analysis of randomized controlled trials. *Medicine, 97*(5).

Wang, Z., Roberts, A. B., Buffa, J. A., Levison, B. S., Zhu, W., Org, E., . . . Culley, M. K. (2015). Non-lethal inhibition of gut microbial trimethylamine production for the treatment of atherosclerosis. *Cell, 163*(7), 1585–1595.

West, N. P., Pyne, D. B., Cripps, A. W., Hopkins, W. G., Eskesen, D. C., Jairath, A., . . . Fricker, P. A. (2011). Lactobacillus fermentum (PCC®) supplementation and gastrointestinal and respiratory-tract illness symptoms: a randomised control trial in athletes. *Nutrition Journal, 10*(1), 1–11.

Xu, R.-y., Wan, Y.-p., Fang, Q.-y., Lu, W., & Cai, W. (2011). Supplementation with probiotics modifies gut flora and attenuates liver fat accumulation in rat nonalcoholic fatty liver disease model. *Journal of Clinical Biochemistry and Nutrition*, 1108190104–1108190104, 1–6.

Yadav, B. S., Yadav, A. K., Singh, S., Singh, N. K., & Mani, A. (2019). Methods in metagenomics and environmental biotechnology. In Gothandam, K. M., Ranjan, S., Dasgupta, N., Lichtfouse, E. (Eds.), *Nanoscience and biotechnology for environmental applications* (pp. 85–113): Springer.

Yang, Q., Liang, Q., Balakrishnan, B., Belobrajdic, D. P., Feng, Q. J., & Zhang, W. (2020). Role of dietary nutrients in the modulation of gut microbiota: a narrative review. *Nutrients, 12*(2), 381.

Yang, B., Ye, C., Yan, B., He, X., & Xing, K. (2019). Assessing the influence of dietary history on gut microbiota. *Current Microbiology, 76*(2), 237–247.

Yang, Y. J., & Sheu, B. S. (2012). Probiotics-containing yogurts suppress Helicobacter pylori load and modify immune response and intestinal microbiota in the Helicobacter pylori-infected children. *Helicobacter, 17*(4), 297–304.

Yılmaz, İ., Dolar, M. E., & Özpınar, H. (2019). Effect of administering kefir on the changes in fecal microbiota and symptoms of inflammatory bowel disease. a randomized controlled trial. *The Turkish Journal of Gastroenterology, 30*(3), 242.

Zanotti, I., Turroni, F., Piemontese, A., Mancabelli, L., Milani, C., Viappiani, A., . . . Elviri, L. (2015). Evidence for cholesterol-lowering activity by Bifidobacterium bifidum PRL2010 through gut microbiota modulation. *Applied Microbiology and Biotechnology, 99*(16), 6813–6829.

Zhou, X., Jin, M., Liu, L., Yu, Z., Lu, X., & Zhang, H. (2020). Trimethylamine N-oxide and cardiovascular outcomes in patients with chronic heart failure after myocardial infarction. *ESC Heart Failure, 7*(1), 189–194.

# 6 Dietary Modulation of the Gut Microbiota by Prebiotics and Other Dietary Nutrients and Relevant Health Effect(s)

*Alison Lacombe and Vivian C.H. Wu*
United States Department of Agriculture

## CONTENTS

## INTRODUCTION

A significant advancement in gastrointestinal microbiology realized the impact diet extends on health status and how gut constituent affects the host's health (David et al. 2014). Within the last 30 years, science has transitioned from viewing the gastrointestinal tract (GIT) as an inert tube to a flourishing ecosystem akin to vibrant and diverse dynamic communities in the Amazon rainforest. Similar to the deepest

DOI: 10.1201/b22970-8

recesses of planet Earth, little is known about the gut community and, more importantly, what inputs keep it thriving. This chapter focuses on the relationship between the gut microbiota, the host diet, and the resulting symbiotic relationship. Evidence accumulated by *in vitro* work and recent evidence from *in vivo* studies and human clinical trials collectively indicate that phytochemicals, fiber, and other nutrients demonstrate prebiotic capabilities (David et al. 2014). Parsing through the panoply of research requires a deep look into the chemical structure of prebiotics in the gut and the metabolic orchestration of the host gut microbiome.

Prebiotic compounds cannot be digested in the human stomach and small intestine and instead pass through to the large intestine. Prebiotics enrich a particular category of bacteria in the large intestine that is proven beneficial to gut health. While numerous bacteria provide health benefits to their host, the families of *Bifidobacteriaceae* and *Lactobacillaceae* specifically dominate the published research even though they merely comprise less than 0.01% of the intestinal microbiome. Before the 1960s, *Bifidobacteria* was known as *Lactobacillus bifidus* because it was observed to ferment carbohydrates into lactic acid. It was later discovered that *Bifidobacteria* employs a unique fructose-6-phosphate phosphoketolase pathway to ferment carbohydrates. This characteristic feature has allowed *Bifidobacteria* to dominate the scientific conversation around prebiotics. Advances in whole genome sequencing technology (see the previous chapters) challenge the conventional consensus of probiotic definition. However, this progress is impeded because many of these species cannot be cultured and subsequently enumerated and characterized outside their host.

## TYPES OF PREBIOTICS

As far back as 1921, several experiments described the enrichment of *Lactobacilli* in humans following the consumption of carbohydrates (Gibson et al. 2017). The first formal definition for prebiotics was established in 1995 as a "nondigestible food ingredient that beneficially affects the host by selectively stimulating the growth and activity of one or a limited number of bacteria already resident in the colon" (Cheplin and Rettger 2011). The definition of prebiotics has expanded over the years as advances in metagenomics and metabolomics have made it possible to take a clearer snapshot of the gastrointestinal environment (Gibson et al. 2017). Genomic technologies have expanded the definitions of nondigestible foods, beneficial bacteria, and the site of interaction (Gibson et al. 2017). This definition continues to evolve, and emerging evidence demonstrates that synergistic activities between microorganisms are not limited to the GIT and nondigestible carbohydrates (Gibson et al. 2017). Here, we will define prebiotics as a food source established to sustain microorganisms. The result is a symbiotic relationship with sustained benefits to the host. Here, we discuss the specific nutrients and microorganisms that support such a beneficial relationship.

The popularity of gut health in the wellness industry has allowed the rapid expansion of products that support beneficial microbes. Several products on the market of undefined composition claim prebiotic capabilities (Hume, Nicolucci, and Reimer 2017). Here, we approach the nondigestible food ingredients/metabolites with an evidence-based approach demonstrating stimulation of the growth and metabolism of beneficial gut microbes. Prebiotics must confer specific positive changes in gut microbial communities and preferentially stimulate the growth of beneficial gut microbes. In addition, prebiotics should be resistant to gastric acidity and mammalian digestive enzymes, allowing them to enter the colon intact.

## CARBOHYDRATE PREBIOTICS

The most common prebiotics with a strong basis of evidence are indigestible carbohydrates (i.e., dietary fiber, such as inulin and oligosaccharides) (Collins and Reid 2016). Although prebiotics are derived from digestible fiber, not all fiber types are prebiotics (Collins and Reid 2016). Bacteria differ in their carbohydrate processing capabilities, and most gut microbiota members selectively metabolize mono- and oligosaccharides. Complex polysaccharides often require multiple microorganisms with specialized enzymatic repertoires for complete digestion to utilizable energy units. Most commercially available prebiotic carbohydrates come from plants; however, emerging research on animals, algae, and bacteria provides promising alternatives (Gurpilhares et al. 2019).

Numerous food compounds are resistant to digestion and are used for fermentation by gut microflora. Saccharolytic fermentation occurs with nondigestible carbohydrates and favors the growth of some specific bacteria genera such as *Bifidobacterium* and *Lactobacillus*. These saccharolytic bacteria produce short-chain fatty acids (SCFA) in the colon, namely acetate, propionate, or butyrate, which contribute calories, absorbed by the gut, and extend the putative effect on systemic inflammation.

### Oligosaccharides

Oligosaccharides are relatively small chains ranging from three to ten simple saccharides, eliciting a variety of functions in cell biology and host immunity. Oligosaccharides are classified by their monosaccharide constituents and linkages to lipids (glycolipids) or amino acids (glycoproteins). Not all oligosaccharides occur as components of glycoproteins or glycolipids. Raffinose is a storage or transport carbohydrate in plants, and maltodextrins result from the microbial breakdown of larger polysaccharides such as starch or cellulose (Fernandes et al. 2017).

In this section, a particular focus is placed on specific examples of oligosaccharides particularly interested in those with a prebiotic function, namely fructooligosaccharides (FOS) and galactooligosaccharides (GOS). FOS elicit between 30% and 50% of the sweetness that sucrose confers. They are different from fructans and inulin, which can be precursors of oligosaccharides, and demonstrate a much higher degree of polymerization than that of FOS and GOS (Figure 6.1).

### Human Milk Oligosaccharides

Intestinal flora plays a crucial role in an infant's physiological postnatal GIT development (Fanaro et al. 2005). Several studies have demonstrated that the mode of delivery influences the infant's gut colonization flora (Fanaro et al. 2005). Maternal milk is arguably an essential source of oligosaccharides for humans since it is delivered during critical development. Human milk contains remarkably more oligosaccharides than bovines, 5.15 vs. 0.05 g/L, respectively. Oligosaccharides are an evolutionary boon to the infant that aids in establishing immunity. Many researchers attempt

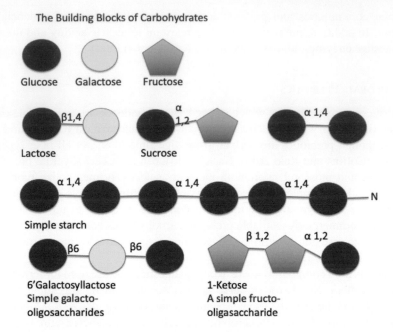

The Building Blocks of Carbohydrates

**FIGURE 6.1** Building blocks of oligosaccharides representing the combinations of simple sugars and glycosidic linkages found in natural products.

to formulate products enriched with human milk oligosaccharides (HMO) to reverse a dysbiotic system. Nevertheless, whether the application of HMO in the adult diet can shift the gastrointestinal microflora and if the shift can indeed produce beneficial downstream effects remains unclear.

For HMO to function as prebiotics, GOS and FOS must enter the colon intact and promote the growth of probiotics given that 10%–80% of the HMO is detected in the infant feces depending on the stage of infant development. These data suggest that the colonized microbiome can utilize more available substrates (Bode 2012) as the infant grows (Kelly 2009; Bode 2012). *In vitro* experiments have proven that both Bifidobacteria and Lactobacilli not merely survive but actually thrive on HMO. The relative abundance of HMO translates to 90% GOS and 10% FOS. Based on the existing data, it could be hypothesized that the 9/1 ratio is ideal for the growth of these bacteria and possibly exerts a symbiotic effect (Kelly 2009). Small *in vitro* pilot trials using the fecal flora obtained from breastfed infants produced the same SCFA profile as isolated HMO with a formula of 9/1 ratio GOS/FOS (Mahovic, Tenney, and Bartz 2007; Fanaro et al. 2005) (Figure 6.2). The results were significantly different from the data obtained from the control group comprised of infants fed a formula supplemented with 0.8 g maltodextrins as a placebo (Fanaro et al. 2005). More recently, it has been demonstrated that both ingredients of the prebiotic mixture are detectable in stools. The experimental data and the results obtained in formula-fed infants indicate that the FOS/GOS mixture can induce the development of an intestinal flora quite similar to that of breastfed infants. While these initial findings are promising, the therapeutic application of HMO still presents many challenges.

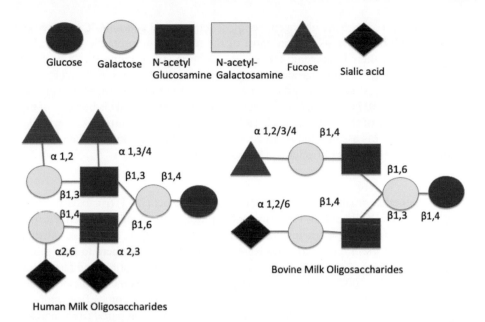

Glucose   Galactose   N-acetyl   N-acetyl-   Fucose   Sialic acid
                       Glucosamine Galactosamine

Human Milk Oligosaccharides

Bovine Milk Oligosaccharides

**FIGURE 6.2**   General structure of milk oligosaccharides and a comparison between human and bovine oligosaccharides.

The advancement of metabolomics and proteomics has allowed for the in-depth analysis of HMO constituents. The findings from these studies suggest that each mother's HMO composition constitutes a unique fingerprint rather than being something homogeneous across the population (Bode 2012; Azad et al. 2018). There are several maternal determinants of the final composition of human breast milk. Lifestyle, exercise, and health status are predictors of the relative abundance of fats, proteins, and oligosaccharides overall (Moossavi et al. 2019; Azad et al. 2018; Addison et al. 2019). However, the relative abundance of individual oligosaccharides is driven primarily by genetics. Principle coordinate analysis of 10,000 human milk samples taken from six continents shows two distinct clusters (Azad et al. 2018). The differences have been linked to a single nucleotide polymorphism (SNP) that encodes for an enzyme called fucosyltransferase II (fucII) that adds L-fucose to the oligosaccharide chain forming a specific α-1,2 linkage (Bode 2012). These SNPs map out geographically, as shown by genome-wide sequence analysis and transcriptomics. For example, 90% of Peruvian women have an active fucII, but that number goes down to 65% on the African continent (Kober, Zehe, and Bode 2013; Bode 2015). Several additional SNPs are associated with the formation of different HMO patterns, and more information can be found at the University of California, San Diego, MOMI Core Institute.

## Polysaccharides

Polysaccharides are heterogeneous macromolecules composed of monosaccharides linked by glycosidic linkages. Typical examples of biologically essential polysaccharides are starches (glucose polymers), a mixture of amylose and amylopectin, and the animal counterpart glycogen, cellulose, chitin, and pectin (O'Connor et al. 2017). As with the previous section, most of the research on prebiotic polysaccharides focuses on their bifidogenic effects. Research is still probing the "tip of the iceberg" regarding polysaccharides and gut microbiota. Not all polysaccharides enter the large intestine intact, but the ones that do tend to have bifidogenic effects (O'Connor et al. 2017). Our current understanding suggests that this is because of the "resistant" nature of the molecule itself and the enzymatic repertoire of bacteria like *Bifidobacteria*. This assumption is not corroborated in human models when investigating in depth the types of bacteria affected by dietary changes.

## Inulin

Inulin is a generic term that covers all linear fructans with beta (2–1) fructosyl-fructose glycosidic bonds (Kelly 2008). The beta configuration of the bonds between fructose monomers and inulin-type fructans resists enzymatic hydrolysis by human salivary constituents and small intestinal digestive enzymes allowing for them to pass to the large intestine intact. As a result, inulin-type fructans are indigestible and fermented in the colon (Kelly 2008). Inulin is present in over 3,000 vegetables and extensively present in plants. Commercially available natural inulin mostly comes from chicory root, dahlia, and Jerusalem artichoke, while synthetic inulin is prepared from sucrose. Inulin is commonly used in processed foods and as a nondigestible carbohydrate to replace sweeteners and is utilized in low-calorie foods (Shoaib et al. 2016).

Inulin stimulates the development and metabolic action of a limited number of bacteria in the colon, particularly *Bifidobacteria* and *Lactobacilli* (Kelly 2008). *In vitro* trials have demonstrated that colonic fermentation depends on inulin's chain length. Fermentation time is dependent on chain length, with longer chain inulin allowing for the initiation of bacterial fermentation in the distal part of the colon. The nutritional utilization of inulin and oligofructose provides a possible way to encourage microbial balance and overcome the difficulties in colonizing the gut mucosa. For this reason, inulin is used to reduce and replace sugar in food products. Inulin has been demonstrated to enhance the growth sustainability of *L. acidophilus*, *L. rhamnosus*, and *B. lactis* when added to milk, yogurt, and ice cream (Kelly 2009).

The consumption of inulin has demonstrated numerous benefits to the host digestive tract. Inulin has improved bowel movements, GI symptoms, quality of life, and increased fecal output in various adult populations (Watson et al. 2019). These shifts are generally attributed to the ability of inulin to reach the colon intact, where inulin is metabolized by bacteria, leading to beneficial byproducts. These improvements have generally been associated with modest changes in gut microbiota composition, specifically *Bifidobacteria*, *Anaerostipes*, and *Clostridium* in constipated subjects (Vandeputte et al. 2017). A recent randomized, double-blind, placebo-controlled cross-over trial with inulin isolated chicory root attempted to elucidate the relationship between diet, bowel movement, and colon microbiota. The study demonstrated that 10 g/d of inulin improved stool frequency and consistency in older adults who experience constipation (<1 bowel movement/day); however, they could not detect a shift in gut microbiota (Watson et al. 2019).

## NON-CARBOHYDRATE PREBIOTICS

Conventional dietary knowledge suggests that a diet high in plant material is beneficial for the host's gut microbiota. As discussed in previous chapters, numerous studies in humans have examined the dietary impact on gut microbiota composition and divided the population into two groups: those that eat fruits and vegetables over a certain level and those that do not. In addition, the relative abundance of one phylum of bacteria relative to another can predict the risk of obesity (Singh et al. 2017). The same phyla are also associated with the consumption of fruits and vegetables. The correlation between health status, diet, and gut composition is putatively linked to nondigestible carbohydrates. However, some ingredients are excluded when examining the relationship between certain foods and gut fermentation.

### POLYPHENOLS

Polyphenols represent a new category of potential prebiotics. Until recently, little was known about the metabolic fate of polyphenols in the intestinal tract. Berries have been used for centuries as elixirs to help with gastrointestinal symptoms. In humans, the intestinal absorption of dietary polyphenols is often slow and largely incomplete; up to 85% of anthocyanins enter the colon intact and can be used as substrates for microbial metabolism (Kahle et al. 2006). The capability for anaerobic digestion of berries in gastrointestinal environments is reflected by increased *Bifidobacteria* populations and other microbes that catabolize the diverse berry compounds available, especially polyphenols (Lacombe et al. 2013).

The use of berries for their prebiotic effect has been tested in clinical trials to improve the clinical picture and the well-being of patients. Promising beneficial effects demonstrated with berries include positive shifts in gut microbiota composition. *In vitro* human fecal batch cultures have demonstrated the enrichment of *Lactobacillus* and *Bifidobacteria* with 1 g/L of gallic acid and 200 mg/L of anthocyanins (Håkansson et al. 2009). These results demonstrate the benefits of dietary enrichment of berries and its impact on bacterial communities with unique functional repertoires by promoting their growth in competitive environments.

Bioprotective effects of polyphenols and other nutrients observed *in vitro* are not entirely transferable to health effects observed *in vivo*; therefore, it is essential to use *in vivo* models to understand mechanisms. Recent studies using the Sprague Dawley (SD) rat model, fed polyphenols extracted from blueberry and blackberry via gavage, demonstrated increased *Lactobacillus* and *Bifidobacteria* (Bò et al. 2009; Vendrame et al. 2013). Actinobacteria, with known impacts on human health, namely *Slackia*, *Bifidobacteria*, and *Coriobacteriaceae* spp, were detected in higher abundance in SD rats fed a blueberry-enriched diet (Lacombe et al. 2013, 2012). In humans, dietary treatment with blueberry increased the population of *Bifidobacteria* more than two-fold, demonstrating the prebiotic activity of berry polyphenols (Vendrame et al. 2013). For clinicians, these findings are significant due to the growing interest in probiotic bacteria and the perceived benefit of increasing their numbers in the GIT to attain their health benefits.

## SHORT-CHAIN FATTY ACIDS

Additional metabolic byproducts created by probiotic bacteria such as *Bifidobacteria* and *Lactobacillus* are discussed below. We specifically look into the saccharolytic and proteolytic byproducts of probiotics such as *Bifidobacteria* and lactic acid–producing bacteria whereby small-chain fatty acids (SCFAs) such as butyrate, acetate, and propionate are produced (Younes et al. 2001). Downstream effects of SCFAs are utilized as energy sources by host epithelial cells, modulate intestinal immunity, enhance barrier function, and inhibit the adhesion of pathogenic bacteria (Younes et al. 2001).

# METABOLISM OF NUTRIENTS BY THE GUT MICROBIOTA

The microbial role in the metabolism of ingested bioactive compounds is not well understood. However, recent evidence suggests that bacterial metabolism has a substantial potential for the bioactivation of essential nutrients and detoxification (Lacombe et al. 2013, 2012). The microbial enzymatic biotransformations may also be relevant for converting many classes of compounds, including flavonoids, isoflavonoids, lignans, phenolic acids, fiber, and tannins (Kahle et al. 2006; Heinonen 2007). Cleavage of the glucosidic bond in the anthocyanin structure is proposed as the first step in bacterial anthocyanin bioconversion, involving β-glucosidase activity (Bò et al. 2009; Pap et al. 2021). New metabolites, including gallic, syringic, and homogentisic acids appeared due to bacterial enzymatic action on malvidin, some of which have been described as more bioavailable and bioactive than the former original molecule (Wu et al. 2004). In addition, recent studies documented a 20% increase in xenobiotic degradation and a two-fold increase in benzoate degradation in the proximal colon of rats fed an 8% blueberry diet (Lacombe et al. 2013). The genome sequence of *Bifidobacterium longum* encodes a large number of predicted proteins (more than 8%) related to the catabolism of nondigestible plant polymers, including enzymes involved in the degradation of complex polysaccharides and xenobiotics (Gill et al. 2006; Claus et al. 2011). In termite hind guts, members of the phylum Actinobacteria have demonstrated their involvement in xenobiotic metabolism (Claus et al. 2011). These microorganisms could contribute to the degradation of benzoate compounds derived from berries. Therefore, the protective anti-inflammatory effect of blueberries may be credited with positive shifts in the composition of the microbiota and concomitant regulation of microbial metabolism (Del Bo' et al. 2010). The downstream effects of a berry-enriched diet are demonstrated by increased plasma antioxidant capacity while protecting the lymphocytes against oxidative DNA damage and lower vascular reactivity and sensitivity to an α-adrenergic agonist in the aorta of SD rats (Vendrame et al. 2011).

## EFFECT OF PREBIOTIC ON IMMUNITY

Prebiotics can improve immune function by increasing the population of beneficial bacteria. Irritable bowel syndrome (IBS) and Crohn's disease (CD) are the most common causes of GIT stress and are directly associated with the nervous system, mucosal barrier, neurotransmitters, hormones, and immune system (Menezes and Da Silva

2017). Interaction of prebiotics with pattern recognition receptor attributes to altering the expression of cytokines. The mechanism of immunomodulation by prebiotics influences pro-inflammatory cytokines, interferons (IFN-γ), and interleukin-2 (IL-2) in the gut lumen (Cavaglieri et al. 2003; Khangwal and Shukla 2019). Prebiotics found in mushrooms such as proteoglycans and polysaccharides are renowned for their antitumor activity (Danneskiold-Samsøe et al. 2019). The available glucans and heteroglycans in mushrooms can activate macrophages, splenocytes, and thymocytes (İspirli, Demirbaş, and Dertli 2018).

What we learn from the infant/mother relationship is essential for application in the adult community. Inflammatory bowel diseases are increasing in the United States' adult population including a significant dietary component (Bode 2009). Macrophages play a significant role in the inflammatory process of ulcerative colitis and CD (Bode 2009). In cell models, HMO and macrophage combined, we see a significant reduction in the inflammatory marker, interleukin-6 (IL-6) (Manthey et al. 2014). When looking at the structure–function relationship between HMO and reduction of IL-6, 3 sialyllactose (3-SL) demonstrates the most significant effect (Bode 2018); however, determining the active binding site is very difficult. RNA-seq studies demonstrated that the lipopolysaccharide-binding site, toll-like receptor 4 (TRL-4), and the sialic acid-binding site lectin are not the target for 3-SL (Manthey et al. 2014). While the receptor for 3-SL is still unknown, the RNA-seq data demonstrate that 90% of genes induced in the presence of 3-SL are involved in lipid metabolism (Manthey et al. 2014). These are the same pathways involved in resolving the inflammatory process in the cell. Even though TRL-4 is not the receptor binding site, HMO acts as an intermediary, switching off the macrophage recruitment significantly faster (Manthey et al. 2014). This has significant implications for other autoimmune diseases as well. Data from cell and rat models suggest that HMO can diminish the progression and symptoms of rheumatoid arthritis using a similar mechanism (Bode and Jantscher-Krenn 2012).

Prebiotics can stimulate the immune response by altering the inflammatory cytokine cascade and decreasing the accumulation of disease-causing pathogens. Various studies on animals and humans have demonstrated that prebiotics inhibit pathogens by enhancing the *Lactobacillus* and *Bifidobacteria* population (Looijer-van Langen and Dieleman 2009). Prebiotic monomers of mannose adhere to the intestinal tract and diminish the infections by *Salmonella* (Revolledo, Ferreira, and Ferreira 2009). In addition, mannose binds to the virulence factor type 1 fimbriae and inhibits the infection (Revolledo, Ferreira, and Ferreira 2009). A study with Wistar rats demonstrated that the inulin as a potential prebiotic, as it increased the population of *Bifidobacterium* and *Lactobacillus* spp., activates toll-like receptors (TLRs) such as TLR-2, TLR-5, and TLR-7, which ultimately improve the immunity (Revolledo, Ferreira, and Ferreira 2009). A mixture of oligofructose and inulin and FOS alone could improve antibody response against viral infections such as influenza and measles (Langkamp-Henken et al. 2004). Apart from this, a supplement of prebiotics reduced the usage of antibiotics and prevented the incidence of febrile seizures in infants (Saavedra and Tschernia 2022). Fructans stimulate the serum IL-4, CD282+/TLR-2+ myeloid dendritic cells, and TLR-2 (Saavedra and Tschernia 2022) and decrease the IL-6 and phagocytosis in monocytes and granulocytes in healthy volunteers (Guigoz et al. 2002). Notably, infants supplemented with FOS have shown a reduced risk of immune diseases (Moro et al. 2006). GOS improves the activity of natural killer cells by increasing the IL-8, IL-10, and C-reactive protein (Vulevic et al. 2013, 2015). It has also been reported to prevent the risks of atopic dermatitis and eczema (Moro et al. 2006).

Necrotizing enterocolitis (NEC) is a severe gastrointestinal necrosis condition in premature neonates. It is one of the most common and often fatal intestinal disorders in preterm infants. Clinical trials have demonstrated a high correlation between HMO in breast milk and positive outcome measures in NEC progression (Bode 2015; Autran et al. 2018). As previously discussed, HMOs have a bifidogenic effect in the gut and protect neonates from NEC and pathogenic bacterial infection (Knol et al. 2005). However, increased levels of bifidogenic oligosaccharides outcompeting pathogens do not entirely describe HMOs' beneficial effects on NEC (Bode 2015). A randomized study revealed that FOS and GOS enhance the population of *Bifidobacteria* but had no significant consequence in controlling the progression of NEC (Srinivasjois, Rao, & Patole, 2009). Research on HMOs has demonstrated improved immunity benefits similar to breastfed infants (Bode 2015). Preclinical research also shows that HMOs reduce intestinal discomfort, reduce food allergy symptoms, and enhance cognition, leading to myriad health benefits for infants (Autran et al. 2018). The link between HMO and necrotizing colitis is associated with competitive binding within the intestinal glycocalyx (Bode 2015). For pathogens to survive in the gut, they must attach to epithelial cells; otherwise, they will be eliminated through excretion. This process occurs through bacterial lectins attaching to glycans on the surface of epithelial cells. In the case of necrotizing colitis, there is a specific oligosaccharide called disialyllacto-N-tetraose (DSLNT), which is associated with protective effects in mouse models (Bode 2006). A human cohort study with preterm infants demonstrated that necrotizing colitis was lower in infants who received higher amounts of DSLNT from their mothers (Bode 2006). DSLNT content in breast milk is a potential noninvasive marker to identify infants at risk of developing NEC and screen high-risk donor milk. In addition, DSLNT could serve as a natural template to develop novel therapeutics against this devastating disorder. This association is significant to note when considering therapeutic applications of HMO in infant formula (Autran et al. 2018).

## PREBIOTICS AS FUNCTIONAL FOODS

Consumers are aware of the potential healing properties of dietary regimens and foods and have fueled the demand for products that promote health. The desire for food that meets nutritional needs and can improve health has led food scientists to develop the concept of functional foods. A formal definition of functional foods was determined by the European Commission Concerted Action on Functional Food Science, which states, "A food can be regarded as 'functional' if it is satisfactorily demonstrated to affect beneficially one or more target functions in the body, beyond adequate nutritional effects, in a way that is relevant to either an improved state of health and well-being and reduction of risk of disease" (Wang et al. 2020b; Bigliardi and Galati 2013). The definition of functional foods can be expanded to include improving general body conditions, reducing the risk of specific diseases, and potential use for the prevention and treatment of illnesses (Bigliardi and Galati 2013). Functional foods differentiate themselves from conventional foods consumed in a standard diet by containing bioactive components whose physiological activity is scientifically proven (Bigliardi and Galati 2013). Categories of functional foods include those that naturally contain one of the bioactive components, fortified foods in which the native bioactive level is enhanced, and processed foods in which the bioactive compound is intentionally added (Bigliardi and Galati 2013).

A typical Western diet contains moderate levels of prebiotics through consuming various fruits and vegetables. However, the number of prebiotics contained in many fruits and vegetables is not sufficient or not consumed in an amount that would significantly alter the composition of intestinal microflora (Jovanovic-Malinovska, Kuzmanova, and Winkelhausen 2014). Therefore, consumers look toward supplementation to increase the effective dose of many prebiotics. This affects the putative mechanism of action by altering the relative abundance of specific nondigestible components in the diet. The mechanism by which prebiotics can attenuate the progression of diseases is of great interest to researchers and clinicians.

Fiber supplementation is one of the most common applications for prebiotics in the Western diet. Most (90%) of the US population does not consume 15 g/d of recommended dietary fiber doses. Many consumers turn to fiber supplements, typically isolated from a single food source (McRorie et al. 2015). However, of the fiber supplements on the market today, only a minority possess the physical characteristics that underlie the mechanisms driving clinically meaningful health benefits. Prebiotics are clinically accepted and recommended as dietary supplements for the treatment of constipation. These carbohydrates and prebiotics are fermented in the large intestine and diminish the transport time of assimilated food by hydrating and increasing acid production (Den Hond, Geypens, and Ghoos 2000). Intestinal-associated diseases like IBS and CD are also thought to benefit from these fermentative processes.

Many prebiotic functional food formulations try to take advantage of the inherent presence of probiotics in the food product. Dairy foods are a popular probiotic food category worldwide and intrinsically contain nutrients that maintain the probiotic organism. Examples of popular probiotic functional foods are yogurt, which represents about 35% of sales overall, followed by cultured drinks, kefir, cheese, ice cream, and infant formula (Tamime et al. 2006; Saavedra and Tschernia 2022). Fermented products, such as yogurt, kefir, and cheese are commonly enhanced probiotic cultures, and more recently, unfermented dairy matrices, such as ice cream and butter, have also been enhanced with probiotic cultures (Koebnick et al. 2003).

Whey protein, which is rich in nutrients and potential prebiotics, has been fortified with probiotics (Tenorio et al. 2010; Suomalainen et al. 2006). The functional use of whey, a byproduct of cheesemaking that is often discarded, has been a focus of functional food development (Tenorio et al. 2010). The commercially available oligosaccharides are usually derived from cow milk, plants, and fermented processes and are very different structurally from what is found in HMO (Bode 2015). Commercial GOS and FOS tend to be linear carbohydrate chains (Vulevic et al. 2013). However, little is known about oligosaccharides' structure–function relationship regarding therapeutic applications (Vulevic et al. 2015).

Current knowledge stems from associated genetic differences from cohort studies and cell/animal models observed within populations. For example, we now know that HMO is not just a preferential food source for *Bifidobacteria* but have antimicrobial properties and can outcompete other bacteria for binding site in the intestinal tract and directly modulate epithelial cell responses (Bode 2015). Applying HMO formulation in the adult population is much more complicated than in infants. Although there are many products on the market that claim they can provide increased gut function, they do not take into account the diversity of HMO (Bode 2015). Adults are not blank slates when it comes to gut microbiota composition, which means its alteration is much more difficult. In addition, diet and lifestyle are very heterogoneous among humans, generating many variations in the human datasets (Bode 2015). This variation makes causal relationships between the structure/function of HMO and the gut microbiota challenging to establish.

Many consumers have allergies to milk proteins, lactose intolerance, and may have adopted diet choices that partially or entirely exclude food of animal origin. In response to the increased market for dairy products of nonanimal origin, plant-based probiotic/prebiotic products are available to consumers. Many raw materials of plant origin often contain prebiotic substances, which can stimulate the growth of probiotic microorganisms both during the processing steps and during storage (Veereman 2007; İspirli, Demirbaş, and Dertli 2018). The use of nuts and grains, such as almonds, rice, and oats, has been widely adopted as animal milk as these products are generally perceived as healthy by the consumer and have an appealing sensory profile (Håkansson et al. 2009; Vulevic et al. 2015). These foods contain additional functional benefits, such as fibers, vitamins, minerals, flavonoids, and antioxidants. Enrichment with probiotic cultures is carried out through osmotic dehydration or vacuum impregnation techniques or by directly adding the microbial cells to juices. A fermentation step may occur in the latter case, creating additional bioactive nutrients.

## NOVEL PREBIOTIC FORMULATIONS

Numerous novel prebiotic formulations are abundantly found in food-processing and agricultural byproducts. The sources of potential prebiotics vary from the agricultural silage from wheat, mushroom, and seaweed products to animal products like dairy effluents (Shoaib et al. 2016; Scott et al. 2011; Danneskiold-Samsøe et al. 2019). Often, disposal of these byproducts confers negative impacts on the ecosystem by burdening the waste stream. Therefore, food-processing byproducts that contain high nutritive values can be used as the primary source of functional or nutraceutical ingredients in a process whereby nutritional valorization of these products is achieved. Manufacturers of prebiotics are shifting the utilization of their raw materials to lower-cost alternative sources. Prominent raw materials or substrates to produce prebiotics are roots of chicory and Jerusalem artichoke and lactose from the agriculture and dairy industries, respectively. However, due to high demand, the cost of these raw materials is exponentially increasing every year. Therefore, various byproducts derived from food processing, including agricultural-based silage, are being developed.

There is a burgeoning market for prebiotic formulations incorporated into various foods such as dairy products, bread, cereals, dietary supplements, and others. For example, soybean whey, a byproduct of tofu manufacturing, contains nondigestible polysaccharides and oligosaccharides. Usually, this product is discarded, but soybean whey may be used as a valuable ingredient in functional foods (Tenorio et al. 2010). The solid wastes that are accumulated in malting industries—namely barley husks, spent grains, and grain fragments—contain oligosaccharides and can be fermented to generate succinate, lactate, formate, acetate, propionate, and butyrate, exhibiting prebiotic potential (Gullón et al. 2021). Wang, Liang, and Liang (2010) studied that mung beans may enhance the growth of *Lactobacillus paracasei*. Gullón, González-Muñoz, and Parajó (2011b) investigated the prebiotic potential of FOS-rich refined product from apple pomace, processed by simultaneous saccharification and solid-state fermentation.

Combining prebiotics and probiotics in the same functional food may present a synergistic effect. The popularity of dairy products fortified with prebiotics and probiotics is also motivated by consumer demand for appropriate texture and flavor. The sensory profile of drinkable yogurts made with prebiotics, namely soluble corn fiber, polydextrose, and chicory inulin, is an acceptable vehicle to deliver the probiotics. Ice cream supplemented with *Lactobacillus casei* and 2.5% inulin demonstrated improved nutritional and sensory properties (Di Criscio et al. 2010). Different dehydrated prebiotic fibers, namely, oat bran, β-glucan, and green banana flour, provided the substratum for adherence, and trehalose acted as a cell protectant prolonging the viability of *L. casei* (Di Criscio et al. 2010). In a sensory evaluation study, the prebiotic oat bran added to a dairy fruit beverage has been well accepted by consumers (Guergoletto et al. 2010). Apple purees enriched with two commercial FOS prebiotics [Beneo GR® (inulin) and HSI®] showed stability for 30-day storage at 4°C (Keenan et al. 2011). However, a large quantity of prebiotics was required to deliver the desired effect, and high hydrostatic pressure posed the risk of certain prebiotic hydrolysis.

## FOOD-PROCESSING EFFECTS ON PROBIOTICS AND PREBIOTICS

Consumers are becoming increasingly health-conscious, leading to consumer demand emphasizing functional foods. The shift of consumer preferences, needs, and acceptances is a dynamic process; hence, the maintenance of food quality via technological innovation is evidently important (Danneskiold-Samsøe et al. 2019). The development of prebiotic food formulations is crucial for the future functional food market. Therefore, there are constant concerns about recovering and maintaining healthy intestines stocked with prebiotic nutrients that support the survival of beneficial health agents. Understanding the molecular details of gut microorganism metabolism of dietary ingredients is essential for creating prebiotic and probiotic formulations that benefit consumers. There is a limited number of quantification methods that analyze complex oligosaccharides and other prebiotic molecules. This had hindered the understanding of probiotic interactions with prebiotics.

In most cases, viable probiotic microorganisms are necessary to deliver the purported health benefits to the host gut. The industry for microbial viability must be high to overcome the hurdles of cellular deterioration over time and adverse conditions of the host gut. Intrinsic features of the food matrix can strongly endanger their viability in food, processing treatments applied, competitive background flora, conditions, and duration of storage. Probiotic microorganisms are relatively sensitive compared to some spoilage microorganisms, and the number of viable bacteria can decrease by 1–2 log CFU (colony-forming unit)/g or even more during production and storage. Minimum values of at least $10^6$–$10^7$ CFU/g are needed for residency in the gut; therefore, the microbial dose in the original product needs to be $10^8$–$10^9$ probiotic cells (Jayamanne and Adams 2006). Since the health effects depend on the conditions of the product at the time of consumption, the maintenance of microbial viability must be ensured over its entire shelf-life.

## FACTORS THAT INFLUENCE PROBIOTIC VIABILITY

The carrier matrix has a significant effect on the quality of probiotic products, as its composition and characteristics can alter the viability and effectiveness of probiotics. One of the main obstacles is represented by the acid pH since *Lactobacilli* have an optimal growth pH of 5.5–6.0 and *Bifidobacteria* of 6.0–7.0 (De Vuyst, 2000). Acidic pH, which is relevant for fermented foods, fruit, and vegetables, leads to an increase in the concentration of organic acids in the undissociated form, therefore increasing the antimicrobial effect of these acids. Furthermore, at low pH values (below 4.5), cells need significant energy to keep the intracellular pH constant, seizing adenosine triphosphate from other cellular needs, causing cell death. Low pH (approx. 3.5) was shown to be the main culprit in the loss of viability of *L. rhamnosus*, *L. plantarum*, and *L. casei* in cherry juice, especially during refrigerated storage (Nematollahi et al. 2016). In fermented milk, *L. acidophilus* tolerates acid conditions better than *Bifidobacteria*, proving the careful selection of the strains used in each probiotic food to be crucial (Tamime et al. 2006).

Water content in food formulations, whether expressed as moisture content or water activity ($a_w$), plays a determining role in the survival of probiotics in food. The $a_w$, i.e., the availability of water for microbial growth, varies based on the product's intended shelf. If a food product has a water activity range above 0.85, it will have to be refrigerated or use another barrier to control pathogen growth (Gomand et al. 2019). At $a_w$ above 0.85, there is a substantial loss of prebiotic viability as other spoilage microorganisms compete for nutrients. In contrast, a food product with a water activity between 0.60 and 0.85 will not require refrigeration but will have a limited shelf-life due to yeasts and molds. Lastly, food with a water activity below 0.60 will have an extended shelf-life, even without refrigeration. With probiotic formulations, food manufacturers can employ several tactics, including drying, freezing, or adding solutes like salt or sugar, helping to reduce their products' water activity levels, extending their shelf-life.

There is a potential benefit to adding probiotics to low moisture or intermediate moisture foods, such as chocolate, peanut butter, cereals, and dried fruit paste because they are stable for prolonged periods (Finn et al. 2013). For example, a viability loss of less than 1 log CFU/g of *L. rhamnosus* was observed in peanut butter ($a_w$ approx. 0.35) stored at 25°C for 27 weeks (Klu et al. 2012). In addition, osmolarity in foods containing high amounts of sugar or salt, such as fruit purees, jams, or aged cheeses, plays a role in the survival of microorganisms in foods. Generally, sugar and salt greatly influence the growth and survival of probiotics in food as their presence increases osmotic pressure. Salt is widely used in foods to prolong its shelf-life, but at high concentrations (~4%–6%), it can put the viability of probiotics at risk. The tolerance to osmotic stress is strain-specific and depends on the phospholipidic composition of the membrane. *Lactobacillus casei* demonstrated slower growth in the presence of high glucose concentrations, as well as *Bifidobacteria*, while *L. plantarum* demonstrated more resistance to osmotic stress (Homayouni et al. 2008).

Since most probiotic species are strictly anaerobic, dissolved oxygen in the matrix is critical for their survival in foods, as hydrogen peroxide is formed through different mechanisms both at intracellular and extracellular levels. Probiotic bacteria are practically devoid of an oxygen scavenging system, which causes the reduction of oxygen to hydrogen peroxide. The toxicity of hydrogen peroxide is due to its ability to block fructose-6-phosphofructoketolase, a key enzyme for sugar metabolism. In addition, superoxide and hydroxyl radicals are formed in dissolved oxygen due to the oxidation of membrane lipids in the cell, which induces DNA damage and causes cell death (Önneby et al. 2013). Different processing steps can contribute to the enrichment of the matrix in dissolved oxygen, such as homogenization, cooling after heat treatment, and mixing with ingredients. Although all probiotics are anaerobic, oxygen tolerance varies enormously between genera and species. Indeed, *Bifidobacteria* tend to be more sensitive than lactic acid bacteria. In the presence of oxygen, the most sensitive bacteria change the profile of membrane fatty acids and show an elongation of the lag phase and a substantial reduction in lactate produced (Looijer-van Langen and Dieleman 2009; Patel and Denning 2013).

Probiotic microorganisms can be exposed to thermal stress when producing food-containing probiotics. When heat treatments are used to inactivate pathogenic and spoiler microorganisms in raw materials, thermal stress on probiotics can be easily avoided by inoculating them downstream of the heat treatment or by using probiotic species other than lactic acid bacteria and *Bifidobacteria*. The genus *Bacillus coagulans* has been successfully used in the processing of various foods such as banana muffins and waffles, brewed coffee, chocolate fudge frosting, and hot fudge topping, and the loss of viability has been less than 1 log CFU/g in all cases (Majeed et al. 2016). However, during fermentation, probiotics may undergo thermal stress. The production of yogurt often requires that the milk is held at temperatures above 40°C–42°C, which can be harmful to probiotics. Therefore, the industry has curated cultivars of probiotics more resistant to thermal treatment. In yogurt making, the incubation temperature can be as high as 44°C, which causes a loss in viability of *L. acidophilus* and *Bifidobacterium* BB-12. At higher fermentation temperatures (e.g., 45°C), more heat-resistant *L. brueckii* subsp. *bulgaricus* becomes the dominant species and produces a large amount of lactic acid, hydrogen peroxide, and sometimes bacteriocins, which causes probiotic growth to stop (Nematollahi et al. 2016). Therefore, to foster the biodiversity of probiotics, some manufacturers inoculate species after the fermentation process.

Freezing is a critical process in the manufacture of ice cream. However, it presents a technical challenge in the development of probiotic-enhancing products. Subzero temperatures are detrimental to microbial viability because as the portion of frozen water increases, the $a_w$ value of the liquid solution decreases. Furthermore, osmotic pressure increases as water diffuses outside the cell, dehydrates, and freezes the extracellular water. The mechanical stress due to ice crystals damages the membranes, the low temperatures shock the cells, the (harmful) solutes concentrate, and the cells become dehydrated. Together with the progressive lowering of the temperature, all this determines the so-called cold shock, which causes cell death. In probiotic ice cream, *L. rhamnosus* loses viability during freezing of about 1.8 log CFU/g, probably due to a combined effect of temperature lowering and oxygen incorporation during mixing (Marino et al. 2017).

Developers of enhanced probiotic products attempt to harness the intrinsic protective substances that protect the viability of probiotics from the stresses accumulated in the food matrix and during the production process and the GIT transit. The compounds most frequently used for this purpose are carbohydrates, and many have additional prebiotic effects. Sugars, especially those with low molecular weight, interact with the polar heads in the cell membranes, replacing the water molecules and stabilizing the membranes themselves during osmotic stresses. Low-molecular-weight sugars, such as trehalose, sucrose, and lactulose, can improve the survival of probiotics during freezing, dehydration, and storage both in products of animal and plant origin (Betoret et al. 2017). Besides, they have also been shown to have direct functional activities, such as a bifidogenic effect and an increase in the hydrophobicity of the surface of probiotic cells, which is related to the ability to adhere to and interact with the intestinal wall (Dlamini et al. 2019).

Even the most complex polysaccharides and fibers can improve the viability of probiotics in food. These are dietary compounds that reach the gut in an undigested form and are selectively fermented by the intestinal microbiota, thus stimulating their growth and activity. However, their stimulation activity also aids the probiotics added to foods. Consequently, the development of functional foods that contain both probiotics and prebiotics (symbiotic foods) can provide a double physiological advantage. Typically, prebiotic substances mainly come from plant food sources. Inulin and FOS, widely used for this purpose, are commonly extracted from onions, bananas, wheat, artichokes, garlic, and other whole foods. Other widely used oligosaccharides, such as GOS and HMO, are of animal origin (Anadón, Martínez-Larrañaga, Arés, & Martínez, 2016).

Even microorganisms are capable of producing extracellular substances that act as prebiotics, such as exopolysaccharide (İspirli, Demirbaş, and Dertli 2018). The effectiveness of prebiotics in the context of functional probiotic foods is linked to the fact that these substances can be metabolized and used as a source of energy by probiotics. Furthermore, owing to their physicochemical characteristics, they can effectively protect cell envelopes, increase the glass transition temperatures in the aqueous phase, retain water, and prevent the formation of ice crystals that may cause mechanical damage to the cells themselves (Tymczyszyn et al. 2011). Due to these activities, the effects essentially protect probiotics against acidity, high temperatures, and dehydration. Their addition to food improves the stability of probiotics during processing, storage, and *in vitro* digestion. In the blended carrot and orange juices, the presence of 2% inulin improved the survival of *L. plantarum* during storage for 30 days at 4°C and during *in vitro* digestion, and a mixture of inulin, FOS, and GOS had a similar effect on *L. casei* in a blended red fruit beverage (Bernal-Castro, Díaz-Moreno, and Gutiérrez-Cortés 2019).

## CONCLUSION

As the concept of prebiotics continues to evolve, researchers investigate the potential benefits of their ingestion. There are many possible sources for prebiotics, which can be found in the natural environment or be synthesized based on research indicating certain functional groups with benefits. However, more work is needed to determine which prebiotic regimen is best for dietary recommendations, while recommendations cannot probably be applied ubiquitously across the population. The future of prebiotic supplementations may rely upon the intended hosts existing microbiome and genetic profile. This opens a fascinating field of inquiry into tailoring probiotic and prebiotic regimens for optimum health.

## REFERENCES

Addison, Ruth, Lauren Hill, Lars Bode, Bianca Robertson, Biswa Choudhury, David Young, Charlotte Wright, Clare Relton, Ada L. Garcia, and David M. Tappin. 2019. "Development of a Biochemical Marker to Detect Current Breast Milk Intake." *Maternal and Child Nutrition*, no. April 2019: 1–8. https://doi.org/10.1111/mcn.12859.

Autran, Chloe A., Benjamin P. Kellman, Jae H. Kim, Elizabeth Asztalos, Arlin B. Blood, Erin C. Hamilton Spence, Aloka L. Patel, Jiayi Hou, Nathan E. Lewis, and Lars Bode. 2018. "Human Milk Oligosaccharide Composition Predicts Risk of Necrotising Enterocolitis in Preterm Infants." *Gut* 67 (6): 1064–70. https://doi.org/10.1136/GUTJNL-2016-312819.

Azad, Meghan B., Bianca Robertson, Faisal Atakora, Allan B. Becker, Padmaja Subbarao, Theo J. Moraes, Piushkumar J. Mandhane, et al. 2018. "Human Milk Oligosaccharide Concentrations Are Associated with Multiple Fixed and Modifiable Maternal Characteristics, Environmental Factors, and Feeding Practices." *Journal of Nutrition* 148 (11): 1733–42. https://doi.org/10.1093/jn/nxy175.

Bernal-Castro, Camila Andrea, Consuelo Díaz-Moreno, and Carolina Gutiérrez-Cortés. 2019. "Inclusion of Prebiotics on the Viability of a Commercial Lactobacillus Casei Subsp. Rhamnosus Culture in a Tropical Fruit Beverage." *Journal of Food Science and Technology* 56 (2): 987. https://doi.org/10.1007/S13197-018-03565-W.

Betoret, E., L. Calabuig-Jiménez, F. Patrignani, R. Lanciotti, and M. Dalla Rosa. 2017. "Effect of High Pressure Processing and Trehalose Addition on Functional Properties of Mandarin Juice Enriched with Probiotic Microorganisms." *LWT – Food Science and Technology* 85 (November): 418–22. https://doi.org/10.1016/J.LWT.2016.10.036.

Bigliardi, Barbara, and Francesco Galati. 2013. "Innovation Trends in the Food Industry: The Case of Functional Foods." *Trends in Food Science and Technology* 31 (2): 118–29. https://doi.org/10.1016/J.TIFS.2013.03.006.

Bode, Lars. 2006. "Recent Advances on Structure, Metabolism, and Function of Human Milk Oligosaccharides." *The Journal of Nutrition*. https://doi.org/10.1093/jn/136.8.2127.

———. 2009. "Human Milk Oligosaccharides: Prebiotics and Beyond." *Nutrition Reviews*. https://doi.org/10.1111/j.1753-4887.2009.00239.x.

———. 2012. "Human Milk Oligosaccharides: Every Baby Needs a Sugar Mama." *Glycobiology* 22 (9): 1147–62. https://doi.org/10.1093/glycob/cws074.

———. 2015. "The Functional Biology of Human Milk Oligosaccharides." *Early Human Development*. https://doi.org/10.1016/j.earlhumdev.2015.09.001.

———. 2018. "Human Milk Oligosaccharides in the Prevention of Necrotizing Enterocolitis: A Journey from In Vitro and In Vivo Models to Mother-Infant Cohort Studies." *Frontiers in Pediatrics*. https://doi.org/10.3389/fped.2018.00385.

Bode, Lars, and Evelyn Jantscher-Krenn. 2012. "Structure-Function Relationships of Human Milk Oligosaccharides." *Advances in Nutrition*. https://doi.org/10.3945/an.111.001404.

Cavaglieri, Claudia R., Anita Nishiyama, Luis Claudio Fernandes, Rui Curi, Elizabeth A. Miles, and Philip C. Calder. 2003. "Differential Effects of Short-Chain Fatty Acids on Proliferation and Production of Pro- and Anti-Inflammatory Cytokines by Cultured Lymphocytes." *Life Sciences* 73 (13): 1683–90. https://doi.org/10.1016/S0024-3205(03)00490-9.

Cheplin, Harry Asber, and Leo Frederick Rettger. 2011. *A Treatise on the Transformation of the Intestinal Flora, with Special Reference to the Implantation of Bacillus Acidophilus. A Treatise on the Transformation of the Intestinal Flora, with Special Reference to the Implantation of Bacillus Acidophilus.* https://doi.org/10.5962/bhl. title.24080.

Claus, Sandrine P., Sandrine L. Ellero, Bernard Berger, Lutz Krause, Anne Bruttin, Jérôme Molina, Alain Paris, et al. 2011. "Colonization-Induced Host-Gut Microbial Metabolic Interaction." *MBio* 2 (2). https://doi.org/10.1128/mBio.00271-10.

Collins, Stephanie, and Gregor Reid. 2016. "Distant Site Effects of Ingested Prebiotics." *Nutrients* 8 (9): 523. https://doi.org/10.3390/nu8090523.

Danneskiold-Samsøe, Niels Banhos, Helena Dias de Freitas Queiroz Barros, Rosangela Santos, Juliano Lemos Bicas, Cinthia Baú Betim Cazarin, Lise Madsen, Karsten Kristiansen, Glaucia Maria Pastore, Susanne Brix, and Mário Roberto Maróstica Júnior. 2019. "Interplay between Food and Gut Microbiota in Health and Disease." *Food Research International.* https://doi.org/10.1016/j.foodres.2018.07.043.

David, Lawrence A., Corinne F. Maurice, Rachel N. Carmody, David B. Gootenberg, Julie E. Button, Benjamin E. Wolfe, Alisha V. Ling, et al. 2014. "Diet Rapidly and Reproducibly Alters the Human Gut Microbiome." *Nature* 505 (7484): 559–63. https://doi.org/10.1038/nature12820.

Del Bo', Cristian, Salvatore Ciappellano, Dorothy Klimis-Zacas, Daniela Martini, Claudio Gardana, Patrizia Riso, and Marisa Porrini. 2009. "Anthocyanin Absorption, Metabolism, and Distribution from a Wild Blueberry-Enriched Diet (Vaccinium Angustifolium) Is Affected by Diet Duration in the Sprague–Dawley Rat." *Journal of Agricultural and Food Chemistry* 58 (4): 2491–97. https://doi.org/10.1021/JF903472X.

Del Bo', Cristian, Daniela Martini, Stefano Vendrame, Patrizia Riso, Salvatore Ciappellano, Dorothy Klimis-Zacas, and Marisa Porrini. 2010. "Improvement of Lymphocyte Resistance against H2O2-Induced DNA Damage in Sprague-Dawley Rats after Eight Weeks of a Wild Blueberry (Vaccinium Angustifolium)-Enriched Diet." *Mutation Research – Genetic Toxicology and Environmental Mutagenesis* 703 (2): 158–62. https://doi.org/10.1016/j.mrgentox.2010.08.013.

Di Criscio, T., A. Fratianni, R. Mignogna, L. Cinquanta, R. Coppola, E. Sorrentino, and G. Panfili. 2010. "Production of Functional Probiotic, Prebiotic, and Synbiotic Ice Creams." *Journal of Dairy Science* 93 (10): 4555–64. https://doi.org/10.3168/JDS.2010-3355.

Dlamini, Ziyanda C., Rashwahla L.S. Langa, Olayinka A. Aiyegoro, and Anthony I. Okoh. 2019. "Safety Evaluation and Colonisation Abilities of Four Lactic Acid Bacteria as Future Probiotics." *Probiotics and Antimicrobial Proteins* 11 (2): 397–402. https://doi.org/10.1007/S12602-018-9430-Y.

Elizabeth Tymczyszyn, E., Esteban Gerbino, Andrés Illanes, and Andrea Gómez-Zavaglia. 2011. "Galacto-Oligosaccharides as Protective Molecules in the Preservation of Lactobacillus Delbrueckii Subsp. Bulgaricus." *Cryobiology* 62 (2): 123–29. https://doi.org/10.1016/J.CRYOBIOL.2011.01.013.

Fanaro, Silvia, Günther Boehm, Johan Garssen, Jan Knol, Fabio Mosca, Bernd Stahl, and Vittorio Vigi. 2005. "Galacto-Oligosaccharides and Long-Chain Fructo-Oligosaccharides as Prebiotics in Infant Formulas: A Review." *Acta Paediatrica, International Journal of Paediatrics, Supplement* 94 (449): 22–26. https://doi.org/10.1080/08035320510043538.

Fernandes, Ricardo, Vinicius A. do Rosario, Michel C. Mocellin, Marilyn G.F. Kuntz, and Erasmo B.S.M. Trindade. 2017. "Effects of Inulin-Type Fructans, Galacto-Oligosaccharides and Related Synbiotics on Inflammatory Markers in Adult Patients with Overweight or Obesity: A Systematic Review." *Clinical Nutrition* 36 (5): 1197–1206. https://doi.org/10.1016/j.clnu.2016.10.003.

Finn, Sarah, Orla Condell, Peter McClure, Alejandro Amézquita, and Séamus Fanning. 2013. "Mechanisms of Survival, Responses and Sources of Salmonella in Low-Moisture Environments." *Frontiers in Microbiology* 4 (Nov). https://doi.org/10.3389/FMICB.2013.00331.

Gibson, Glenn R., Robert Hutkins, Mary Ellen Sanders, Susan L. Prescott, Raylene A. Reimer, Seppo J. Salminen, Karen Scott, et al. 2017. "Expert Consensus Document: The International Scientific Association for Probiotics and Prebiotics (ISAPP) Consensus Statement on the Definition and Scope of Prebiotics." *Nature Reviews Gastroenterology & Hepatology* 14 (8): 491. https://doi.org/10.1038/nrgastro.2017.75.

Gill, Steven R., Mihai Pop, Robert T. DeBoy, Paul B. Eckburg, Peter J. Turnbaugh, Buck S. Samuel, Jeffrey I. Gordon, David A. Relman, Claire M. Fraser-Liggett, and Karen E. Nelson. 2006. "Metagenomic Analysis of the Human Distal Gut Microbiome." *Science* 312 (5778): 1355–59. https://doi.org/10.1126/SCIENCE.1124234.

Gomand, Faustine., Frederic Borges, Jennifer Burgain, Justine Guerin, Anne Marie Revol-Junelles, and Claire Gaiani. 2019. "Food Matrix Design for Effective Lactic Acid Bacteria Delivery." *Annual Review of Food Science and Technology* 10 (March): 285–310. https://doi.org/10.1146/ANNUREV-FOOD-032818-121140.

Guergoletto, Karla Bigetti, Marciane Magnani, Juca San Martin, Celia Guadalupe Tardeli de Jesus Andrade, and Sandra Garcia. 2010. "Survival of Lactobacillus Casei (LC-1) Adhered to Prebiotic Vegetal Fibers." *Innovative Food Science and Emerging Technologies* 11 (2): 415–21. https://doi.org/10.1016/J.IFSET.2009.11.003.

Guigoz, Yves., Florence Rochat, Gregoire Perruisseau-Carrier, Inez Rochat, and Eduardo. Schiffrin, 2002. "Effects of Oligosaccharide on the Faecal Flora and Non-Specific Immune System in Elderly People."

Gullón, Patricia, Pablo G. del Río, Beatriz Gullón, Diana Oliveira, Patricia Costa, and José Manuel Lorenzo. 2021. "Pectooligosaccharides as Emerging Functional Ingredients: Sources, Extraction Technologies, and Biological Activities." *Sustainable Production Technology in Food* (January): 71–92. https://doi.org/10.1016/B978-0-12-821233-2.00004-6.

Gurpilhares, Daniela de Borba, Leonardo Paes Cinelli, Naomi Kato Simas, Adalberto Pessoa, and Lara Durães Sette. 2019. "Marine Prebiotics: Polysaccharides and Oligosaccharides Obtained by Using Microbial Enzymes." *Food Chemistry.* https://doi.org/10.1016/j.foodchem.2018.12.023.

Håkansson, Åsa, Camilla Bränning, Diya Adawi, Göran Molin, Margareta Nyman, Bengt Jeppsson, and Siv Ahrné. 2009. "Blueberry Husks, Rye Bran and Multi-Strain Probiotics Affect the Severity of Colitis Induced by Dextran Sulphate Sodium." *Scandinavian Journal of Gastroenterology* 44 (10): 1213–25. https://doi.org/10.1080/00365520903171268.

Heinonen, Marina. 2007. "Antioxidant Activity and Antimicrobial Effect of Berry Phenolics - A Finnish Perspective." *Molecular Nutrition and Food Research* 51 (6): 684–91. https://doi.org/10.1002/MNFR.200700006.

Homayouni, Alireza, Mohammand Reza Ehsani, Azizi Azizi, Shahab Razavi, and Mohammad. Yarmand. 2008. "Growth and Survival of Some Probiotic Strains in Simulated Ice Cream Conditions." *Journal of Applied Sciences* 8 (2): 379–82. https://doi.org/10.3923/JAS.2008.379.382.

Hond, Elly Den, Benny Geypens, and Yvo Ghoos. 2000. "Effect of High Performance Chicory Inulin on Constipation." *Nutrition Research* 20 (5): 731–36. https://doi.org/10.1016/S0271-5317(00)00162-7.

Hume, Megan P., Alissa C. Nicolucci, and Raylene A. Reimer. 2017. "Prebiotic Supplementation Improves Appetite Control in Children with Overweight and Obesity: A Randomized Controlled Trial." *The American Journal of Clinical Nutrition* 105 (4): 790–99. https://doi.org/10.3945/ajcn.116.140947.

İspirli, Hümeyra, Fatmanur Demirbaş, and Enes Dertli. 2018. "Glucan Type Exopolysaccharide (EPS) Shows Prebiotic Effect and Reduces Syneresis in Chocolate Pudding." *Journal of Food Science and Technology* 55 (9): 3821–26. https://doi.org/10.1007/S13197-018-3181-3.

Jayamanne,Vijith, and Steve Munyard Adams. 2006. "Determination of Survival, Identity and Stress Resistance of Probiotic Bifidobacteria in Bio-Yoghurts." *Letters in Applied Microbiology* 42 (3): 189–94. https://doi.org/10.1111/J.1472-765X.2006.01843.X.

Jovanovic-Malinovska, Ruzica, Slobodanka Kuzmanova, and Eleonora Winkelhausen. 2014. "Oligosaccharide Profile in Fruits and Vegetables as Sources of Prebiotics and Functional Foods." 17 (5): 949–65. https://doi.org/10.1080/10942912.2012.680221.

Kahle, Kathrin, Michael Kraus, Wolfgang Scheppach, Matthias Ackermann, Friederike Ridder, and Elke Richling. 2006. "Studies on Apple and Blueberry Fruit Constituents: Do the Polyphenols Reach the Colon after Ingestion?" *Molecular Nutrition and Food Research* 50: 418–23. https://doi.org/10.1002/mnfr.200500211.

Keenan, Derek F., Nigel Brunton, Francis Butler, Rudy Wouters, and Ronan Gormley. 2011. "Evaluation of Thermal and High Hydrostatic Pressure Processed Apple Purees Enriched with Prebiotic Inclusions." *Innovative Food Science and Emerging Technologies* 12 (3): 261–68. https://doi.org/10.1016/J.IFSET.2011.04.003.

Kelly, Greg. 2008. "Inulin-Type Prebiotics – A Review: Part 1." *Alternative Medicine Review: A Journal of Clinical Therapeutic* 13 (4): 315–29.

———. 2009. "Inulin-Type Prebiotics: A Review (Part 2)." *Alternative Medicine Review.* https://doi.org/10.1519/SSC.0b013e318281f689.

Khangwal, Ishu, and Pratyoosh Shukla. 2019. "Potential Prebiotics and Their Transmission Mechanisms: Recent Approaches." *Journal of Food and Drug Analysis* 27 (3): 649–56. https://doi.org/10.1016/J.JFDA.2019.02.003.

Klu, Yaa Asantewaa Kafui, Jonathan H. Williams, Robert D. Phillips, and Jinru Chen. 2012. "Survival of Lactobacillus Rhamnosus GG as Influenced by Storage Conditions and Product Matrixes." *Journal of Food Science* 77 (12). https://doi.org/10.1111/J.1750-3841.2012.02969.X.

Knol, Jan, Petra Scholtens, Corinna Kafka, Jochem Steenbakkers, Sabine Groß, Klaus Helm, Malte Klarczyk, Helmut Schöpfer, Heinz Michael Böckler, and John Wells. 2005. "Colon Microflora in Infants Fed Formula with Galacto- and Fructo-Oligosaccharides: More like Breast-Fed Infants." *Journal of Pediatric Gastroenterology and Nutrition* 40 (1): 36–42. https://doi.org/10.1097/00005176-200501000-00007.

Kober, Lars, Christoph Zehe, and Juergen Bode. 2013. "Optimized Signal Peptides for the Development of High Expressing CHO Cell Lines." *Biotechnology and Bioengineering.* https://doi.org/10.1002/bit.24776.

Koebnick, Corinna, Irmtrud Wagner, Peter Leitzmann, Udo Stern, and H. J.Franz Zunft. 2003. "Probiotic Beverage Containing Lactobacillus Casei Shirota Improves Gastrointestinal Symptoms in Patients with Chronic Constipation." *Canadian Journal of Gastroenterology=Journal Canadien de Gastroenterologie* 17 (11): 655–59. https://doi.org/10.1155/2003/654907.

Lacombe, Alison, Robert. Li, Dorothy Klimis-Zacas, ALekzandra Kristo, Shravani Tadepalli, Emily Krauss, Ryan Young, and Vivian C.H.. Wu. 2012. "Lowbush Blueberries, Vaccinium Angustifolium, Modulate the Functional Potential of Nutrient Utilization and DNA Maintenance Mechanisms in the Rat Proximal Colon Microbiota." *Functional Foods in Health and Disease* 2 (6). https://doi.org/10.31989/ffhd.v2i6.87.

———. 2013. "Lowbush Wild Blueberries Have the Potential to Modify Gut Microbiota and Xenobiotic Metabolism in the Rat Colon." *PLoS One* 8 (6). https://doi.org/10.1371/journal.pone.0067497.

Langkamp-Henken, Bobbi, Bradley S. Bender, Elizabeth M. Gardner, Kelli A. Herrlinger-Garcia, Michael J. Kelley, Donna M. Murasko, Joseph P. Schaller, Joyce K. Stechmiller, Debra J. Thomas, and Steven M. Wood. 2004. "Nutritional Formula Enhanced Immune

Function and Reduced Days of Symptoms of Upper Respiratory Tract Infection in Seniors." *Journal of the American Geriatrics Society* 52 (1). 3–12. https://doi.org/10.1111/J.1532-5415.2004.52003.X.

Looijer-van Langen, Mirjam A.C., and Levinus A. Dieleman. 2009. "Prebiotics in Chronic Intestinal Inflammation." *Inflammatory Bowel Diseases* 15 (3): 454–62. https://doi.org/10.1002/IBD.20737.

Mahovic, Michael J., Joel D. Tenney, and Jerry A. Bartz. 2007. "Applications of Chlorine Dioxide Gas for Control of Bacterial Soft Rot in Tomatoes." *Plant Disease* 91 (10): 1316–20. https://doi.org/10.1094/pdis-91-10-1316.

Majeed, Muhammed, Shaheen Majeed, Kalyanam Nagabhushanam, Sankaran Natarajan, Arumugam Sivakumar, and Furqan Ali. 2016. "Evaluation of the Stability of Bacillus Coagulans MTCC 5856 during Processing and Storage of Functional Foods." *International Journal of Food Science & Technology* 51 (4): 894–901. https://doi.org/10.1111/IJFS.13044.

Manthey, Carolin F., Chloe A. Autran, Lars Eckmann, and Lars Bode. 2014. "Human Milk Oligosaccharides Protect against Enteropathogenic Escherichia Coli Attachment in Vitro and EPEC Colonization in Suckling Mice." *Journal of Pediatric Gastroenterology and Nutrition.* https://doi.org/10.1097/MPG.0000000000000172.

McRorie, Johnson W. 2015. "Evidence-Based Approach to Fiber Supplements and Clinically Meaningful Health Benefits, Part 2: What to Look for and How to Recommend an Effective Fiber Therapy." *Nutrition Today* 50 (2): 90–97. https://doi.org/10.1097/NT.0000000000000089.

Menezes, Fabiano P, and Rosane S Da Silva. 2017. "Chapter 22 – Caffeine." Edited by Ramesh C. Gupta. *Reproductive and Developmental Toxicology (Second Edition),* Elsevier 399–411

Moossavi, Shirin, Shadi Sepehri, Bianca Robertson, Lars Bode, Sue Goruk, Catherine J. Field, Lisa M. Lix, et al. 2019. "Composition and Variation of the Human Milk Microbiota Are Influenced by Maternal and Early-Life Factors." *Cell Host and Microbe.* https://doi.org/10.1016/j.chom.2019.01.011.

Moro, G., S. Arslanoglu, B. Stahl, J. Jelinek, U. Wahn, and G. Boehm. 2006. "A Mixture of Prebiotic Oligosaccharides Reduces the Incidence of Atopic Dermatitis during the First Six Months of Age." *Archives of Disease in Childhood* 91 (10). 814–19. https://doi.org/10.1136/ADC.2006.098251.

Nematollahi, Amene, Sara Sohrabvandi, Amir Mohammad Mortazavian, and Sahar Jazaeri. 2016. "Viability of Probiotic Bacteria and Some Chemical and Sensory Characteristics in Cornelian Cherry Juice during Cold Storage." *Electronic Journal of Biotechnology* 21 (May): 49–53. https://doi.org/10.1016/J.EJBT.2016.03.001.

O'Connor, Sarah, Sarah Chouinard-Castonguay, Claudia Gagnon, and Iwona Rudkowska. 2017. "Prebiotics in the Management of Components of the Metabolic Syndrome." *Maturitas.* https://doi.org/10.1016/j.maturitas.2017.07.005.

Önneby, Karin, Leticia Pizzul, Joakim Bjerketorp, Denny Mahlin, Sebastian Håkansson, and Per Wessman. 2013. "Effects of Di- and Polysaccharide Formulations and Storage Conditions on Survival of Freeze-Dried Sphingobium Sp." *World Journal of Microbiology and Biotechnology* 29 (8): 1399–1408. https://doi.org/10.1007/S11274-013-1303-7.

Pap, Nora, Marina Fidelis, Luciana Azevedo, Mariana Araújo Vieira do Carmo, Dongxu Wang, Andrei Mocan, Eliene Penha Rodrigues Pereira, et al. 2021. "Berry Polyphenols and Human Health: Evidence of Antioxidant, Anti-Inflammatory, Microbiota Modulation, and Cell-Protecting Effects." *Current Opinion in Food Science* 42: 167–86. https://doi.org/10.1016/j.cofs.2021.06.003.

Patel, Ravi Mangal, and Patricia Wei Denning. 2013. "Therapeutic Use of Prebiotics, Probiotics, and Postbiotics to Prevent Necrotizing Enterocolitis: What Is the Current Evidence?" *Clinics in Perinatology* 40 (1): 11–25. https://doi.org/10.1016/J.CLP.2012.12.002.

Revolledo, Lillana., C. S.A. Ferreira, and Antonio J.P. Ferreira. 2009. "Prevention of Salmonella Typhimurium Colonization and Organ Invasion by Combination Treatment in Broiler Chicks." *Poultry Science* 88 (4): 734–43. https://doi.org/10.3382/PS.2008-00410.

Saavedra, Lucas., and A. Tschernia. 2022. "Human Studies with Probiotics and Prebiotics: Clinical Implications." https://doi.org/10.1079/BJN/2002543.

Scott, Karen P., Jenny C. Martin, Christophe Chassard, Marlene Clerget, Joanna Potrykus, Gill Campbell, Claus Dieter Mayer, et al. 2011. "Substrate-Driven Gene Expression in Roseburia Inulinivorans: Importance of Inducible Enzymes in the Utilization of Inulin and Starch." *Proceedings of the National Academy of Sciences of the United States of America* 108 (Suppl. 1): 4672–79. https://doi.org/10.1073/pnas.1000091107.

Shoaib, Muhammad, Aamir Shehzad, Mukama Omar, Allah Rakha, Husnain Raza, Hafiz Rizwan Sharif, Azam Shakeel, Anum Ansari, and Sobia Niazi. 2016. "Inulin: Properties, Health Benefits and Food Applications." *Carbohydrate Polymers*. https://doi.org/10.1016/j.carbpol.2016.04.020.

Singh, Rasnik K., Hsin Wen Chang, Di Yan, Kristina M. Lee, Derya Ucmak, Kirsten Wong, Michael Abrouk, et al. 2017. "Influence of Diet on the Gut Microbiome and Implications for Human Health." *Journal of Translational Medicine* 15 (1): 1–17. https://doi.org/10.1186/S12967-017-1175-Y.

Tamime, AdnanY., Maria Saarela, A. Korslund Søndergaard, V.V. Mistry, and N.P. Shah. 2006. "Production and Maintenance of Viability of Probiotic Micro-Organisms in Dairy Products." *Probiotic Dairy Products* (November): 39–72. https://doi.org/10.1002/9780470995785.CH3.

Tenorio, María Dolores, Irene Espinosa-Martos, Guadalupe Préstamo, and Pilar Rupérez. 2010. "Soybean Whey Enhance Mineral Balance and Caecal Fermentation in Rats." *European Journal of Nutrition* 49 (3): 155–63. https://doi.org/10.1007/S00394-009-0060-8.

Vandeputte, Doris, Gwen Falony, Sara Vieira-Silva, Jun Wang, Manuela Sailer, Stephan Theis, Kristin Verbeke, and Jeroen Raes. 2017. "Prebiotic Inulin-Type Fructans Induce Specific Changes in the Human Gut Microbiota." *Gut* 66 (11): 1968–74. https://doi.org/10.1136/gutjnl-2016-313271.

Veereman, Gigi. 2007. "Pediatric Applications of Inulin and Oligofructose." *The Journal of Nutrition* 137 (11): 2585S–2589S. https://doi.org/10.1093/JN/137.11.2585S.

Vendrame, Stefano, Allison Daugherty, Aleksandra S. Kristo, Patrizia Riso, and Dorothy Klimis-Zacas. 2013. "Wild Blueberry (Vaccinium Angustifolium) Consumption Improves Inflammatory Status in the Obese Zucker Rat Model of the Metabolic Syndrome." *Journal of Nutritional Biochemistry* 24 (8): 1508–12. https://doi.org/10.1016/j.jnutbio.2012.12.010.

Vendrame, Stefano, Simone Guglielmetti, Patrizia Riso, Stefania Arioli, Dorothy Klimis-Zacas, and Marisa Porrini. 2011. "Six-Week Consumption of a Wild Blueberry Powder Drink Increases Bifidobacteria in the Human Gut." *Journal of Agricultural and Food Chemistry* 59 (24): 12815–20, https://doi.org/10.1021/jf2028686.

Vulevic, Jelena, Aleksandra Juric, George Tzortzis, and Glenn R. Gibson. 2013. "A Mixture of Trans-Galactooligosaccharides Reduces Markers of Metabolic Syndrome and Modulates the Fecal Microbiota and Immune Function of Overweight Adults 1–3." *Journal of Nutrition* 143 (3): 324–31. https://doi.org/10.3945/jn.112.166132.

Vulevic, Jelena, Aleksandra Juric, Gemma E. Walton, Sandrine P. Claus, George Tzortzis, Ruth E. Toward, and Glenn R. Gibson. 2015. "Influence of Galacto-Oligosaccharide Mixture (B-GOS) on Gut Microbiota, Immune Parameters and Metabonomics in Elderly Persons." *The British Journal of Nutrition* 114 (4): 586–95. https://doi.org/10.1017/S0007114515001889.

Wang, Shumin, Yue Xiao, Fengwei Tian, Jianxin Zhao, Hao Zhang, Qixiao Zhai, and Wei Chen. 2020a. "Rational Use of Prebiotics for Gut Microbiota Alterations: Specific Bacterial Phylotypes and Related Mechanisms." *Journal of Functional Foods* 66 (September 2019). https://doi.org/10.1016/j.jff.2020.103838.

———. 2020b. "Rational Use of Prebiotics for Gut Microbiota Alterations: Specific Bacterial Phylotypes and Related Mechanisms." *Journal of Functional Foods*. Elsevier Ltd. https://doi.org/10.1016/j.jff.2020.103838.

Watson, Anthony W., David Houghton, Peter J. Avery, Christopher Stewart, Elaine E. Vaughan, P. Diederick Meyer, Minse J.J. de Bos Kuil, Peter J.M. Weijs, and Kirsten Brandt. 2019. "Changes in Stool Frequency Following Chicory Inulin Consumption, and Effects on Stool Consistency, Quality of Life and Composition of Gut Microbiota." *Food Hydrocolloids*. https://doi.org/10.1016/j.foodhyd.2019.06.006.

Wu, Xianli, Liwei Gu, Ronald L. Prior, and Steve McKay. 2004. "Characterization of Anthocyanins and Proanthocyanidins in Some Cultivars of Ribes, Aronia, and Sambucus and Their Antioxidant Capacity." *Journal of Agricultural and Food Chemistry* 52 (26): 7846–56. https://doi.org/10.1021/JF0486850.

Younes, Hassan, Charles Coudray, Jacques Bellanger, Christian Demigné, Yves Rayssiguier, and Christian Rémésy. 2001. "Effects of Two Fermentable Carbohydrates (Inulin and Resistant Starch) and Their Combination on Calcium and Magnesium Balance in Rats." *British Journal of Nutrition* 86 (4): 479–85. https://doi.org/10.1079/bjn2001430.

# Section III

## T2–3 Effectiveness Trials in General Population and Regulatory Limitations

# 7 Gut Microbiota and Polyphenols: Discussing a Powerful Interplay and Its Effect on Health

*Aleksandra S. Kristo*
California Polytechnic State University

*Dorothy Klimis-Zacas*
University of Maine

## CONTENTS

## INTRODUCTION

Gut microbiota and polyphenols, each in their own right, constitute research areas of increasing interest due to accumulating scientific evidence indicating their significant potential benefits and functions in human health and longevity. While polyphenols have been investigated separately as bioactive compounds that can confer notable health benefits in an array of metabolic conditions, the association and interaction with the gut microbiome is less studied while is gaining increasing interest lately.

Polyphenols, as plant-secondary metabolites minimally processed by human metabolism, rely heavily on the metabolic capacities of the gut microbiota for their absorption and potential biological actions. By producing bioactive polyphenol-derived compounds through enzymatic activities of a diverse community of microorganisms, gut microbiota can affect human health in a variety of ways. Polyphenols can shape gut microbiota composition and function, thereby eliciting beneficial changes in the gut ecosystem (Vendrame et al., 2011; Lacombe et al., 2013). Elucidation of the specific bacterial populations and the metabolic processes involved in producing the polyphenol-derived bioactive compounds, the specific metabolites, and their mechanisms of action is deemed necessary to understand the microbiota–polyphenol interplay and consequently implications for human health. In this sense, one could argue that the current state of affairs in polyphenol and microbiota interplay research is found in its "infancy."

Presently, human studies of microbial metabolism on polyphenols or polyphenol-induced modification of microbiota are limited. Further, the evidence generated in the available studies is inconsistent, owing to methodological challenges including the variations in chemical nature, doses, single compounds or mixtures of polyphenols under study, the dissimilar health status or the inherent interindividual microbiota variations of the participants, the small study size, or the insufficient endpoints investigated. Therefore, drawing definite associations between the polyphenol–microbiota interplay and health effects on the host as a result of such interplay can be daunting. The multitude of polyphenols with different structures, signaling capabilities, synergies, pathways involved, and physiological roles, makes it challenging to fully elucidate their short- and long-term health effects both positive and potentially negative, let alone any additional effects due to interactions such as those with the microbiota.

The reported health benefits of plant-based diets, which to a significant degree have been shown by the scientific literature, cannot be attributed to any specific phytochemical(s). Rather benefits derive from the combined effects of various phytochemicals including fiber, carotenoids, phytosterols, or polyphenols. The latter has gained special research attention initiated by their early recognition as antioxidants along with evidence indicating oxidative stress as the underlying cause of chronic disease. Before realizing the function, metabolic capacity, and potential role of microbiota in human health, the bioavailability of polyphenols was often overlooked in earlier *in vitro* studies of polyphenol compounds that employed native compounds and pharmacological doses, highly unlikely to represent tissue exposure post-polyphenol consumption, augmenting a limited view of polyphenols as mere antioxidants and in general leading to inconsistencies in results and conclusions.

Polyphenols' capacity to chelate metals and scavenge free radicals renders them their antioxidant potential. Notably, however, the potency of polyphenol antioxidant activity highly depends on their chemical structure and more specifically the number of hydroxyl groups augmenting, while glycosylation reducing their antioxidant potential (Di Meo et al., 2018). In this regard, factors that would alter the chemical structure of polyphenols could affect the latter's ability to function as antioxidants. There is a significant body of literature suggesting the beneficial health effects of polyphenols due to their antioxidant capacity. Early evidence indicated reduced capillary resistance and permeability in the case of human blood vessels as a result of the activity of citrus flavonoids, hesperidin, and rutin (Bentsath et al., 1936).

As relevant research is being conducted for a number of decades now, a significant body of literature currently exists to support cardiovascular and other potential health effects of polyphenols. More specifically, consumption of plant-based food items such as apples, berries, citrus fruits, plums, beans, nuts, cocoa, tea, coffee, and wine are considered good sources of polyphenols and have been to a greater or lesser degree documented to confer health benefits related to chronic conditions including cardiovascular disease (CVD) and type 2 diabetes mellitus (T2DM) (Williamson, 2017), along with neurodegenerative diseases (Renaud and Martinoli, 2019). While polyphenols gained early recognition for their antioxidant capacity, mechanistic studies employing individual compounds are increasingly documenting their signaling properties via multiple cell signaling mechanisms, commonly related to oxidative or inflammatory status (Vendrame et al., 2015).

Recently, more emphasis has been placed on the potential interplay of polyphenols and the microbiome. More specifically, work is being conducted to investigate mechanisms of action involving microbiota-derived metabolites, as these relate to polyphenol action. The gut microbiome can convert polyphenols into secondary compounds that may extend health benefits.

Notably, the global polyphenol market, which includes a variety of their uses in foods, beverages, pharmaceuticals, and cosmetics, was estimated to have exceeded 700 million USD in 2015 and is projected to reach 1.1 billion USD by 2022. Interestingly, however, there is currently no uniform regulatory framework or recommendation consensus regarding polyphenol consumption and/or supplementation or fortification in functional foods (Cory et al., 2018).

## OVERVIEW OF POLYPHENOLS

### CLASSIFICATION AND GENERAL DESCRIPTION

Polyphenols constitute the largest group of phytochemicals, i.e., chemicals naturally occurring in plants. Produced as secondary metabolites, polyphenols serve to defend the plant from environmental stress related to oxidative damage, ultraviolet radiation, extreme temperatures, pathogens, parasites, or plant predators. Additionally, the bright colors of fruits and vegetables are attributed to polyphenols (Zhang, 2015). While not considered essential nutrients, such substances may considerably affect human health, especially with regard to chronic diseases including CVD, diabetes, and cancer. A plethora of evidence indicates potential health benefits of plant-based diets and polyphenol dietary sources, including fruits, vegetables, whole grains, legumes, nuts, and seeds, as well as tea, coffee, and wine (Kristo et al., 2016). While originally classified as "vegetable tannins" because of their tanning action on animal skin, polyphenols are currently moderately estimated to comprise over 8,000 unique chemical compounds that extend pharmacological and/or therapeutic action (Renaud and Martinoli, 2019). From a chemistry standpoint, it is primarily the presence of hydroxylated phenol (aromatic) rings that characterizes this large heterogeneous group of naturally occurring compounds (D'Archivio et al., 2007).

According to the number of phenolic rings and relative substitution groups, polyphenols are classified as flavonoid and non-flavonoid molecules. Flavonoids, which are the largest subgroup in terms of the number of identified compounds, are further classified into flavanones, flavones, dihydroflavonols, flavonols, flavan-3-ols, or flavonols, isoflavones, anthocyanidins, and proanthocyanidins (PACs). Non-flavonoids on the other hand include phenolic acids and other various phenolics (Cardona et al., 2013).

Along with flavonoids, phenolic acids (derived from benzoic and cinnamic acid) and stilbenes constitute the main subclasses (Williamson and Clifford, 2017). Interestingly, most polyphenols, particularly flavonoids, occur in glycosylated forms (i.e., with a sugar moiety attached to the main polyphenolic structure), while esterified and/or polymerized versions are fairly common modifications also. Moreover, flavonols, flavanones, and anthocyanins are typically found in planta as glycosides with glucose and rhamnose units being the main saccharides attached. Flavanols primarily occur in their free native form or alternatively in polymerized forms, while finally can be found as galloylated versions such as in the case of green tea. Polymerized flavonols, also referred to as PACs, constitute a widespread group of compounds found in a variety of food items including cocoa. Phenolic acids are typically attached to quinic acid or other organic acids and are found in plant-based foods specifically coffee and most fruits at very high and moderate levels, respectively (Williamson and Clifford, 2017).

## FOOD SOURCES AND CONSUMPTION

The type, variety, and number of polyphenols as well as concentrations in a particular food item can vary depending on where (soil/climate conditions), when the food is grown (seasonality), how it is farmed and transported, how ripe it is, and how it is cooked and/or prepared. Overall, polyphenols are the best food sources and hence provide the most abundant antioxidants to our diet and are found as widespread constituents of fruits (particularly apples, citrus fruits, plums, and berries), vegetables (such as broccoli, celery, parsley, onion, and leek), cereal, olive, dry legumes, nuts, chocolates, and beverages, such as tea, coffee, and wine (D'Archivio et al., 2007). Not surprisingly, the differences in the dietary patterns among populations reflect the differences in the type and amount of polyphenol intake. As a result, there is significant variation in terms of both the type and amount of polyphenol intake among humans as reasonably expected.

More specifically, Edmands and colleagues compared the polyphenol metabolome from urine samples of 481 participants from four European countries as part of the European Prospective Investigation on Cancer and Nutrition cohort. The researchers concluded that the metabolome approach mapped the dietary intake, which, however, is significantly diverse and produced variable results based on the type and amount of polyphenol intake of the participants (Edmands et al., 2015). Similarly, in a separate experiment conducted in the framework of the Adventist Health Study, different dietary patterns were associated with notable differences in polyphenol intake, their main classes, or sources of dietary polyphenols, corroborating the findings of others. More specifically, high flavonoid intake was stated to signify vegetarian diets, while phenolic acid intake, primarily due to significant coffee consumption, was found higher in nonvegetarian diets (Burkholder-Cooley et al., 2016).

In an earlier comprehensive review of the evidence, Scalbert and Williamson concluded that the main polyphenol dietary sources are fruits and beverages (fruit juice, wine, tea, coffee, chocolate, and beer) and, to a lesser extent vegetables, dry legumes,

**TABLE 7.1**

**Dietary Polyphenols: Their Characteristic Bioactive Compounds and Typical Food Sources**

| Dietary Polyphenol Type | Characteristic Bioactive Compound(s)[a] | Dietary Source(s) |
| --- | --- | --- |
| Phenolic acids | Chlorogenic, caffeic, gallic, ferulic acids | Coffee, berries, kiwi, apple, cherry |
| Phenolic alcohols | Hydroxytyrosol | Olive |
| Stilbenes | Resveratrol | Grapes, red wine (primarily) |
| Lignans | Secolariciresinol | Linseed |
| Flavonoids | Genistein, daidzein (isoflavones), | Soy, miso |
| | Luteolin, apigenin (flavones) | Celery, parsley |
| | Hesperetin, naringenin (flavanones) | Oranges, lemon |
| | Quercetin, kaempferol, myricetin (flavonols) | Onion, leek, broccoli |
| | (Epi)catechins (flavanols) | Grapes, wine, cocoa, apricots |
| | (Epi)gallocatechins (flavanols) | Beans, green tea |
| | Epigallocatechin gallate (flavanols) | Berries, aubergine |
| | Delphinidin, cyanidin, malvidin (anthocyanins) | |
| Tannins | Procyanidins (condensed tannins) | Cocoa, chocolate, apples, grapes |
| | Gallotannins, ellagitannins (hydrolyzable tannins) | Mango, pomegranate |

[a] Polyphenol subclass designation in parentheses when applicable

and cereals, while the total intake was estimated to be 1 g/d. Nonetheless, significant uncertainties were due to the lack of accurate and comprehensive data on the content of some main polyphenol classes in foods (Scalbert and Williamson, 2000). More recently, the estimated intake of polyphenols through dietary sources and herbal medicines and/or supplements combined was at 2 g/d, a higher amount than initially anticipated (Espin et al., 2017). The types of dietary polyphenols, with characteristic bioactive compounds and typical dietary sources, can be viewed in Table 7.1, while the classification of compounds can be seen in Figure 7.1.

## OVERALL METABOLISM/BIOAVAILABILITY AND EXCRETION

Certain plant bioactive compounds can be absorbed in their native form by the stomach or gut, but the majority of the glycosylated, polymeric, or esterified native plant compounds must be hydrolyzed prior to absorption, a step partly performed by the gut microbiota. For the intestinal uptake of the bioactive compounds, both passive and active mechanisms have been reported, as well as efflux transporters, which lower the absolute influx of bioactive compounds through intestinal absorption. Nevertheless, our knowledge of the carriers involved in the various compounds is still very scarce. When absorbed, hydrophilic plant food compounds typically undergo first-pass metabolism in the intestine and liver with phase 1 (oxidation/

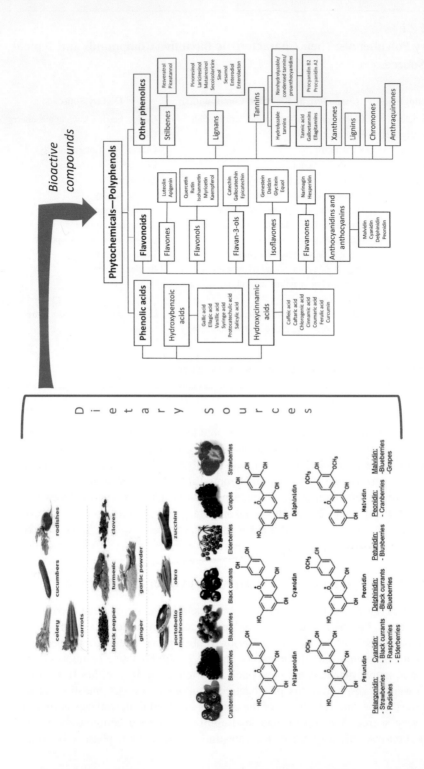

**FIGURE 7.1** Main bioactive compounds as they pertain to polyphenols and respective dietary sources displayed (Modified from: Kristo et al., 2016).

reduction reactions) and predominantly phase II (β-glucuronidation, sulfation, methylation, and glutathione conjugation) biotransformations.

In general, however, the metabolism of polyphenols is rather well understood due to the xenobiotic nature of these compounds. Polyphenols specifically undergo metabolism in the small intestine, liver, and finally the colon by colonic microbes. While significant metabolism and uptake of polyphenol derivatives occur in the colonic environment, phenolic compounds are glucuronidated and sulfated in the liver and intestinal tissues, with those metabolites detected in body fluids. More specifically, absorbed metabolites produced by microbial transformation (enterolignans and dihydroxylated compounds) such as methylcatechol can be subjected to further glucuronidation, methylation, sulfation, or glycination in the liver. While there is a significant lag time from the interplay between the colon and the liver in terms of blood residence time, ultimately, phenolic microbial metabolites are distributed to tissues and finally excreted via urine, primarily as hepatic conjugates or in their free form (Bohn et al., 2015). This is an interesting interplay that deems further research and understanding of its kinetics. An interesting point is that small colon-derived phenolic acids may not be accounted for in analyses of human or cell fluids due to their hydrophilic nature and the challenges posed in terms of their identification and quantification.

Furthermore, gut microbiota-driven polyphenol metabolism also occurs via the opening of carbon rings, breaking of C–C bonds, demethylation, reduction, and hydrogenation/de-hydrogenation, all of which can eventually modulate their bioavailability and/or biological activity. Therefore, whenever considering the effects of polyphenols as they relate to the gut microbiome, metabotype characterization emerges as the key toward interpreting those effects (Tressera-Rimbau et al., 2018), while the individual epigenome needs to be also considered even though the role of the individual epigenome in the variation of responses to plant food bioactive compounds is still unexplored.

As previously mentioned, in human studies, there is often a significant interindividual variation observed in terms of microbially derived metabolites and bioavailability of polyphenols, echoed by different plasma concentrations and urinary excretion levels of bioactive compounds or their metabolites in individuals with similar dietary intake (Manach et al., 2017).

Notably, in clinical trials of soy isoflavones and ellagitannins, the observed health effect of those polyphenols was associated with certain gut metabotypes. Polyphenol compounds, or by the same token polyphenol-rich foods, produce a positive impact on desirable microbial species such as *Akkermansia muciniphila*, *Faecalibacterium prausnitzii*, and *Roseburia* spp. Oligomeric and polymeric polyphenols reaching the colonic environment unmodified interestingly demonstrate probiotic-like effects (Williamson and Clifford, 2017; Duenas et al., 2015). More specifically, polyphenols and polyphenol-like compounds, as well as polyphenol-rich foods, have been demonstrated to significantly induce the population *of A. muciniphila*, *F. prausnitzii*, and *Roseburia* spp., bacterial species associated with positive health effects (Tressera-Rimbau et al., 2018).

Observed inter-participant differences could arise due to variances in absorption, metabolism, tissue distribution and turnover, excretion, or a combination of these parameters. In nutrition, this intra-participant variation in the response of supplementation of carotenoids for example has been demonstrated, thus leading researchers to introduce the concept of responsiveness degree, alluding to the classification of low, medium, and high responders to nutrient supplementation either through the diet or other types of oral supplementation (Tressera-Rimbau et al., 2018). Interestingly, a series of pharmacogenomics studies have demonstrated that for specific drugs, including some phytochemicals of the alkaloid family like codeine, individuals can be categorized into poor, intermediate, or extensive, and ultra-rapid metabolizers, and dosing must be adapted to achieve equivalent plasma or tissue concentration of the active metabolite (Filipski et al., 2016).

An interesting example of the approach toward a better understanding of the role of genetic polymorphisms in the variability of the response to diet can be seen in the case of the Mediterranean diet (MedDiet). More specifically, the benefit of the Mediterranean diet on cardiovascular-related outcomes has been shown to depend significantly on genetic variants of the transcription factor 7-like 2 (*TCF7L2*) gene (Corella et al., 2013). This specific gene encodes for a protein functioning as a transcription factor, and the TCF7L2-rs7903146 polymorphism is known as a strong genetic determinant of T2DM risk and fasting plasma glucose concentration regulation (Palmer et al., 2011). More specifically, the prevalence of the 7903146T allele is associated with higher T2DM risk. In an elegant study, Corella et al. demonstrated that intervention with the MedDiet was more beneficial toward significantly attenuating cardiovascular risk factors and stroke incidence for individuals with the 7903146T allele (Corella et al., 2013). Nonetheless, it must be underlined that the majority of nutrigenetics studies thus far are observational and association studies, while obtained results have not been fully confirmed in follow-up intervention experimental studies.

## MICROBIOTA METABOLISM OF POLYPHENOLS AND HEALTH EFFECTS

### GUT-DERIVED METABOLITES

The biological properties of dietary polyphenols as they relate to health benefits and relevant effects are determined to a large extent by the bioavailability of their gut-derived metabolites. The human microbiota, composed of bacteria, fungi, archaea, viruses, and protozoans, can be found throughout the body; as it colonizes the skin, mouth, vagina, gastroenteric tube, and/or respiratory system. Over 70% of microbiota colonizes the gastrointestinal tract and contains more than 100 trillion microbes.

The human microbiome, a synergistic community of microorganisms often considered an independent endocrine organ in a symbiotic relationship with the host, is comprised of two primary phyla, namely Bacteroidetes and Firmicutes. These two phyla represent 98% of the gut microbiota and are typically found in a ratio favoring Bacteroidetes over Firmicutes (B/F >1) when we consider a healthy/desirable gut phenotype. Notably, however, a universal definition of "healthy microbiota" as it would pertain to a specific microbial profile is still lacking. Other phyla include Proteobacteria, Verrucomicrobia, Fusobacteria, Cyanobacteria, and Actinobacteria. Firmicutes can be grouped into three major classes: Clostridia, Negativicutes, and Bacilli, while Firmicutes overall consist of over 200 genera, including *Staphylococcus*, *Lactobacillus*, *Ruminococcus*, and *Clostridium*. The relevant phyla consist primarily of gram-positive bacteria, except for those belonging to the Negativicutes class.

Interestingly, Negativicutes possess an outer membrane with lipopolysaccharides (LPS), making them stain gram-negative (Sikalidis and Maykish, 2020). Bacterial species of the genera *Lactobacillus* and *Bifidobacterium* are considered beneficial; thus, they are commonly used as probiotics, whereas the *Clostridium*, *Eubacterium*, and *Bacteroides* genera are implicated in adverse health outcomes (Nash et al., 2018). Eubiosis (from the Greek words ευ/eu: good and βίος/bios: life) refers to the normal/ healthy profile of gut microflora, as opposed to dysbiosis (from the Greek words δυς/ dys: nonfavorable/difficult and βίος/bios: life) which produces a profile that in turn induces the risk for certain diseases; hence, in a healthy microbiome–host relationship promoting the well-being of the host, the condition would be a eubiotic one. Notably, the profile of gut microbiota is highly amenable to a variety of external factors including diet, antibiotic use, hygiene, pharmaceuticals, exercise frequency, climate, geographical region, pollution level, toxins, and physiological and/or psychological stress potentially resulting in dysbiosis, which is shown to be associated with increased risk for a plethora of diseases particularly chronic ones such as inflammatory bowel disease, CVD, and T2DM. Endogenous factors, such as age, genetics, birth gestational date, mode of delivery at birth, infant feeding method, weaning period, hormonal changes, and health status, may also influence the microbiota composition (profile). The microbiota composition may finally also vary depending on the colonization location in the gut. Moreover, a significant body of literature discusses the differential antimicrobial properties of polyphenols and their capacity to adversely affect pathogenic bacteria (Ozdal et al., 2016; Maharjan et al., 2018; Luca et al., 2020).

Notably, a small fraction of polyphenol molecules can be absorbed in the small intestine (namely the smaller molecules), while glycosylated and polymeric forms (estimated at 90–95% of total ingested polyphenols) reach the colon in their native form. Microbes of the gut then convert polyphenols into phenolic compounds of low molecular weight, hence increasing absorption by intestinal epithelial cells (Pasinetti et al., 2018; Aura, 2008).

Moreover, conjugation reactions, such as methylation, sulfation, and glucuronidation, increase the hydrophilicity of polyphenolics, hence facilitating absorption by the gut, in addition to biliary and urinary elimination (Filosa et al., 2018). A noteworthy variety of gut bacteria can perform enzymatic reactions such as deglycosylations, while the production of certain metabolites such as urolithin by *Gordonibacter urolithinfaciens* and *Gordonibacter pamelaeae*, and S-equol by *Bifidobacterium breve* is a characteristic of gut bacteria with significant potential to support health (Marin et al., 2015). In this context, it is important to develop a better and more accurate understanding of this polyphenolic biotransformation, and it is important to grasp the significant breadth of catalytic abilities for the various bacterial species. From an absorption standpoint, interestingly, the best absorbed among flavonoids appear to be isoflavones, followed by catechins, flavanones, and flavonol glycosides, while the least absorbed are PACs, flavan-3-ol gallates, and anthocyanins (Crozier et al., 2010). A conceptual schematic of the main biotransformations of dietary polyphenols can be seen below (Figure 7.2).

In general, phenolic compounds are typically found conjugated to glycosides, glucuronides, and organic acids, which can be hydrolyzed by gut microbiota, resulting in aglycones. Subsequently, post-colonic absorption, transformation into phase II

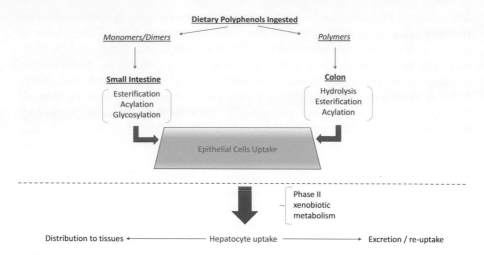

**FIGURE 7.2** Conceptual schematic depicting the major bio-transformations and relevant locations of dietary polyphenols (the blue dashed line represents separation between the intestinal lumen and the internal organismal space).

conjugates occurs (sulfated and glucuronidated conjugates) in the intestinal tissues and the liver. Conjugated compounds are excreted into the gut as biliary constituents via enterohepatic recirculation, and before being reabsorbed or transformed, microbial enzymes deconjugate these compounds (Plamanda and Vondar 2021). Fecal microbial enzymes—β-glucosidase, α-rhamnosidase, esterase, β-glucuronidase—catalyze the deconjugation in the gut, while reactions such as ring and lactone fission, dehydroxylation, reduction, decarboxylation, demethylation, and isomerization are also induced by the gut microbiota. The degree and type of microbial transformations are significantly influenced by the phenolic structure, flavonoid and nonflavonoid factors, polymerization degree, and spatial configuration (Makarewicz et al., 2021).

Flavonols, flavanones, flavan-3-ols, isoflavones, and anthocyanins, all belonging to the flavonoid category, share the common basic structure: two benzene rings (ring A and B), linked by a heterocyclic pyrone C-ring. In foods, they are found as glycosides, O-glycosides, C-glycosides, and flavan-3-ols, which are not conjugated. Flavan-3-ols can form either PACs or condensed tannins, and either procyanidins, prodelphinidins, or propelargonidins, when they are solely comprised of one single compound—epicatechin, epigallocatechin, epiafzelechin. Simple phenolics derived from the A and B rings are released after the gut microbiota disrupts the C-ring at different positions. The resulting type of phenolic compounds is affected by the hydroxylation pattern and the position of the B-ring. Thus, in phenolic compounds, such as flavonols, flavan-3-ols, PACs, rendering hydroxyphenyl-propionic acids and hydroxyphenyl acid, the C-ring cleavages are produced at 1–2 and 4–10 bonds or 1–2 and 3–4 bonds. In flavanone and isoflavone groups, the resulting metabolites indicate that the C-ring cleavage is produced at either position 1 and 2, or 4 and 10. Subsequent steps of flavonoid metabolism involving the gut microbiota include demethylation and dehydroxylation reactions, while the majority of the resulting metabolites are acid or aldehyde phenolics with one, two, or three hydroxyl and methyl ester radicals, for example, 3-(3,4-dihydroxyphenyl)-propionic acid from the flavonol quercetin and equol from the isoflavone daidzein (Plamanda and Vondar 2021; Makarewicz et al., 2021).

Moreover, the gut microbiota is also able to transform gallic acid and ellagic acid. More specifically, gallic acid is prone to decarboxylation and dihydroxylation reactions, while ellagic acid is more susceptible to dehydroxylation. Following the dihydroxylation of ellagic acid, nasutin metabolites are produced, which are compounds characterized by the removal of the two hydroxyl units. After ellagic acid is transformed by way of lactone ring cleavage, decarboxylation, and dehydroxylation reactions, the urolithin metabolites are formed (Catalkaya et al., 2020). After lactonases open one of the lactone rings, luteic acid is produced, which is in turn converted by decarboxylases in the gut, to produce pentahydroxyurolithin, a critical stage in the production of different types of urolithins. Further, after dehydroxylations of pentahydroxyurolithin, tetrahydroxyurolithins, and trihydroxyurolithins are created, compounds that lead to the principal metabolites are typically detected *in vivo*, namely dihydroxy-urolithins urolithin-A (Uro-A), isourolithin-A (IsoUro-A), and the hydroxyurolothin (Uro-B) (Catalkaya et al., 2020; Plamanda and Vondar 2021).

In summary, the inherently markedly low bioavailability of polyphenols is essentially greatly improved through a variety of gut microbial enzymatic reactions (dihydroxylation, deglycosylation, demethylation) that produce structurally simpler metabolites such as aglycones and monomers that are well absorbed in the intestine and can be subsequently detected in the systemic circulation for a longer time (Shortt et al., 2018). Generally, extensive microbial metabolism ultimately truncates the structural diversity of the native polyphenols to a limited number of mainly simple aromatic metabolites. Other major metabolites that have been seen to be by-products of microbial metabolism in the gut also associated with health effects are short-chain fatty acids (SCFAs) with butyrate being the most prominent and well-studied, branched-chain amino acids (BCAAs) with established signaling properties/functions and LPS (Sikalidis and Maykish, 2020). The SCFAs and BCAAs are typically reported to extend positive health effects by promoting eubiosis, especially in metabolic syndrome, CVD, and cancer, whereas LPS on the contrary appears to have a negative impact through dysbiosis. While these are not derivatives of polyphenols, however, they add to the complexity of the health effects extended to the host as a result of gut microbiome metabolism and the interactions with dietary constituents of naturally consumed mixed diets.

While human studies indicate an increasing number of metabolites appearing at high concentrations in the colon and systemic circulation, interestingly, the biological relevance for most of these metabolites is largely unknown (van Duynhoven et al., 2011). Synergistic deployment of *in vitro* and *in vivo* (humanized mouse) models, as well as human intervention trials, is required in order to unlock the complex metabolic fate of dietary polyphenols.

## Health Effects of Polyphenol/Metabolite-Microbiota Interaction

A variety of common phenolic compounds have been investigated in the context of studies conducted on berries. After their extraction and chemical characterization typically through high-performance liquid chromatography, compounds such as anthocyanins, flavonols, caffeic acid derivatives, ellagic acid derivatives, or ellagitannins were identified. An in-depth study conducted in 2020 by Baenas et al. analyzed polyphenols from raspberry through an *in vitro* fermentation model and metabolites, such as SCFAs. The results showed that the identified polyphenols were mainly hydrolyzable polyphenols found in the insoluble fraction of fibers, and those were identified as the primary compounds responsible for the raspberries' prebiotic effect. The study by Baenas et al. concluded that, through their antimicrobial and antioxidant effects, raspberry and/or raspberry extracts could be utilized as a prebiotic substrate in foods, functional foods, as well as in dietary supplements. In another work focusing on berries' polyphenols and their impact on gut microbiota, the authors reported that a high quantity of polyphenols can effectively reach the colon, thus actively further producing a host of metabolites. Berries' polyphenols were shown to produce changes in the bacteria population, specifically enhancing the growth of *Bifidobacterium*, *Lactobacillus*, *Akkermansia*, *Bacteroides*, and *Eubacterium*, while simultaneously decreasing the extent of the populations for *Pseudomonas*, *Salmonella*, *Staphylococcus*, or *Bacillus*. The mechanism whereby *in vitro* approaches are followed in studies to identify the effects of polyphenols on gut microbiota still requires deeper understanding; however, the ability for high production of SCFAs has been identified repeatedly and corroborated by several studies and as such could lend strong support illustrating the prebiotic-like effect polyphenols seem to extend (Plamanda and Vondar 2021).

A food particularly rich in polyphenols is grapes. Polyphenols in grapes can be found mainly in the fruit in native form, but also wine or wine by-products, through the grape pomace. The most common polyphenols identified in grapes are quercetin, anthocyanins, anthocyanosides, anthocyanidins, catechins, and PACs. Previous studies conducted on the fruit, wine, wine industry by-products, and grape extracts have demonstrated the ability of polyphenols to influence the intestinal bacteria, with significant stimulation of the *Lactobacillus* and *Bifidobacterium* genera. Polyphenols were able to be used as a carbon source by these beneficial bacteria. Another manuscript published in 2018 showed modifications in the bacteria ratio from gut microbiota (Gil-Sánchez et al., 2018). There was an increase of *Enterococcus*, *Prevotella*, *Bacteroides*, *Bifidobacterium*, *Bacteroides uniformis*, *Eggerthella lenta*, *Blautia coccoides–Eubacterium rectale* groups, as well as a decrease of *Actinobacteria*, *Clostridium* spp., *C. histolyticum* group. In the case of dealcoholized wine intake, an increase in the *Fusobacteria/Firmicutes* population and a decrease in the *Actinobacteria* population (Gil-Sánchez et al., 2018; Sáyago-Ayerdi et al., 2019) were noted. In general, gram-positive (gram+) bacteria are prone to be enriched in the gut rather than gram negatives (gram−) when polyphenols are ingested because of the difference in their cell wall composition. Gram-negative bacteria are more impervious to flavan-3-ols than gram-positive bacteria.

Recent evidence from research on the gut microbiome has prompted a shift of focus on health and disease, highlighting the idea that consumption of a healthier diet reduces disease risk at the microbiota level which in turn reduces the disease risk further, utilizing eubiotic mechanisms not yet fully understood. While the protective role of polyphenols depends, to some extent, on interindividual variations of metabolism by gut microbiota, polyphenol consumption is associated with protection against CVD, metabolic syndrome, and cognitive decline (Derrien et al., 2017). Specific polyphenols such as isoflavones, lignans, and ellagitannins are biotransformed by gut microbes to equol, enterolignans (enterolactone or enterodiol), and urolithins, respectively. The binding of the produced phytoestrogens to estrogen receptors can confer protection against breast and prostate cancer by suppressing oncogenes. Moreover, glucosinolates, typically received via consumption of cruciferous plants of the Brassicaceae family, are the precursors of isothiocyanates. Furthermore, bacterial or plant myrosinases convert glucosinolates into isothiocyanates, and glucosinolates, post-ingestion of cooked crucifers, are converted into isothiocyanates by gut microbial myrosinases. These transformations produce metabolites that extend further protection against tumorigenesis (Derrien et al., 2017).

There is evidence to suggest that fruits, vegetables, cereals, and coffee contain conjugated hydroxycinnamates, and antioxidant and anti-inflammatory compounds that are activated post-microbial biotransformation. Interestingly, members of *Bifidobacterium*, *Lactobacillus*, and *Escherichia* in the human gut have been shown to hydrolyze esters of caffeic and ferulic acids, hence transforming the ester conjugates naturally found in plants to the respectively active compounds of caffeic acid, ferulic acid, and p-coumaric acid that are shown to yield health benefits pertinent to their antioxidant potential (Carmody and Turnbaugh, 2014). Other similar examples of microbial biotransformation of dietary-derived compounds producing bioactives include the production of the nonsteroidal estrogen equol from the soy-derived isoflavonoid daidzein and liberation of aglycones with anticancer properties from anthocyanins (Tsuji et al., 2012; Selma et al., 2009). An important aspect to be considered is that the polyphenols are catabolized in the colon by the gut microbiota into metabolites, which have greater bioavailability and more potent anti-inflammatory properties compared to their precursors.

Studies have proposed potential mechanisms via which the polyphenol microbiota interaction may reduce the risk for carcinogenesis, i.e., via a reduction of inflammation and/or abrogation of cell proliferation signaling combined with the induction of apoptosis. The anti-inflammatory action of resveratrol for example involves inhibition of pro-inflammatory moderators, modification of eicosanoid synthesis, and inhibition of enzymes, such as COX-2, NF-κB, AP-1, TNF-α, IL-6, and VEGF. In cells, several phenolic compounds impede COX-2 function, probably by complexing with the enzyme (Namasivayam N, 2011). Notably, both urolithins A and B, being the most representative microbial metabolites of dietary ellagitannins, have demonstrated estrogenic function in a dose-dependent manner, even at high concentrations (40 microM), without antiproliferative or toxic effects toward MCF-7 breast cancer cells (Cardona et al., 2013). In an LT97 human adenoma cell line, it was demonstrated that certain intestinal polyphenol metabolites 3,4-dihydroxyphenylacetic acid and 3-(3,4-dihydroxyphenyl)-propionic acid, metabolites of quercetin and chlorogenic acid/caffeic acid upregulate GSTT2 and downregulate COX-2, a combined effect that could plausibly contribute to the chemopreventive potential of polyphenols, post-gut biotransformation (Cardona et al., 2013).

Markedly, in a study by Monagas et al., the authors observed that dihydroxylated phenolic acids (3,4-dihydroxyphenylpropionic acid, 3-hydroxyphenylpropionic acid, and 3,4-dihydroxyphenylacetic acid) derived from microbial metabolism of PACs, presented marked *In vitro* anti inflammatory properties, reducing the secretion of TNF-α, IL-1b, and IL-6 in LPS-stimulated peripheral blood mononuclear cells from healthy participants (Monagas et al., 2009). It has been advocated that these microbial metabolites could be among the new generation of therapeutic agents for the management of immunoinflammatory diseases such as atherosclerosis, but also for stifling the inflammatory response to bacterial antigens, which plausibly extends significant implications in terms of chronic inflammatory or autoimmune diseases such as inflammatory bowel disease (Cardona et al., 2013).

Interestingly, Beloborodova *et al.* analyzed the role of phenolic acids of microbial origin as biomarkers in the progress of sepsis. They reported that *p*-hydroxyphenylacetic acid was able to prevent reactive oxygen species production in neutrophils. By acting on neutrophils, there is retardation of immune responses, however, when acting on mitochondria, there is preclusion or attenuation of multiple organ failure. Thus, during the development of bacteremia and purulent foci of infection associated with *P. aeruginosa* and *Acinetobacter baumanii*, their metabolite, *p*-hydroxyphenylacetic acid, can directly enter the systemic blood flow and inhibit the phagocytic activity of neutrophils (Beloborodova et al., 2012).

While limited studies are investigating these relationships in humans, some representative characteristic examples are discussed below. In healthy men, a single intake of approximately 240 g of fresh blueberries, rich in polyphenols such as anthocyanins, was shown to increase flow-mediated dilation (FMD), accompanied by increases in plasma concentrations of phenolic metabolites such as vanillic acid, homovanillic acid, benzoic acid, hippuric acid, and hydroxyhippuric acid. Hence, sufficient residence time of blueberry metabolites in the circulation allows for their vascular activity to be exerted. In addition, blueberries induced a dose-dependent and biphasic increase in FMD, while the elevation in plasma polyphenol metabolites occurred in tandem with FMD improvement (Rodriguez-Mateos et al., 2013).

Dietary intervention with 66 healthy men consuming polyphenols from Aronia berry (extract or fruit) for 12 weeks demonstrated significant associations between changes in endothelial function, plasma metabolites of Aronia berry polyphenols, and specific gut microbial genera. FMD, used to assess endothelial function, increased alongside changes in the gut microbiota. Aronia (poly)phenol-rich extract (116 mg, 75 g berries) was shown to increase the growth of Anaerostipes and whole fruit powder (12 mg, 10 g berries) caused a notable increase in Bacteroides, without any changes in the diversity of gut microbiota in either treatment (Istas et al., 2019). The authors concluded that in healthy men, Aronia consumption resulted in improved endothelial function and positively modulated gut microbiota composition, indicating a potential benefit for maintaining cardiovascular health (Istas et al., 2019).

Moreover, *A. muciniphila* was reported to be induced post-consumption of pomegranate extract (rich in hydrolyzable ellagitannins) in 16 out of the 20 healthy participants that were producing urolithin-A (Li et al., 2015). Nevertheless, in a separate study with 49 healthy overweight or obese participants consuming a higher dose of a different pomegranate extract, no significant alterations were observed for *A. muciniphila* (Gonzalez-Sarrias et al., 2017). A clinical trial with obese insulin-resistant patients showed that resveratrol, a natural phenolic compound, increased the abundance of *A. muciniphila* in Caucasians but not in other ethnic groups (Verhoog et al., 2019). In conclusion, there is a variety of gut bacteria that can produce metabolic by-product compounds when exposed to polyphenols and may promote health in humans.

There is a series of recent human studies that aimed to use different approaches to delineate the effects of plant polyphenols on the gut microbiota. Basak et al. recently studied the efficacy of curcumin on tumor suppression. More specifically, a double-blind, randomized, placebo-controlled phase 1 clinical trial was conducted with APG-157 in 13 normal subjects and 12 patients with oral cancer. Two doses of 100 or 200 mg were delivered transorally every hour for 3 hours. Blood and saliva were collected before and 1, 2, 3, and 24 hours after treatment. Electrocardiograms and blood tests did not demonstrate any toxicity. Curcumin was found in the blood and tumor tissues. Inflammatory markers and Bacteroides species were found to be decreased in the saliva, and immune T-cells were increased in the tumor tissue. APG-157 is absorbed well, reduces inflammation, and attracts T-cells to the tumor, suggesting its potential use in combination with immunotherapy drugs. Though endowed with properties of tumor cell suppression due to its antioxidant and anti-inflammatory actions, curcumin is poorly absorbed when administered orally and consequently less effective. APG-157, a botanical drug containing curcumin among other polyphenols, on the other hand, is absorbed well and is reported to be potentially beneficial when combined with immunotherapy by reducing inflammation and increasing T-cell concentration in the tumor (Basak et al., 2020).

Vetrani and colleagues showed that a diet naturally rich in polyphenols and/or long-chain $n-3$ polyunsaturated fatty acids (LCn3) increased the diversity of the predominant fecal bacteria; the polyphenols increased *Clostridium leptum* (clostridial cluster IV), which was directly associated with good glucose tolerance, by early secretion of insulin. More specifically, 78 individuals with high waist circumference and at least one additional component of the metabolic syndrome were randomized to an isoenergetic 8-week diet: (a) low LCn3 and polyphenols; (b) high LCn3; (c) high polyphenols; or (d) high LCn3 and polyphenols. Microbiota analysis was performed on feces collected before and after the intervention. Denaturing gradient gel electrophoresis (DGGE) analysis of the predominant bacteria, *Eubacterium rectale* and *Blautia coccoides* group (Lachnospiraceae, EREC), *C. leptum* (Ruminococcaceae, CLEPT), *Bacteroides* spp., *Bifidobacteria*, and *Lactobacillus* group was performed. A quantitative real-time PCR was performed for the same group additionally including the Atopobium cluster (*Coriobacteriaceae*). Before and after the intervention, participants underwent a 75 g oral glucose tolerance test and a high-fat test meal to evaluate glucose and lipid response. The authors reported that polyphenols significantly increased microbial diversity and CLEPT but reduced EREC. LCn3 significantly increased the numbers of Bifidobacteria. Thus, it was concluded that diets naturally rich in polyphenols or LCn3 influenced gut microbiota composition in individuals at high cardiometabolic risk, with these modifications associated with changes in glucose/lipid metabolism (Vetrani et al., 2020).

In an *in vitro* colon system study, polyphenol-rich fractions of blueberry-containing anthocyanins/flavonol glycosides (ANTH/FLAV), PACs, sugar/acid fraction (S/A), and total polyphenols (TPP) had a distinct effect on fecal microbiota composition. Effective promotion of microbiome alpha diversity was observed with ANTH/FLAV, and PAC fractions as opposed to the S/A and TPP fractions, which has been attributed to the differentially responsive taxa. Older compared to the younger group showed an abundance of gut microbiota diversity with blueberry consumption, which correlated with increased plasma antioxidant activity (Ntemiri et al., 2020).

Flavonoid-rich orange juice treatment, in contrast to flavonoid-low treatment, resulted in an abundance of Lachnospiraceae family—namely Lachnospiraceae_uc, Eubacterium_g4, Roseburia_uc, Coprococcus_g_uc, and Agathobacter_uc—and showed a positive correlation with brain-derived neurotrophic factor. Treatment with flavonoids also improved depression in young adults, probably due to an alteration of the stool microbiome (Park et al., 2020).

A randomized, double-blinded, crossover clinical trial, comparing urinary excretion of isoflavones and their metabolites, after a soybean meal and fermented soybean meal (FSBM) consumption, suggested a benefit for FSBM, in terms of higher excretion of all metabolites, a higher (67%) urinary recovery of isoflavones, and prevalence of O-demethylangolensin-producer metabotype (72%), while that of equol producer was similar (11%) and nonproducer was low (17%). The findings suggest an improvement in the bioavailability of isoflavones and a reduction in the impact of gut microbiota on its metabolism following fermentation (de Oliveira Silva et al., 2020).

A crossover interventional trial studying the impact of increased intestinal permeability on the bioavailability of polyphenols and results showed a significant difference in the urinary levels of phase II and microbiota-derived metabolites in participants with healthier barrier integrity and those with disrupted integrity. The disturbance in the gut microbial metabolism and phase II methylation process and the microbiota-derived metabolites were found to be responsible for the biological activity of dietary polyphenols against age-related intestinal permeability disruption (Hidalgo-Liberona et al., 2020).

In a study comparing the efficacy of green tea and its extract epigallocatechin-3-gallate (EGCG) as an antimicrobial in mouthwash in children, the results showed a significant reduction in the two mutants of streptococci and lactobacilli in the oral cavity after rinsing with EGCG solution. Even though ECGC demonstrated a better antimicrobial activity, both EGCG and green tea were found to be alternatives to chlorhexidine-based mouthwashes (Vilela et al., 2020).

An improved insulin sensitivity consequent to an increase in the phosphorylation of adenosine monophosphate protein kinase in the skeletal muscles of obese participants was observed with consumption of genistein for 2 months. The improvement in insulin sensitivity is also attributed to an increase in *A. muciniphila,* following a decrease in gut microbiota dysbiosis and metabolic endotoxemia, after genistein treatment (Guevara-Cruz et al., 2020).

A placebo-controlled interventional study in athletes elucidated a beneficiary effect of a daily intake of 5 g of cocoa (425 mg of flavanols), with a significant reduction of body fat percentage, especially in the trunk, viscera, and lower limbs, associated with an elevation of plasma follistatin and decrease in leptin, while the myostatin levels remained static. Despite the reduction in body fat, the performance status of these athletes remained status quo (Ángel García-Merino et al., 2020).

Daily consumption of orange juice showed improvement in the blood biochemical parameters including low-density lipoprotein cholesterol, insulin sensitivity, and glucose in young women. It also showed a positive and beneficial change in the composition and metabolic activity of the microbiota and an increase in the population of fecal *Bifidobacterium* spp. and *Lactobacillus* spp. A PCR-DGGE of the microbiota found that the composition of total bacteria was similar. A reduction in ammonia and an increase in the production of SCFAs were also elucidated. The study implies a positive effect on the daily consumption of orange juice in young women (Lima et al., 2019).

Consumption of an olive pomace-enriched biscuit formulation (OEP), which delivers $17.1 \pm 4.01$ mg/100 g of hydroxytyrosol and its derivative on analysis, showed an upregulation of the microbial polyphenol biotransformation in the intestine, as evidenced by a significant increase in the excretion of small phenolic acids in urine. OEP also significantly elevated homovanillic acid and 3,4-dihydroxyphenylacetic acid in fasted plasma samples, indicating clearance of these compounds from blood and an extended release and uptake from the intestine. However, the study failed to show any change in ox-LDL or urinary isoprostane (Conterno et al., 2019).

A study on the targets of curcumin natural polyphenols on nonalcoholic fatty liver disease determined amino acids, TCA cycle, bile acids, and gut microbiota. Phospholipid curcumin supplement led to a significant reduction in 3-methyl-2-oxovaleric acid, 3-hydroxyisobutyrate, kynurenine, succinate, citrate, $\alpha$-ketoglutarate, methylamine, trimethylamine, hippurate, indoxyl sulfate, chenodeoxycholic acid, taurocholic acid, and lithocholic acid (Chashmniam et al., 2019).

Dietary intervention with functional foods in patients with T2DM who exhibit intestinal dysbiosis, characterized by an increase in *Prevotella copri*, showed a reduction in *P. copri* and increased species with anti-inflammatory effects, namely *Faecalibacterium prausnitzii* and *A. muciniphilia*. A significant reduction in area under curve for glucose, total and LDL cholesterol, FFA, HbA1c, triglyceride, and CRP, as well as an increase in antioxidant activity was also observed. The study suggested a beneficial effect on fecal microbiota, pointing to novel avenues for improving glycemic control, dyslipidemia, and inflammation with long-term adherence to high-fiber, polyphenol-enriched, vegetable-protein-based diet (Medina-Vera et al., 2019).

In another study, Kim and colleagues showed that mango (*Mangifera indica* L.) polyphenols reduce IL-8, growth-related oncogene (GRO), and GM-SCF plasma levels and increase Lactobacillus species in a pilot study in patients with inflammatory bowel disease (Kim et al., 2020). In this study, ten participants received a daily dose of 200–400 g of mango pulp for 8 weeks. Mango intake significantly improved the primary outcome, Simple Clinical Colitis Activity Index score, and decreased the plasma levels of pro-inflammatory cytokines including interleukin-8 (IL-8), GRO, and granulocyte macrophage colony-stimulating factor by 16.2% ($p = 0.0475$), 25.0% ($p = 0.0375$), and 28.6% ($p = 0.0485$), all factors related to neutrophil-induced inflammation, respectively. Mango intake beneficially altered fecal microbial composition by significantly increasing the abundance of *Lactobacillus* spp., *Lactobacillus plantarum*, *Lactobacillus reuteri*, and *Lactobacillus lactis*, which was accompanied by increased fecal butyric acid production. Therefore, an enriching diet with mango fruits or potentially other gallotannin-rich foods seems to be a promising adjuvant therapy combined with conventional medications in the management of IBD via reducing biomarkers of inflammation and modulating the intestinal microbiota (Kim et al., 2020).

Yang and colleagues studied the effect of standardized grape powder consumption, a rich source of polyphenols and fiber, on the gut microbiome of healthy participants. More specifically, 46 g of whole grape powder, providing the equivalent of two servings of California table grapes, were assessed as per their effects on the gut microbiome in healthy adults. The study included a 4-week standardization to a low-polyphenol diet, followed by 4 weeks of 46 g of grape powder consumption while continuing the low-polyphenol diet. Compared to the baseline, 4 weeks of grape powder consumption significantly increased the alpha diversity index of the gut microbiome. The authors concluded that grape powder consumption significantly modified the gut microbiome (Yang et al., 2021).

In separate experiments through a small-scale pilot study, Ezzat-Zadeh and coworkers reported that California strawberry consumption increased the abundance of gut microorganisms related to lean body weight, health, and longevity in healthy participants (Ezzat-Zadeh et al., 2021). More specifically, 15 healthy adults consumed a beige diet + 26 g of freeze-dried strawberry powder (SBP) for 4 weeks, followed by 2 weeks of beige diet only. Stool samples were collected at 0, 4, and 6 weeks. Fecal microbiota was analyzed by 16S rRNA sequencing. Fecal cholesterol, bile acid (BA), and microbial metabolites were assessed via gas chromatography. Daily SBP altered the abundance of 24 operational taxonomic units (OTUs). Comparing week 4 to baseline, the most significant increases were observed for one OTU from Firmicutes\Clostridia\Christensenellaceae\NA, one OTU from Firmicutes\Clostridia\Mogibacteriacea\NA, one OTU from Verrucomicrobia\Verrucomicrobiaceae\Akkermansia muciniphila, one OTU from Actinobacteria\Bifidobacteriaceae\Bifidobacterium\NA, and one OTU from Bacteroidetes\Bacteroidia\Bacteroidaceae\Bacteroides and a decrease of one OTU from Proteobacteria\Betaproteobacteria\Alcaligenaceae\Sutterella. Comparing weeks 4–6, we observed a reversal of the same OTUs from C Christensenellaceae, V muciniphilia, and C Mogibacteriaceae. Fecal SCFAs and most of the fecal markers including cholesterol, coprostanol, and primary and secondary BAs were not changed significantly except for lithocholic acid, which was increased significantly at week 6 compared to baseline (Ezzat-Zadeh et al., 2021).

Wilson and collaborators investigated SunGold kiwi fruit supplementation of individuals with prediabetes and demonstrated that such supplementation alters gut microbiota and improves vitamin C status as well as anthropometric and clinical markers. More specifically, two SunGold kiwifruit per day over 12 weeks were consumed by participants ($n = 24$). Venous blood samples were collected at each study visit (baseline, 6, and 12 weeks) to determine glycemic indices, plasma vitamin C concentrations, hormones, lipid profiles, and high-sensitivity CRP. Participants provided a fecal sample at each study visit. DNA was extracted from the fecal samples and a region of the 16S ribosomal RNA gene was amplified and sequenced to determine fecal microbiota composition. Compared to a baseline measurement, the results of 12 weeks showed a significant increase in plasma vitamin C (14 μmol/L, $p < 0.001$). There was a significant reduction in both diastolic (4 mmHg, $p = 0.029$) and systolic (6 mmHg, $p = 0.003$) blood pressure and a significant reduction in waist circumference (3.1 cm, $p = 0.001$) and waist-to-hip ratio (0.01, $p = 0.032$). Results also showed a decrease in HbA1c (1 mmol/mol, $p = 0.005$) and an increase in fasting glucose (0.1 mmol/L, $p = 0.046$); however, these changes were small and were not clinically significant (Wilson et al., 2018).

An interesting study investigating the effects of a dietary supplement on the gut microbiota was a recent study by Shin and colleagues (Shin et al., 2021). The researchers evaluated the effects of *Saengshik* supplementation on the gut microbial composition among healthy Korean adults in a pilot study. *Saengshik* is a type of meal replacement product or dietary supplement comprising an uncooked and dried plant-based food mixture with various health-promoting properties, such as anti-diabetic, anti-dyslipidemic, antioxidant, and anticancer properties. The researchers conducted a single-group design trial involving 102 healthy men and women who received a 40 g/day dose of *Saengshik* powder as a dietary supplement for 8 weeks, during which stool samples were collected at two fixed time points (baseline and the endpoint) for gut microbiota profiling analysis. The authors reported a significant decrease in the α-diversity of gut microbiota after *Saengshik* consumption ($p$ <0.05), with significant changes evident in the composition of major microbial taxa, such as *Bacteroidetes* ($p$ <0.0001), *Proteobacteria*, *Actinobacteria*, as well as *Verrucomicrobia* ($p$ <0.0001). Markedly, the gut microbial response was strongly related to the interindividual variability of habitual dietary intake and enterotype at baseline (Shin et al., 2021). The obtained results suggest that individual habitual diet patterns, as well as gut microbial shapes, should be considered as key aspects when supplementation strategies are aimed at the optimization of gut microflora as designed.

Recent research and clinical trials have identified the beneficial effects of a plant-based diet to increase bacterial diversity and ameliorate various disorders, including intestinal disorders, obesity-related endotoxemia, and cardiovascular disorders (Vazhappilly et al., 2019, 2021; Guglielmetti et al., 2020).

## Considerations on Limitations of Human Studies, Novel Metabolic Approaches, and Metabotypes

Even though there is a significantly large body of evidence in support of the gut microbiome's role and specific enzymes in the biotransformation of polyphenols, there are still significant aspects of the interplay between the microbiome and polyphenol metabolism that need to be unlocked. It appears that gut bacteria possess innate mechanisms, allowing them to generate *de novo* and potentially highly bioactive compounds when exposed to dietary polyphenols.

In this regard, innovative approaches are essential to reveal the precise activities of certain bacteria and the exact role they play in the biotransformation of polyphenols. One such approach entails gut bacterial population characterization, using metagenomic binning of bacterial DNA methylation to create bacterial barcodes for efficient identification of unique bacterial strains. Other efforts employ gnotobiotic and germ-free mice to manipulate bacterial populations so as to better understand host metabolism. Such novel approaches can enhance identification of the distinctive metabolism of gut microbiota, different among individuals, as well as elucidate how this may regulate bioavailability and modulate the bioactivity of polyphenolic metabolites (Pasinetti et al., 2018). These approaches could provide more insights as to the interpersonal variation usually observed in the microbiome and metabolite types in human trials. Such complex polyphenol–microbiota interactions, which are determined notably by interindividual variability leading to different polyphenol-metabolizing phenotypes or "metabotypes", may be the key in terms of a more personalized approach for the optimization of diet and health with the involvement of the microbiome (Bolca et al., 2013). The term "metabotype" refers to a particular metabolic phenotype with specific gut microbiome-derived metabolites, which characterize metabolism of the parent compound (i.e., nutrient, pharmaceutical, and toxin) (Espin et al., 2017).

In general, limited human studies have studied metabotypes. More specifically, a pilot study assessed the phenolic compound capsaicin and reported stronger effects on metabolic and inflammatory markers in healthy participants of the Bacteroides enterotype compared to those of the Prevotella enterotype (Kang et al., 2016). Other researchers reported that an interaction was observed between gut bacterial profiles and enterolignan production in response to lipid levels after 1 week of intervention in healthy normal-weight participants (Lagkouvardos et al., 2015). Interestingly, even though the ability to stratify the population based on their capacity to produce specific microbial-derived metabolites in response to certain polyphenols and the impact of this differential on health has not been investigated significantly, most available evidence pertains to the correlation of certain metabotypes to isoflavones and ellagitannins. More specifically, randomized clinical trials have demonstrated that patients' capacity to produce the microbial metabolites equol and O-desmethylangolesin (ODMA) has been shown to reduce the risk for CVD (Espin et al., 2017). Ellagitannins represent another interesting example of a nexus between a specific metabotype and a polyphenolic compound(s). In this regard, there are three distinct metabotypes: (a) type A which is characterized by excretion of Uro-A and related conjugates as the final urolithin; (b) type B which produces Uro-B and/or IsoUro-A additionally to Uro-A; and (c) type 0 which does not produce any of these urolithins. Interestingly, metabotype B has been correlated with obesity, metabolic syndrome, and colorectal cancer, hence suggesting a potential role in dysbiosis for this metabotype (Espin et al., 2017). Furthermore, in certain human trials with overweight participants, while metabotype A was positively associated with HDL cholesterol, metabotype B was associated with VLDL (Selma et al., 2009). These interesting results could at least partly contribute to a potential explanation for mixed and nonconclusive results in the case of polyphenol-rich dietary supplementations such as the earlier case of the pomegranate study, for example. Interindividual variability regarding the improvement of cardiovascular risk in 49 healthy overweight or obese participants consuming pomegranate was explained by urolithin metabotypes (Gonzalez-Sarrias et al., 2017). Although the exact mechanisms explaining the gut microbiota/polyphenol interplay-related impact on human health remains under investigation, it appears that microbiota-derived bioactive metabolites from dietary polyphenols are primarily involved in such effects.

Finally, it is important to consider the overall diet in addition to the interventions made in terms of polyphenols when microbiota is considered. There is strong evidence supporting the plasticity of the microbiome and it is significantly influenced by the dietary regimen of the individual regardless of other factors. For example, in a cross-sectional study, Noh et al. investigated the association of habitual dietary intake with the taxonomic composition and diversity of the human gut microbiota among 222 Koreans aged 18–58 years (Noh et al., 2021). Gut microbiota data were obtained by 16S rRNA gene sequencing on DNA extracted from fecal samples. The habitual dict for the year previous to the study was evaluated through a food frequency questionnaire. After multivariable adjustment, intake of several food groups, including vegetables, fermented legumes, legumes, dairy products, processed meat, and nonalcoholic beverages, were associated with major phyla of the gut microbiota. A dietary pattern related to higher α-diversity (HiαDP) derived by reduced rank regression was characterized by higher intakes of fermented legumes, vegetables, seaweeds, and nuts/seeds and lower intakes of nonalcoholic beverages. The HiαDP was found to be positively associated with several genera of *Firmicutes* such as *Lactobacillus*, *Ruminococcus*, and *Eubacterium* ($p$ <0.05). Among enterotypes identified by principal coordinate analysis based on the β-diversity, the *Ruminococcus* enterotype exhibited higher HiαDP scores and was strongly positively associated with the intake of vegetables, seaweeds, and nuts/seeds, compared to the two other enterotypes. The authors concluded that a plant- and fermented food-based diet was positively associated with certain genera of Firmicutes indicative of improved gut microbial health. Their conclusions indicate that diet is a very strong determinant, in its own right, of the microbiota profile in humans, which should be appreciated and considered as such in studies and therapeutic approaches.

Moreover, significant in size, human studies with long-term assessment of diet also support further the point discussed above. More specifically, Yu et al. showed that long-term diet quality is associated with gut microbiome diversity and composition in urban Chinese adults (Yu et al., 2021). The studies comprised 1,920 men and women, enrolled in two prospective cohorts (baseline 1996 2006), who remained free of CVDs, diabetes, and cancer at stool collection (2015–2018) and had no diarrhea or antibiotic use in the last 7 days before stool collection. The microbiome was profiled by 16S rRNA sequencing. Long-term diet was assessed by repeated surveys at baseline and follow-ups (1996–2011), with intervals of 5.2–20.5 years between dietary surveys and stool collection. Associations of dietary variables with microbiome diversity and composition were evaluated by linear or negative binomial hurdle models, adjusting for potential confounders. False discovery rate (FDR) <0.1 was considered significant. Diet quality was positively associated with microbiome α-diversity and abundance of *Firmicutes, Actinobacteria, Tenericutes*, and genera/species within these phyla, including *Coprococcus, Faecalibacterium/Faecalibacterium prausnitzii, Bifidobacterium/ Bifidobacterium adolescentis*, and order RF39 (all FDRs <0.1). Significant associations were also observed for intakes of dairy, fish/seafood, nuts/legumes, refined grains, and processed meat, including a positive association of dairy with *Bifidobacterium* and inverse associations of processed meat with *Roseburia/Roseburia faecis*. Most associations were similar, with or without adjustment for BMI and hypertension status or excluding participants with antibiotic use in the past 6 months (Yu et al., 2021).

Overall, there are limited studies in humans, typically with a small number of participants examining the effect of polyphenols on the configuration and activity of the gut microbiome. This represents an important gap in our understanding regarding the polyphenol–microbe interactions in humans. Nonetheless, there is some evidence mostly in the form of *in vitro, in vivo* studies, while more rarely clinical studies, suggesting that particular doses of specific polyphenols do extend modulation of the gut microbial populations; hence, as certain bacterial groups can be inhibited, others can thrive. While this concept carries biological plausibility, further research is warranted and more results need to be obtained for such a relationship to be established and most critically a mechanistic explanation to be derived.

In conclusion, all the findings suggest that in addition to the dietary polyphenols, their microbial metabolites must also be taken into consideration when assessing the impact of polyphenols on the host's health. Despite the recent surge of interest in their relationship and our increased appreciation of this dynamic cross talk between dietary polyphenols and gut microbiota, we are far from fully grasping their therapeutic potential for employing informed strategies in medical nutrition therapy and/or microbial therapeutic interventions. However, smartly manipulating the gut microbiota through dietary interventions for the prevention or treatment of disorders might lead to the enrichment of "personalized nutrition" to be more comprehensive in its considerations and help better understand the effects of dietary bioactive compounds on the host microbiome.

From a clinical perspective and through a lens of developing therapeutic pharmaceuticals and schemes, there is strong evidence from human studies that polyphenols contribute to disease prevention and the overall properties (antioxidant, anti-inflammatory) contribute to the favorable health outcomes documented (Safe et al., 2021). However, it is equally evident from mechanistic *in vitro* and *in vivo* studies that individual compounds as well as their mixtures modulate activity and/or expression of multiple genes and downstream responses at various levels and degrees. For example, similarly to other flavonoids, genistein interacts directly with multiple tyrosine kinases, G-protein coupled receptors, and intracellular receptors alike. Therefore, a potential clinical application utilizing genistein that would target a single gene/pathway is rather complicated due to its diverse activities and highly possible off-target effects. Discerning the successful development of clinical applications of polyphenols, a series of requirements pertinent to mechanistic precision medicine approaches need to be considered and include the following aspects:

I. Development of improved overall and tissue-specific delivery methods to enhance the overall bioavailability of flavonoids.
II. Response-specific mechanisms for inflammatory and age-related diseases need to be identified and utilized for treatment.
III. After successfully identifying mechanism-based intracellular targets required for specific polyphenol-mediating responses, structure–activity studies need to be conducted to identify the optimally most active (ideal) compound.
IV. Applications need to be maximized using optimal combinations of compounds, thus creating powerful and effective cocktails.
V. Consider incorporation of bioengineering to positively influence cellular and community dynamics which could amplify desirable therapeutic responses.

Another limitation in phenolic compound-related research and potential applications in human health is that typically, existing studies have generally ignored the effect of food matrix and processing conditions. Food components interact, not uncommonly highly selectively, with different forms (e.g., free, bound, and polymerized) of polyphenols. Such interactions significantly affect the bioaccessibility and subsequently the bioavailability that ultimately affect the phenolic compounds and their metabolites. They can directly act on the epithelium to modulate local immune system functions and absorb metabolites into the systemic circulation to have systemic effects on the host. It is a very challenging task for the research community to grasp the relationship fully and delineate the various interplays among the complex gut microbiota, the diverse types, and forms of dietary polyphenols, the varied immunomodulatory ability of the hosts, and connections with gut–brain functions.

Innovative approaches such as that of Foodomics, driven by the integration of the use of advanced-omics technologies, such as transcriptomics, proteomics, and metabolomics, together with biostatistics, chemometrics, and bioinformatics, to allow the evaluation of complex biological systems, as well as the mechanisms of bioactive food compounds that may affect them, are emerging (Valdés et al., 2022). The utilization of such methods has brought a significant change in the field of food science, as the performed research may be redirected to ascertain newfangled associations. For example, by way of Foodomics-related applications, our knowledge regarding the binomial between food/diet and health has widened. Foodomics expand the possibilities toward unraveling the enormous complexity of the Foodome, which has been defined as the pool of all compounds present in a food item and/or in a biological system interacting with the investigated food at a given time (Valdés et al., 2022). The investigation in foods of bioactive compounds which widely vary in chemical structure, including polyphenols, can be meaningfully supported by Foodomics toward understanding function, but also investigating the presence, bioavailability, and biological characteristics (such as toxicity, antioxidant, antiproliferative, or anti-inflammatory properties) of these interesting molecules, while considering different food matrices and processing influences (Valdés et al., 2022). Such approaches may constitute an important and most helpful tool toward advancing our current understanding of those interactions and their effects.

# REFERENCES

Ángel García-Merino J, Moreno-Pérez D, de Lucas B, Montalvo-Lominchar MG, Muñoz E, Sánchez L, Naclerio F, Herrera-Rocha KM, Moreno-Jiménez MR, Rocha-Guzmán NE, Larrosa M. Chronic flavanol-rich cocoa powder supplementation reduces body fat mass in endurance athletes by modifying the follistatin/myostatin ratio and leptin levels. *Food Funct.* 2020;11(4):3441–3450. doi: 10.1039/d0fo00246a.

Aura A. Microbial metabolism of dietary phenolic compounds in the colon. *Phytochem Rev.* 2008;7:407–429. doi: 10.1007/s11101-008-9095-3.

Baenas N, Nuñez-Gómez V, Navarro-González I, Sánchez-Martínez L, García-Alonso J, Periago MJ, González-Barrio R. Raspberry dietary fibre: Chemical properties, functional evaluation and prebiotic in vitro effect. *LWT.* 2020;134:110140. doi: 10.1016/j.lwt.2020.110140.

Basak SK, Bera A, Yoon AJ, Morselli M, Jeong C, Tosevska A, Dong TS, Eklund M, Russ E, Nasser H, Lagishetty V, Guo R, Sajed D, Mudgal S, Mehta P, Avila L, Srivastava M, Faull K, Jacobs J, Pellegrini M, Shin DS, Srivatsan ES, Wang MB. A randomized, phase 1, placebo-controlled trial of APG-157 in oral cancer demonstrates systemic absorption and an inhibitory effect on cytokines and tumor-associated microbes. *Cancer.* 2020;126(8):1668–1682. doi: 10.1002/cncr.32644.

Beloborodova N, Bairamov I, Olenin A, Shubina V, Teplova V, Fedotcheva N. Effect of phenolic acids of microbial origin on production of reactive oxygen species in mitochondria and neutrophils. *J Biomed Sci.* 2012;19:89. doi: 10.1186/1423-0127-19-89.

Bentsáth A, Rusznyák S, Szent-Györgyi A. Vitamin nature of flavones. *Nature.* 1936;138:798. doi: 10.1038/138798a0.

Bohn T, McDougall GJ, Alegría A, et al. Mind the gap-deficits in our knowledge of aspects impacting the bioavailability of phytochemicals and their metabolites – A position paper focusing on carotenoids and polyphenols. *Mol Nutr Food Res.* 2015;59(7): 1307–1323. doi: 10.1002/mnfr.201400745.

Bolca S, Van de Wiele T, Possemiers S. Gut metabotypes govern health effects of dietary polyphenols. *Curr Opin Biotechnol.* 2013;24(2):220–225. doi: 10.1016/j.copbio.2012.09.009.

Burkholder-Cooley N, Rajaram S, Haddad E, Fraser GE, Jaceldo-Siegl K. Comparison of polyphenol intakes according to distinct dietary patterns and food sources in the adventist health Study-2 cohort. *Br J Nutr.* 2016;115(12):2162–2169. doi: 10.1017/ S0007114516001331.

Cardona F, Andrés-Lacueva C, Tulipani S, Tinahones FJ, Queipo-Ortuño MI. Benefits of polyphenols on gut microbiota and implications in human health. *J Nutr Biochem.* 2013;24(8):1415–1422. doi: 10.1016/j.jnutbio.2013.05.001.

Carmody RN, Turnbaugh PJ. Host-microbial interactions in the metabolism of therapeutic and diet-derived xenobiotics. *J Clin Invest.* 2014;124:4173–4181.

Chashmniam S, Mirhafez SR, Dehabeh M, Hariri M, Azimi Nezhad M, Nobakht M Gh BF. A pilot study of the effect of phospholipid curcumin on serum metabolomic profile in patients with non-alcoholic fatty liver disease: A randomized, double-blind, placebo-controlled trial. *Eur J Clin Nutr.* 2019;73(9):1224–1235. doi: 10.1038/s41430-018-0386-5.

Conterno L, Martinelli F, Tamburini M, Fava F, Mancini A, Sordo M, Pindo M, Martens S, Masuero D, Vrhovsek U, Dal Lago C, Ferrario G, Morandini M, Tuohy K. Measuring the impact of olive pomace enriched biscuits on the gut microbiota and its metabolic activity in mildly hypercholesterolaemic subjects. *Eur J Nutr.* 2019;58(1):63–81. doi: 10.1007/ s00394-017-1572-2.

Corella D, Carrasco P, Sorlí JV, Estruch R, Rico-Sanz J, Martínez-González MÁ, Salas-Salvadó J, Covas MI, Coltell O, Arós F, Lapetra J, Serra-Majem L, Ruiz-Gutiérrez V, Warnberg J, Fiol M, Pintó X, Ortega-Azorín C, Muñoz MÁ, Martínez JA, Gómez-Gracia E, González JI, Ros E, Ordovás JM. Mediterranean diet reduces the adverse effect of the TCF7L2-rs7903146 polymorphism on cardiovascular risk factors and stroke incidence: A randomized controlled trial in a high-cardiovascular-risk population. *Diabetes Care.* 2013 Nov;36(11):3803–3811. doi: 10.2337/dc13-0955.

Catalkaya G, Venema K, Lucini L, Rocchetti G, Delmas D, Daglia M, De Filippis A, Xiao H, Quiles JL, Xiao J, et al. Interaction of dietary polyphenols and gut microbiota: Microbial metabolism of polyphenols, influence on the gut microbiota, and implications on host health. *Food Front.* 2020;1.109–133. doi: 10.1002/fft2.25.

Cory H, Passarelli S, Szeto J, Tamez M, Mattei J. The role of polyphenols in human health and food systems: A mini-review. *Front Nutr.* 2018;5:87. doi: 10.3389/fnut.2018.00087.

Crozier A, del Rio D, Clifford MN. Bioavailability of dietary flavonoids and phenolic compounds. *Mol Aspects Med.* 2010;31(6):446–467. doi: 10.1016/j.mam.2010.09.007.

D'Archivio M, Filesi C, Di Benedetto R, Gargiulo R, Giovannini C, Masella R. Polyphenols, dietary sources and bioavailability. *Ann Ist Super Sanita.* 2007;43(4):348–361.

de Oliveira Silva F, Lemos TC, Sandôra D, Monteiro M, Perrone D. Fermentation of soybean meal improves isoflavone metabolism after soy biscuit consumption by adults. *J Sci Food Agric.* 2020;100(7):2991–2998. doi: 10.1002/jsfa.10328.

Derrien M, Veiga P. Rethinking diet to aid human-microbe symbiosis. *Trends Microbiol.* 2017;25(2):100–112. doi: 10.1016/j.tim.2016.09.011.

Di Meo F, Donato S, Di Pardo A, Maglione V, Filosa S, Crispi S. New therapeutic drugs from bioactive natural molecules: The role of gut microbiota metabolism in neurodegenerative diseases. *Curr Drug Metab.* 2018;19:478–489.

Dueñas M, Muñoz-González I, Cueva C, Jiménez-Girón A, Sánchez-Patán F, Santos-Buelga C, Moreno-Arribas MV, Bartolomé B. A survey of modulation of gut microbiota by dietary polyphenols. *Biomed Res Int.* 2015;2015:850902. doi: 10.1155/2015/850902.

Edmands WM, Ferrari P, Rothwell JA, Rinaldi S, Slimani N, Barupal DK, Biessy C, Jenab M, Clavel-Chapelon F, Fagherazzi G, Boutron-Ruault MC, Katzke VA, Kühn T, Boeing H, Trichopoulou A, Lagiou P, Trichopoulos D, Palli D, Grioni S, Tumino R, Vineis P, Mattiello A, Romieu I, Scalbert A. Polyphenol metabolome in human urine and its association with intake of polyphenol-rich foods across European countries. *Am J Clin Nutr.* 2015;102(4):905–913. doi: 10.3945/ajcn.114.101881.

Espín JC, González-Sarrías A, Tomás-Barberán FA. The gut microbiota: A key factor in the therapeutic effects of (poly)phenols. *Biochem Pharmacol.* 2017;139:82–93. doi: 10.1016/j.bcp.2017.04.033.

Ezzat-Zadeh Z, Henning SM, Yang J, Woo SL, Lee RP, Huang J, Thames G, Gilbuena I, Tseng CH, Heber D, Li Z. California strawberry consumption increased the abundance of gut microorganisms related to lean body weight, health and longevity in healthy subjects. *Nutr Res.* 2021;85:60–70. doi: 10.1016/j.nutres.2020.12.006.

Filipski KK, Pacanowski MA, Ramamoorthy A, Feero WG, Freedman AN. Dosing recommendations for pharmacogenetic interactions related to drug metabolism. *Pharmacogenet Genomics.* 2016 Jul;26(7):334–339. doi: 10.1097/FPC.0000000000000220.

Filosa S, Di Meo F, Crispi S. Polyphenols-gut microbiota interplay and brain neuromodulation. *Neural Regen Res.* 2018;13(12):2055–2059. doi: 10.4103/1673-5374.241429.

Gil-Sánchez I, Cueva C, Sanz-Buenhombre M, Guadarrama A, Moreno-Arribas MV, Bartolomé B. Dynamic gastrointestinal digestion of grape pomace extracts: Bioaccessible phenolic metabolites and impact on human gut microbiota. *J. Food Compos. Anal.* 2018; 68:41–52. doi: 10.1016/j.jfca.2017.05.005.

González-Sarrías A, García-Villalba R, Romo-Vaquero M, et al. Clustering according to urolithin metabotype explains the interindividual variability in the improvement of cardiovascular risk biomarkers in overweight-obese individuals consuming pomegranate: A randomized clinical trial. *Mol Nutr Food Res.* 2017;61(5). doi: 10.1002/mnfr.201600830.

Guevara-Cruz M, Godinez-Salas ET, Sanchez-Tapia M, Torres-Villalobos G, Pichardo-Ontiveros E, Guizar-Heredia R, Arteaga-Sanchez L, Gamba G, Mojica-Espinosa R, Schcolnik-Cabrera A, Granados O, López-Barradas A, Vargas-Castillo A, Torre-Villalvazo I, Noriega LG, Torres N, Tovar AR. Genistein stimulates insulin sensitivity through gut microbiota reshaping and skeletal muscle AMPK activation in obese subjects. *BMJ Open Diabetes Res Care.* 2020;8(1):e000948. doi: 10.1136/bmjdrc-2019-000948.

Guglielmetti S, Bernardi S, Del Bo' C, Cherubini A, Porrini M, Gargari G, Hidalgo-Liberona N, Gonzalez-Dominguez R, Peron G, Zamora-Ros R, Winterbone MS, Kirkup B, Kroon PA, Andres-Lacueva C, Riso P. Effect of a polyphenol-rich dietary pattern on intestinal permeability and gut and blood microbiomics in older subjects: Study protocol of the MaPLE randomised controlled trial. *BMC Geriatr.* 2020;20(1):77. doi: 10.1186/s12877-020-1472-9.

Hidalgo-Liberona N, González-Domínguez R, Vegas E, Riso P, Del Bo' C, Bernardi S, Peron G, Guglielmetti S, Gargari G, Kroon PA, Cherubini A, Andrés-Lacueva C. Increased intestinal permeability in older subjects impacts the beneficial effects of dietary polyphenols by modulating their bioavailability. *J Agric Food Chem.* 2020;68(44):12476–12484. doi: 10.1021/acs.jafc.0c04976

Istas G, Wood E, Le Sayec M, Rawlings C, Yoon J, Dandavate V, Cera D, Rampelli S, Costabile A, Fromentin E, Rodriguez-Mateos A. Effects of aronia berry (poly)phenols on vascular function and gut microbiota: A double-blind randomized controlled trial in adult men. *Am J Clin Nutr.* 2019;110(2):316–329. doi: 10.1093/ajcn/nqz075.

Kang C, Zhang Y, Zhu X, et al. Healthy subjects differentially respond to dietary capsaicin correlating with specific gut enterotypes. *J Clin Endocrinol Metab.* 2016;101(12): 4681–4689. doi: 10.1210/jc.2016-2786.

Kim H, Venancio VP, Fang C, Dupont AW, Talcott ST, Mertens-Talcott SU. Mango (Mangifera indica L.) polyphenols reduce IL-8, GRO, and GM-SCF plasma levels and increase Lactobacillus species in a pilot study in patients with inflammatory bowel disease. *Nutr Res.* 2020;75:85–94. doi: 10.1016/j.nutres.2020.01.002.

Kristo AS, Klimis-Zacas D, Sikalidis AK. Protective role of dietary berries in cancer. *Antioxidants (Basel).* 2016;5(4):37. Published 2016 Oct 19. doi: 10.3390/antiox5040037.

Lacombe A, Li RW, Klimis-Zacas D, Kristo AS, Tadepalli S, Krauss E, Young R, Wu VC. Lowbush wild blueberries have the potential to modify gut microbiota and xenobiotic metabolism in the rat colon. *PLoS One.* 2013;8(6):e67497. doi: 10.1371/journal. pone.0067497.

Lagkouvardos I, Kläring K, Heinzmann SS, et al. Gut metabolites and bacterial community networks during a pilot intervention study with flaxseeds in healthy adult men. *Mol Nutr Food Res.* 2015;59(8):1614–1628. doi: 10.1002/mnfr.201500125.

Li Z, Henning SM, Lee RP, et al. Pomegranate extract induces ellagitannin metabolite formation and changes stool microbiota in healthy volunteers. *Food Funct.* 2015;6(8): 2487–2495. doi: 10.1039/c5fo00669d.

Lima ACD, Cecatti C, Fidélix MP, Adorno MAT, Sakamoto IK, Cesar TB, Sivieri K. Effect of daily consumption of orange juice on the levels of blood glucose, lipids, and gut microbiota metabolites: Controlled clinical trials. *J Med Food.* 2019;22(2):202–210. doi: 10.1089/jmf.2018.0080.

Luca SV, Macovei I, Bujor A, Miron A, Skalicka-Woźniak K, Aprotosoaie AC, Trifan A. Bioactivity of dietary polyphenols: The role of metabolites. *Crit Rev Food Sci Nutr.* 2020; 60(4):626–659.

Mahajan R, Attri S, Mehta V, Udayabanu M, Goel G. Microbe-bio-chemical insight: Reviewing interactions between dietary polyphenols and gut microbiota. *Mini Rev Med Chem.* 2018;18(15):1253–1264. doi: 10.2174/1389557517666170208142817.

Makarewicz M, Drożdż I, Tarko T, Duda-Chodak A. The interactions between polyphenols and microorganisms, especially gut microbiota. *Antioxidants (Basel).* 2021;10(2):188. doi: 10.3390/antiox10020188.

Manach C, Milenkovic D, Van de Wiele T, Rodriguez-Mateos A, de Roos B, Garcia-Conesa MT, Landberg R, Gibney ER, Heinonen M, Tomás-Barberán F, Morand C. Addressing the inter-individual variation in response to consumption of plant food bioactives: Towards a better understanding of their role in healthy aging and cardiometabolic risk reduction. *Mol Nutr Food Res.* 2017;61(6). doi: 10.1002/mnfr.201600557.

Marín L, Miguélez EM, Villar CJ, Lombó F. Bioavailability of dietary polyphenols and gut microbiota metabolism: Antimicrobial properties. *Biomed Res Int.* 2015;2015:905215. doi: 10.1155/2015/905215.

Medina-Vera I, Sanchez-Tapia M, Noriega-López L, Granados-Portillo O, Guevara-Cruz M, Flores-López A, Avila-Nava A, Fernández ML, Tovar AR, Torres N. A dietary intervention with functional foods reduces metabolic endotoxaemia and attenuates biochemical abnormalities by modifying faecal microbiota in people with type 2 diabetes. *Diabetes Metab.* 2019;45(2):122–131. doi: 10.1016/j.diabet.2018.09.004.

Monagas M, Khan N, Andrés-Lacueva C, et al. Dihydroxylated phenolic acids derived from microbial metabolism reduce lipopolysaccharide-stimulated cytokine secretion by human peripheral blood mononuclear cells. *Br J Nutr.* 2009;102(2):201–206. doi: 10.1017/S0007114508162110.

Namasivayam N. Chemoprevention in experimental animals. *Ann N Y Acad Sci.* 2011;1215: 60–71. doi: 10.1111/j.1749-6632.2010.05873.x.

Nash V, Ranadheera CS, Georgousopoulou EN, et al. The effects of grape and red wine polyphenols on gut microbiota – A systematic review. *Food Res Int.* 2018;113:277–287. doi: 10.1016/j.foodres.2018.07.019.

Noh H, Jang HH, Kim G, Zouiouich S, Cho SY, Kim HJ, Kim J, Choe JS, Gunter MJ, Ferrari P, Scalbert A, Freisling H. Taxonomic composition and diversity of the gut microbiota in relation to habitual dietary intake in Korean adults. *Nutrients.* 2021;13(2):366. doi: 10.3390/nu13020366.

Ntemiri A, Ghosh TS, Gheller ME, Tran TTT, Blum JE, Pellanda P, Vlckova K, Neto MC, Howell A, Thalacker-Mercer A, O'Toole PW. Whole blueberry and isolated polyphenol-rich fractions modulate specific gut microbes in an in vitro colon model and in a pilot study in human consumers. *Nutrients.* 2020;12(9):2800. doi: 10.3390/nu12092800.

Ozdal T, Sela DA, Xiao J, Boyacioglu D, Chen F, Capanoglu E. The reciprocal interactions between polyphenols and gut microbiota and effects on bioaccessibility. *Nutrients.* 2016;8(2):78. doi: 10.3390/nu8020078.

Palmer ND, Hester JM, An SS, Adeyemo A, Rotimi C, Langefeld CD, Freedman BI, Ng MC, Bowden DW. Resequencing and analysis of variation in the TCF7L2 gene in African Americans suggests that SNP rs7903146 is the causal diabetes susceptibility variant. *Diabetes.* 2011;60(2):662–668. doi: 10.2337/db10-0134.

Park M, Choi J, Lee HJ. Flavonoid-rich orange juice intake and altered gut microbiome in young adults with depressive symptom: A randomized controlled study. *Nutrients.* 2020;12(6):1815. doi: 10.3390/nu12061815.

Pasinetti GM, Singh R, Westfall S, Herman F, Faith J, Ho L. The role of the gut microbiota in the metabolism of polyphenols as characterized by gnotobiotic mice. *J Alzheimers Dis.* 2018;63(2):409–421. doi: 10.3233/JAD-171151.

Plamada D, Vodnar DC. Polyphenols-gut microbiota interrelationship: A transition to a new generation of prebiotics. *Nutrients.* 2021;14(1):137. doi: 10.3390/nu14010137.

Renaud J, Martinoli MG. Considerations for the use of polyphenols as therapies in neurodegenerative diseases. *Int J Mol Sci.* 2019;20(8):1883. doi:10.3390/ijms20081883.

Rodriguez-Mateos A, Rendeiro C, Bergillos-Meca T, Tabatabaee S, George TW, Heiss C, Spencer JP. Intake and time dependence of blueberry flavonoid-induced improvements in vascular function: A randomized, controlled, double-blind, crossover intervention study with mechanistic insights into biological activity. *Am J Clin Nutr.* 2013;98(5):1179–1191.

Safe S, Jayaraman A, Chapkin RS, Howard M, Mohankumar K, Shrestha R. Flavonoids: Structure-function and mechanisms of action and opportunities for drug development. *Toxicol Res.* 2021;37(2):147–162. doi: 10.1007/s43188-020-00080-z.

Sáyago-Ayerdi SG, Zamora-Gasga VM, Venema K. Prebiotic effect of predigested mango peel on gut microbiota assessed in a dynamic in vitro model of the human colon (TIM-2). *Food Res Int.* 2019;118:89–95. doi: 10.1016/j.foodres.2017.12.024.

Scalbert A, Williamson G. Dietary intake and bioavailability of polyphenols. *J Nutr.* 2000;130(8S Suppl):2073S-85S. doi: 10.1093/jn/130.8.2073S.

Selma MV, Espin JC, Tomas-Barberan FA. Interaction between phenolics and gut microbiota: Role in human health. *J Agr Food Chem.* 2009;57(15):6485–6501. doi: 10.1021/jf902107d.

Shin JH, Ahn YJ, Chung WH, Lim MY, Hong S, Kim JH, Park MH, Nam YD. Effect of Saengshik supplementation on the gut microbial composition of healthy Korean Adults: A single-group pilot study. *Front Nutr.* 2021;8:743620. doi: 10.3389/fnut.2021. 743620.

Shortt C, Hasselwander O, Meynier A, et al. Systematic review of the effects of the intestinal microbiota on selected nutrients and non-nutrients. *Eur J Nutr.* 2018;57(1):25–49. doi: 10.1007/s00394-017-1546-4.

Sikalidis AK, Maykish A. The gut microbiome and Type 2 diabetes mellitus: discussing a complex relationship. *Biomedicines* 2020;8(1):8.

Tresserra-Rimbau A, Lamuela-Raventos RM, Moreno JJ. Polyphenols, food and pharma. Current knowledge and directions for future research. *Biochem Pharmacol.* 2018;156:186–195. doi: 10.1016/j.bcp.2018.07.050.

Tsuji H, Moriyama K, Nomoto K, Akaza H. Identification of an enzyme system for daidzein-to-equol conversion in Slackia sp. strain natts. *Appl Environ Microbiol.* 2012;78(4): 1228–1236. doi: 10.1128/AEM.06779-11.

Valdés A, Álvarez-Rivera G, Socas-Rodríguez B, Herrero M, Ibáñez E, Cifuentes A. Foodomics: Analytical opportunities and challenges. *Anal Chem.* 2022;94(1):366–381. doi: 10.1021/acs.analchem.1c04678.

van Duynhoven J, Vaughan EE, Jacobs DM, Kemperman RA, van Velzen EJ, Gross G, Roger LC, Possemiers S, Smilde AK, Doré J, Westerhuis JA, Van de Wiele T. Metabolic fate of polyphenols in the human superorganism. *Proc Natl Acad Sci U S A.* 2011;108(Suppl 1): 4531–4538 doi: 10.1073/pnas.1000098107.

Vazhappilly CG, Amararathna M, Cyril AC, Linger R, Matar R, Merheb M, Ramadan WS, Radhakrishnan R, Rupasinghe HPV. Current methodologies to refine bioavailability, delivery, and therapeutic efficacy of plant flavonoids in cancer treatment. *J Nutr Biochem.* 2021;94:108623. doi: 10.1016/j.jnutbio.2021.108623.

Vendrame S, Guglielmetti S, Riso P, Arioli S, Klimis-Zacas D, Porrini M. Six-week consumption of a wild blueberry powder drink increases bifidobacteria in the human gut. *J Agric Food Chem.* 2011;59(24):12815–12820.

Vendrame S, Klimis-Zacas D. Anti-inflammatory effect of anthocyanins via modulation of nuclear factor-κB and mitogen-activated protein kinase signaling cascades. *Nutr Rev.* 2015;73(6):348–358. doi: 10.1093/nutrit/nuu066.

Verhoog S, Taneri PE, Roa Díaz ZM, et al. Dietary factors and modulation of bacteria strains of Akkermansia muciniphila and Faecalibacterium prausnitzii: A systematic review. *Nutrients.* 2019;11(7):1565. Published 2019 Jul 11. doi: 10.3390/nu11071565.

Vetrani C, Maukonen J, Bozzetto L, Della Pepa G, Vitale M, Costabile G, Riccardi G, Rivellese AA, Saarela M, Annuzzi G. Diets naturally rich in polyphenols and/or long-chain n-3 polyunsaturated fatty acids differently affect microbiota composition in high-cardiometabolic-risk individuals. *Acta Diabetol.* 2020;57(7):853–860. doi: 10.1007/s00592-020-01494-9.

Vilela MM, Salvador SL, Teixeira IGL, Del Arco MCG, De Rossi A. Efficacy of green tea and its extract, epigallocatechin-3-gallate, in the reduction of cariogenic microbiota in children: A randomized clinical trial. *Arch Oral Biol.* 2020;114:104727. doi: 10.1016/j.archoralbio.2020.104727.

Williamson G. The role of polyphenols in modern nutrition. *Nutr Bull.* 2017;42(3):226–235. doi:10.1111/nbu.12278.

Williamson G, Clifford MN. Role of the small intestine, colon and microbiota in determining the metabolic fate of polyphenols. *Biochem Pharmacol.* 2017;139:24–39. doi: 10.1016/j.bcp.2017.03.012.

Wilson R, Willis J, Gearry RB, Hughes A, Lawley B, Skidmore P, Frampton C, Fleming E, Anderson A, Jones L, Tannock GW, Carr AC. SunGold kiwifruit supplementation of individuals with prediabetes alters gut microbiota and improves vitamin c status, anthropometric and clinical markers. *Nutrients.* 2018;10(7):895. doi: 10.3390/nu10070895.

Yang J, Kurnia P, Henning SM, Lee R, Huang J, Garcia MC, Surampudi V, Heber D, Li Z. Effect of standardized grape powder consumption on the gut microbiome of healthy subjects: A pilot study. *Nutrients.* 2021;13(11):3965. doi: 10.3390/nu13113965.

Yu D, Nguyen SM, Yang Y, Xu W, Cai H, Wu J, Cai Q, Long J, Zheng W, Shu XO. Long-term diet quality is associated with gut microbiome diversity and composition among urban Chinese adults. *Am J Clin Nutr.* 2021;113(3):684–694. doi: 10.1093/ajcn/nqaa350.

Zhang PY. Polyphenols in health and disease. *Cell Biochem Biophys.* 2015;73(3):649–664. doi: 10.1007/s12013-015-0558-z.

# 8 Diet, Obesity, and Gut Microbiome

*Yu-Chieh Cheng*
Academia Sinica

*Alison Lacombe and Vivian C.H. Wu*
United States Department of Agriculture

## CONTENTS

## INTRODUCTION

Obesity and overweight have become serious public health issues worldwide. The population of obese individuals has shown rapid growth over the past four decades. From 1975 to 2016, obesity prevalence demonstrated nearly tripling growth. In 2016, more than 1.9 billion adults (18 years and older) were defined as overweight, and

DOI: 10.1201/b22970-11

650 million adults were obese (World Health Organization, 2020). Overweight and obesity issues also reflect human physiological conditions that represent abnormal or excessive fat accumulation. To define overweight and obesity in adults, body mass index (BMI) is a typical approach that calculates the ratio of a person's weight expressed in kilograms divided by the square of his/her height expressed in meters. For the BMI scale, according to the World Health Organization definition, overweight in adults is a BMI greater than or equal to 25, whereas obesity in adults is a BMI greater than or equal to 30. BMI provides a useful and standardized measure that only needs simple and physiological data to readily classify overweight and obese populations in adults (World Health Organization, 2020).

While there are complex and multiple reasons for obesity, the fundamental cause of obesity is an energy imbalance when energy intake exceeds energy expenditure. Macronutrients from dietary intake are used as a metabolic fuel and for maintaining physiological function, while any excess calories promote the accumulation of adipose tissue, leading to obesity. The most common obesogenic dietary pattern is that of a high-fat and high-sugar diet. High–energy–density foods provide few portions with extremely high calories, a condition that, when combined with lower levels of physical activity due to an increase in sedentary behavior, leads to obesity. Excessive energy intake is a cause of obesity but not the single obesogenic factor (Chooi et al., 2019). Alterations in dietary and physical activity patterns are often linked to environmental and societal changes as well as a lack of policies to support health and agriculture, change the mode of transportation, urban planning, food overprocessing, and lack of education.

Overweight and obesity have a detrimental relationship with human health, which may lead to metabolic disorders such as type 2 diabetes, dyslipidemia, and hypertension. Other systemic complications, cardiovascular diseases, and musculoskeletal disorders are also related to obesity and overweight. There is evidence that obesity may increase the risk of liver, gallbladder, and pancreatic cancers, as well as hematological cancers and aggressive prostate cancer (Calle and Kaaks, 2004). Previous reports revealed that obese patients exhibit a higher risk for hospitalization and mechanical ventilation support due to insufficient expiratory reserve volume, functional capacity, and respiratory system compliance. Thus, these functional disorders can lead to significant increases in morbidity and mortality from COVID-19 (Caussy et al., 2020; Dietz and Santos-Burgoa, 2020; Popkin et al., 2020).

Currently, the mortality of obese and overweight individuals is higher than underweight individuals in the world. The high prevalence of obesity develops serious social problems and may squander unnecessary medical resources in society. Fortunately, obesity and overweight rates could be attenuated through a healthy diet and lifestyle, as well as increasing physical activity. According to the World Health Organization suggestions, limiting energy intake from sugars and fats; increasing fruit, vegetable, legume, whole grain, and nuts consumption; and enhancing regular physical activity frequency are advised to individuals to prevent overweight and obesity. With obesity becoming a worldwide epidemic, insights into how obesity contributes to metabolism and human homeostasis, as well as new interventions, are urgently needed. Nowadays, numerous research teams are dedicated to inquiry on the mechanism to provide more efficient resolutions for obesity.

The human gastrointestinal (GI) tract is colonized by abundant microorganisms from the external environment, including bacteria, archaea, eukarya, and viruses that form an ecosystem so-called the "gut microbiota." The gut microbiota has the largest number of bacteria and the most diversity among other parts of the body, which number approximately 100 trillion. (Rinninella et al., 2019; Thursby and Juge, 2017). Previous studies have estimated that the density of bacterial cells in the colon is between $10^{11}$ and $10^{12}$/mL, making the colon one of the most intensive microbial habitats on Earth (Ley et al., 2006). The formation of the gut microbiota is exogenous. Infants are born to be uninhabited with gut microflora, but they receive exogenous microbes and establish gut microflora in the GI tract from the environment and mother, developing into a complex microbial ecosystem gradually (Nejrup et al., 2017). The establishment of the gut microbiome and its stability in the GI tract requires approximately 2 years. Thus, the first colonizers of the human gut are crucial to the host's early life and are in turn linked to a range of diseases, immune system development, and energy metabolism. The diversity of microorganisms in the gut is increased from breastfeeding and kept stable when transferred to solid food due to reduced food diversity (Zmora et al., 2019). Various studies have also demonstrated that there is a correlation between the childhood gut microbiota composition and immune and metabolic disorders later in life (Milani et al., 2017; Rao et al., 2021).

The composition of the gut microbiota is dynamic; microbial communities are a complex dynamical system and change promptly following host lifestyle, gestational age, host intestinal epithelium, immune ontogeny, environments, medication, and diet (Gonze et al., 2018). Variations in the gut microbiota communities benefit host health conditions by modulating host immunity, strengthening gut integrity, shaping the intestinal epithelium, and protecting the pathogen invasion (Thursby and Juge, 2017). Moreover, the gut microbiota has been reported to have a clear influence on human energy homeostasis, aging, exercise performance, circadian rhythm, and brain function (Foster and Neufeld, 2013; O'Toole and Jeffery, 2015; Scheiman et al., 2019; Voigt et al., 2016). If the commensal microflora is disrupted, known as microbial dysbiosis, the host immune system would be damaged easily and develop intestinal disorders such as irritable bowel syndrome and inflammatory bowel disease (IBD). Microbial dysbiosis has been a serious consequence that leads to the pathogenesis of colon, gastric, pancreatic, laryngeal, breast, hepatic, and gallbladder carcinomas as well (Kaakoush et al., 2012; Rinninella et al., 2019; Sobhani et al., 2011; Xuan et al., 2014). Moreover, numerous studies have proven the correlation between the gut microbiota and host energy metabolism, which could separate into multiple parts, such as satiety modulation, fat accumulation, and energy production. When dysbiosis occurs, the risks of metabolic disorders such as obesity, type 2 diabetes, nonalcoholic liver disease, cardiometabolic diseases, and malnutrition are increased significantly (Bäckhed et al., 2004; Fan and Pedersen, 2021). At present, scientists are gaining knowledge concerning the interplay between the microbial community and host physiology in order to develop promising therapeutic interventions. In this chapter, the relationship between the gut microbiota and obesity is discussed. The chapter focuses on critical factors that influence the bacteria–gut–host physiology system in order to gain a clear understanding of the potential of the bacterium to improve host metabolic health.

# GUT MICROBIOTA FORMATION AND CHARACTERISTIC

## GUT MICROBIAL COMPOSITION, DYNAMICS, AND FUNCTION

The gut microbiota composition is unique and has large diversity, which plays a vital role in host metabolism, immunomodulation, and biosynthesis. The gut microbiota involves not only nutrient absorption but also metabolite production, including lipids, amino acids, bile acids, and short-chain fatty acids (SCFAs). Moreover, resident bacteria inhibit pathogen invasion by maintaining intestinal epithelium integrity, competing for nutrients and space with pathogens by pH modification and antimicrobial peptide secretions (Coyte and Rakoff-Nahoum, 2019). Microorganisms are classified into phyla, classes, orders, families, genera, and species by using the taxonomy. The dominant phyla in the gut microbes are Firmicutes, Bacteroidetes, Actinobacteria, Proteobacteria, Fusobacteria, and Verrucomicrobia. Firmicutes and Bacteroidetes account for the vast majority of microorganisms which are approximately 97% of the gut microbiota. Over 200 genera of Firmicutes are found in this phylum, including *Lactobacillus*, *Bacillus*, *Clostridium*, *Enterococcus*, and *Ruminicoccus*. In addition, the *Clostridium* genus constituted 95% of the Firmicutes phylum. Bacteroides are the most abundant and variable genera which contain *Bacteroides* and *Prevotella*. The predominant genera in Bacteroidetes are *Bacteroides* and *Prevotella*. For Actinobacteria, the most abundant genus is *Bifidobacterium* (Arumugam et al., 2011; Rinninella et al., 2019; Rosenbaum et al., 2015).

## DIVERSITY AND COMPOSITION OF GUT MICROORGANISMS IMPLICATED IN HOST HEALTH MAINTENANCE

The first understanding of this interaction relied on germ-free (GF) mice, which exist in a sterile environment completely without microorganisms. It is illustrated that GF animals had a lower body weight and had poorer intestinal function than conventionally raised mice. An enlarged liver and lower concentrations of amino acids in the gut were observed as well. Scientists used GF mice to colonize microbiota from conventionally raised mice, and the results showed a significant increase in body weight, fat accumulation, and relative insulin resistance (Bäckhed et al., 2004). Interestingly, although body weight was increased, the energy expenditure grew by approximately 30%, whereas energy intake declined by 30% approximately after GF mice received a microbial community. Many GF animal studies proved resident microbes are implicated in the energy balance equation (Bäckhed et al., 2007; Rosenbaum et al., 2015). An additional study mentioned that GF animals are protected against diet-induced obesity such as Western-style, high-sugar, and high-fat diets (HFDs) (Bäckhed et al., 2007). Supporting this notion, increased expression of glucagon-like peptide-1 (GLP-1), which is an obesity-related peptide in the brain and can reduce food intake, was observed (Uzbay, 2019).

The species variation of gut microbiota is dynamic. The colonization of microbes in the GI tract begins postpartum. Infants are born to be uncolonized with the gut microbiota and then develop an unstable microflora receiving from the environment and the maternal microbial reservoir. Infants temporarily acquire microbes and form microflora from the maternal skin and vagina and then persistently accumulate from the maternal gut, and it has been proven that the strains are more adapted than other sources (Ferretti et al., 2018). Many factors, such as types of birth delivery, gestational age at birth, methods of milk feeding, and antibiotic medications, impact the composition of the neonatal gut microbiota. These pioneering microbes utilize lactose, galactose, and sucrose as their energy sources; after infants switch diet into solid food, the gut microbiome alternates to the pathway of carbohydrate fermentation and vitamin biosynthesis (Zmora et al., 2019). However, dysbiosis has been revealed to be related to several diseases during the early stage, such as allergies, asthma, type 1 diabetes, Crohn's disease, IBD, necrotizing enterocolitis, and inflammation (Ferretti et al., 2018; Renz and Skevaki, 2021). Developing a healthy gut microbial community in the early stage is crucial for later life. Conversely, studies have indicated that the human gut microbiome can be altered and develop into maturity over the different life stages. Scientists have observed a decline in microbiota diversity during aging in elderly people. There is a trend whereby saccharolytic bacteria decrease while proteolytic bacteria increase (Bischoff, 2016). Elderly individuals have higher levels of *Escherichia coli*, Bacteroidetes, and Proteobacteria than adults and infants but a lower ratio of Firmicutes to Bacteroidetes than younger adults (Mariat et al., 2009). The dominant population has been replaced by subdominant species, which may be due to an age-related decrease in immune function and aging-associated pathologies (Vaiserman et al., 2017).

Additionally, more factors alter the composition of the gut microbiome. Circadian rhythms modulate daily events that affect feeding, sleeping, hormone secretion, metabolism, and temperature, which rely on the oscillation of light during the 24 h cycle (Liang and FitzGerald, 2017; Mu et al., 2016). The functions of the intestine, gut motility, and nutrient absorption are also affected by the circadian rhythm (Hussain and Pan, 2009). The gut microbiota shows diurnal variations modulated by circadian rhythms. Bacteroidetes, Firmicutes, and Proteobacteria are reported to be related to oscillation. Bacteroidetes were discovered to be the most sensitive phylum that exhibited circadian rhythmicity. During the daytime, Bacteroidetes are more copious than nighttime with abundance oscillations which impacts the gut microbiome assembly (Liang et al., 2015; Zmora et al., 2019). In addition, disruption of the host circadian clock drives loss of microbiota rhythms and dysbiosis which facilitates glucose intolerance and obesity in humans and mice (Thaiss et al., 2014).

Previous studies have recently shown the association between microbial profiles and numerous human diseases, such as cardiovascular disease, IBD, irritable bowel syndrome, obesity, and type 2 diabetes. Furthermore, accumulating evidence suggests that the gut microbiota is involved in maintaining brain health. It has been reported that the gut microbiota impacts the central nervous system homeostasis indirectly by modulating neurotransmitter and host immune function and blood–brain barrier integrity. Thus, the alterations react to stress responsivity, anxiety-like behaviors, sociability, and cognition (Luczynski et al., 2016). Increasing validation for the essential role of microbial metabolism in maintaining the host immune system has been found in recent research analyzing the composition and function of individual microbial species and complex microbial communities. The crosstalk between the gut microbiome and host immune system is complex and has systemic impacts on the whole body. In general, resident bacteria produce metabolites by undigested nutrients, as well as endogenous compounds to modulate the host immune system and lead to immune reactions or dysfunction. The GI tract has a single layer of epithelial cells that boost microbial-produced compounds that can easily interact with host cells (Rooks and Garrett, 2016). One of the factors that leads to gut immune system development and functional maturation is the gut microbiota. Resident bacteria can interact with gut-associated lymphoid tissue, T helper 17 cells, inducible regulatory T cells, IgA-producing B cells, and innate lymphoid cells. Furthermore, the gut microbiota prevents pathogen invasion by direct competition for nutrients, indirect innate immunity enhancement, and adaptive immunity promotion (Kamada et al., 2013). One of the most direct and crucial elements that changes the gut microbiome is the dietary pattern. Many studies have demonstrated that different dietary styles produce varying gut microbial profiles and could be modified by changing the dietary pattern in just a few days. The change in accurate time depends on individuals, which is approximately 1–4 days (Zmora et al., 2019). Variations in the gut microbiome with dietary conversion can have synergistic or opposing effects on the host health. The details of food modulation will be further discussed later.

Resident bacteria in the gut produce a large number of metabolites from the fermentation of undigested carbohydrate and host-derived products, and it can mediate host physiology by signaling, stimulatory, and inhibitory. These bacterial metabolomes can interact with host metabolomes and can be detected in host feces, urine, and blood (Flint et al., 2015; Martin et al., 2007). The metabolites induce and mediate host homeostasis in multiple ways, inducing both local and systemic effects. In the gut lamina propria, these metabolites can affect barrier function and immune cell populations. Additionally, metabolites may affect downstream organ systems as well. Actively or passively transported metabolites can cross the intestinal epithelium and directly affect distal organ functions or diseases. Moreover, the metabolites produced by groups of microbes can impact other members of the microbiota or pathogens, altering their composition or function. Changes both locally and systemically can have indirect consequences for the host (McCarville et al., 2020).

SCFAs are a major product generated by microbial from the fermentation of undigested fibers, including acetic acid, butyric acid, and propionic acid. Most of SCFAs are produced at the distal colon and absorbed mostly (Topping and Clifton, 2001). Various species have been reported that have the ability to produce SCFAs. Dietary patterns with rich fermentable fiber or microbe-accessible carbohydrates provide a critical source for the bacteria that produce SCFAs (Sonnenburg et al., 2016). In general, acetate and butyrate are the major energy providers in all body tissues, while propionate participates in the gluconeogenic pathway which occurs in the liver. Additionally, acetate can be used for lipogenesis and is associated with satiety-regulating hormones. In colonocytes, approximately 60–70% of the energy is from butyrate, and it is a preferential energy resource for colon cells by using diffusion or plasma membrane transporters (Blaut, 2015; McCarville et al., 2020). SCFAs have been reported to possess anti-inflammatory and antiapoptotic abilities and act as histone deacetylase inhibitors that induce colon cancer cell cycle arrest, differentiation, and apoptosis. Thus, SCFAs promote intestinal integrity and play an important role in colorectal cancer and colitis prevention. G protein-coupled receptors are integral membrane proteins on the surface of epithelial cells and immune cells. SCFAs bind to G protein-coupled receptors to induce signal transduction into host cells, resulting in the promotion of immune tolerance and gut homeostasis. The SCFAs–G protein-coupled receptors interaction enhances forkhead box P3 expression, transforming growth factor-β and interleukin-10, which are pivotal anti-inflammatory activities in the host body (Rooks and Garrett, 2016). Moreover, inhibition of nuclear factor-κB and modulation of interleukin-8 have also been reported to represent mediating mechanisms of SCFA-induced effects on host immunity. In response to SCFAs, enhanced mucin gene transcription by intestinal goblet cells and altered tight junction permeability of intestinal epithelial cells are observed to enforce epithelial barrier integrity, thereby preventing pathogen invasion (Rooks and Garrett, 2016; Willemsen et al., 2003). Butyrate has been demonstrated *in vitro* to play an important role in maintaining the gut barrier function, stabilizing transcription factors, assembling tight junction proteins, and keeping mucin secreted even under anaerobic conditions. Enhancing the integrity of the gut barrier can block the translocation of lipopolysaccharide (LPS), which has been associated with insulin resistance, inflammation, adiposity, hepatic fat, and metabolic endotoxemia (Cani et al., 2008). In addition, SCFAs also participate in appetite control (Byrne et al., 2015).

However, high levels of SCFAs are linked with obesity but inversely correlated with gut microbiota diversity. Metagenomic studies have shown that the obese human gut microbiome exhibits upregulation of the pathways related to the processing of carbohydrates and SCFAs production (Turnbaugh et al., 2009). SCFAs overexcretion demonstrates a positive correlation with gut dysbiosis, gut permeability, excess adiposity, and cardiometabolic risk factors (la Cuesta-Zuluaga et al., 2019). This contradictory situation may indicate the involvement of additional particular bacteria or metabolites that may trigger multiple metabolic mechanisms into a systemic result. LPSs are microbial metabolites produced by gram-negative bacteria particularly. They are found in the outer membrane of bacteria and consist of lipids and polysaccharides. For the host, LPSs are endotoxins that pass through the gut barrier into circulation and induce inflammation (Manco et al., 2010). A high concentration of LPS in circulation is closely related to metabolic disorders. Moreover, HFDs alter the gut microbiota composition and induce LPS absorption, resulting in elevated LPS levels in circulation (Heiss and Olofsson, 2018).

## ENERGY METABOLISM AND GUT MICROBIOTA

### GUT MICROBIOTA IN OBESITY

Gut microbiota composition has been linked to BMI class and diet. The ratio of Bacteroidetes and Firmicutes phyla shows variation in obese adults, in which Bacteroidetes decrease dramatically and enrich the proportions of Firmicutes as well as Proteobacteria. A clinical trial supports this notion. The individuals were separated into two groups and received an underfeeding or overfeeding diet. The results revealed that the energy intake has a positive correlation with the relative amount of Firmicutes but a negative correlation with the relative abundance of Bacteroidetes. These studies validated the gut microbiota is responsive to host energy balance (Jumpertz et al., 2011). Moreover, scientists have discovered that differences at the genus and species level are more relevant to obesity. For example, the relative amount of *Bifidobacterium* decreased while *Lactobacillus* increased conversely in overweight to obese individuals (Million et al., 2012). Erysipelotrichaceae, the predominant family, has four groups of closely related species-level phylotypes that were revealed to have different responses during dietary changes and metabolic phenotypes (Zhao, 2013). Previous studies indicated lower proportions of *Bifidobacterium vulgatus* in obese humans than in lean individuals (Bervoets et al., 2013; Rinninella et al., 2019). These variations are very sensitive to energy balance and can be recovered along with weight loss based on a healthy diet.

Similarly, the gene richness and diversity of the gut microbiome declines significantly in obese adults compared to lean individuals and is enhanced after dietary weight loss (Rosenbaum et al., 2015; Torres-Fuentes et al., 2017). Low microbial richness also has a relationship with host metabolic parameters, including serum insulin, homeostasis model assessment insulin resistance, triglyceride levels, and free fatty acids in plasma (Le Chatelier et al., 2013). This means that the variation in the gut microbiota in obese populations results in dysbiosis and affects host metabolism and health, which may lead to detrimental comorbidities and complications such as diabetes and metabolic syndrome. The low diversity of the gut microbiome also has a high correlation with trunk fat mass and comorbidities such as type 2 diabetes and hypertension (Aron-Wisnewsky et al., 2019). Furthermore, the obese microbiome is transmittable. GF mice inoculated with bacteria from obese mice's cecum exhibited significant weight gain compared with those received from a lean donor. A decline in fecal energy excretion is observed in colonization with microbiota from an obese donor, and it has been illustrated that the gut microbiome from obese individuals can enhance energy harvest capacity from the diet (Turnbaugh et al., 2006).

## REGULATION ON HOST METABOLISM

The crosstalk between the gut microbiome and host is implicated in metabolism and energy homeostasis. Scientists have found this phenomenon by using the GF mouse model. GF mice lacking gut microbiota are protected against diet-induced obesity with an HFD. GF mice fed a lard-based HFD showed increased energy expenditure, fecal fat content, and energy excretion, which led to diet-induced obesity. It has also been observed that mice with microbiota depletion have more browning of the inguinal subcutaneous and perigonadal visceral adipose tissue. This metabolic improvement can enhance the volume of brown adipose tissue, improve insulin sensitivity, and decrease white fat and adipocyte size (Suárez-Zamorano et al., 2015). In short, these results indicate the reason why GF mice have the resistance to diet-induced obesity.

Additionally, accumulating evidence suggests that gut microbiome composition and host metabolism are highly correlated. The alteration of the Bacteroidetes and Firmicutes ratio in the gut depends on the difference in the host metabolism status and it is illustrated that related to carbohydrate degradation and fermentation (Ley et al., 2006). Moreover, scientists monitored the relationship between resting energy expenditure, body composition, and the gut microbiome. The population of Firmicutes has demonstrated a positive correlation with fat mass, whereas the opposite relationship with resting energy expenditure and the maximal oxygen consumption ($VO_2$max) has been observed (Kocełak et al., 2013). The gut microbiome composition can be altered by probiotics and prebiotic intervention. By using inulin-type fructo-oligosaccharides as a supplement, an increase in health-promoting species such as *Bifidobacterium*, *Lactobacillus*, *Roseburia*, and *Faecalibacterium* has been observed. This alteration has been proven to decrease postprandial plasma glucose responses after a standardized meal, also enhancing plasma GLP-1 and peptide YY (PYY) concentrations which may contribute to host satiation and glucose homeostasis (Cani et al., 2009).

Accumulating evidence proves that there are specific relevant functions in each phylum. In Firmicutes, some species transfer indigested fiber into butyrate and join symbiosis with pathogens. The other predominant phylum, Bacteroidetes, has been reported to degrade polysaccharides and ferment fiber, and its major energy sources are protein and grain-rich diets. Actinobacteria, which account for approximately 3% of the total gut bacteria, have been illustrated to work on host vitamin biosynthesis. In addition, although other minor phyla account for less than 1%, they are also implicated in host metabolisms, such as iron degradation, vitamin synthesis, and carbohydrate fermentation (Consortium, 2012; Turnbaugh et al., 2009). Specific bacteria may inhibit circulating lipoprotein lipase inhibitors in the intestinal epithelia, resulting in host weight gain due to enhanced triglyceride synthesis, promoted fat accumulation as well as reduced insulin sensitivity (Sun et al., 2018).

Furthermore, metabolites produced by resident microorganisms comprehensively affect host energy homeostasis function. SCFAs, bacterial metabolites, provide an important energy source for intestinal epithelial cells. The major consortiums of bacteria that produce SCFAs were *Faecalibacterium prausnitzii* and *Eubacterium*, *Lactobacillus*, and *Bifidobacterium* species. Bacteria produce SCFAs throughout carbohydrate fermentation, and increased energy harvesting accounts for a substantial part of energy uptake. The gut microbiome also protects against Western diet–induced obesity and metabolic disorders by SCFAs production. According to previous studies, the intervention with butyrate and succinate in mouse models improved glucose sensitivity and glucose tolerance and enhanced energy expenditure (De Vadder et al., 2016; Gao et al., 2009). Type 2 diabetes patients have been discovered with the α lower relative ratio of SCFA-producing bacteria in the gut microbiota. Clinically, a high-fiber diet alters gut microbiota composition and improves patients' glycated hemoglobin A1c (HbA1c) via induced GLP-1 production (Zhao et al., 2018). Conversely, some studies have indicated that there is a negative correlation between host metabolism and SCFAs, especially acetate and propionate. In the rodent model, circulating acetate which is enriched by altering gut microbiota leads to activation of the parasympathetic nervous system, which may drive insulin secretion and increase the risk of obesity (Perry et al., 2016). Studies in humans have revealed that a diet with propionate may induce insulin resistance and obesity. One of the reasons may be that SCFAs are ligands of free fatty acid receptors (FFAR2 and FFAR3). Free fatty acid receptors activation has a high correlation with satiety and insulin sensitivity (Tirosh et al., 2019). Hence, the beneficial effect of SCFAs on host metabolism is controversial and inconsistent.

Accumulating evidence suggests the implication between obesity and LPS which are produced by gram-negative bacteria. A number of Enterobacteriaceae and Desulfovibrionaceae families which belong to the phylum Proteobacteria were enhanced in the obese population. These families are known to produce high concentrations of LPS (Zhao, 2013). LPS is recognized by toll-like receptor 4 which induces cholecystokinin (CCK) secretion to impact the host gastrointestinal system. Additionally, LPS has been reported as a triggering factor for insulin resistance in adipose tissue. By consumption of HFDs, LPS levels increase intestinal permeability, resulting in elevated systemic LPS levels and low-grade inflammation (Blaut, 2015).

## MODULATING FEED BEHAVIOR AND SATIETY

Regulating feeding behavior is extremely complicated and could be separated into homeostatic control and nonhomeostatic control. Both controls could respond to host energy status and react to feeding behavior. Communication between the brain and viscera relies on the vagus nerve, which is the longest cranial nerve in the body. The vagus nerve participates as a coordinator in the regulation of the homeostatic and nonhomeostatic feeding systems by connecting gastrointestinal hunger and satiety signals and bidirectionally regulating higher-order brain regions. According to previous studies, the microorganisms that inhabit the host gut have the capacity to modulate appetite via the intestinal satiety pathway and consequently impact obesity and eating disorders. In this mechanism, bacterial components and microbiota-derived metabolites play major roles in modulating host satiety (Yu and Hsiao, 2021). In animal models, accumulating evidence suggests that gut microbiota has the ability to influence host dietary preference (Alcock et al., 2014). The possible mechanisms may be that the gut microbiome affects oral and intestinal taste receptors, while endocannabinoid signaling is also discussed as a possible avenue (Méndez-Díaz et al., 2012). By using the intervention of prebiotics, the composition of the gut microbiome has been changed, which affects host food intake by regulating hedonic and motivational drives for a food reward. Thus, prebiotics alleviates dysbiosis of the gut microbiome and increases the sensitivity of sweet taste, which suggests a high correlation between gut microbiota composition and taste (Bernard et al., 2019).

The hypothalamus has an important function to integrate external stimulation and sensory, hormonal, and nutrient signals into regulating feeding behavior. In particular, the hypothalamus has been divided functionally into two parts to control appetite which are anorexigenic arcuate pro-opiomelanocortin (POMC) neurons and orexigenic agouti-related protein/neuropeptide Y (AgRP/NPY)–coexpressing neurons. POMC neurons, located in the arcuate nucleus of the hypothalamus, are activated by energy surplus and inhibited by energy deficits. When POMC is activated, the cells decrease appetite and promote weight loss (Rau and Hentges, 2019). Conversely, AgRP/NPY neurons act as an anabolic promotor, producing peptides to promote food intake and enhance body weight. In particular, AgRP/NPY neurons express leptin and insulin receptors and are inhibited by these two hormones. When leptin and insulin levels are decreased, AgRP/NPY neurons can be activated (Morrison et al., 2005; Morton and Schwartz, 2001). Furthermore, the hypothalamus provides connective function between many brain regions, ensuring coordinated responses to metabolic state and demand (Wright et al., 2016). Several animal studies have proven that variations in the gut microbiota may implicate hypothalamic gene expression, neuropeptide and neurotransmitter levels, and neuronal activity. One of the animal trials revealed a decrease in *Npy* and *Agrp* expression but increased the *Pomc* expression compared with GF mice. Moreover, conventionally raised mice have less brain-derived neurotrophic factor expression which is an anti-obesity neuropeptide (Schéle et al., 2013). In contrast, another study indicated that conventionally raised mice have lower hypothalamic *Pomc* and suppressor of cytokine signaling 3 expression than GF mice. The discrepancy between these results and influences on the hypothalamus may be caused by the variability of the diet and other rearing conditions. The potential mechanisms are discussed, and microbial metabolism and microbiota metabolites are involved in the potential modulation. SCFAs are regarded as modulators that affect host feeding behavior via hypothalamic neurons. Acetate has been demonstrated to be an anorectic signal by directly inducing hypothalamic neuronal activation, while propionate and butyrate are reported to influence peripheral circuits that innervate the hypothalamus (Blaak et al., 2020; Byrne et al., 2015). The gut microbiota also has modulating ability on the host brainstem, which bidirectionally processes both descending neural signals from the midbrain and forebrain and ascending signals from the vagus nerve, hormones, microbes, and host metabolites (Liu and Kanoski, 2018). The brainstem is divided into two nuclei, the nucleus of the solitary tract and the dorsal raphe nucleus. Previous reports have proven that both the nucleus of the solitary tract and dorsal raphe nucleus can be modulated by the gut microbiota and lead to feeding behavior alterations (Campos et al., 2016; Minaya et al., 2020; Vaughn et al., 2017).

It has also been reported that variations in gut microbiota composition caused by different nutritional status and physical activity could affect appetite-regulating hormones such as leptin and ghrelin. Leptin, a hormone generated from adipose tissue, is highly correlated with body fat mass. Leptin is transferred by blood circulation and then passes through the blood-brain barrier to the hypothalamus, the place that has leptin receptors and stimulates appetite suppression. This chain reaction results in reduced food intake, inhibited fat accumulation, and ultimately reduced body weight (Zhou and Rui, 2013). In the GF mouse model, lower levels of leptin were shown compared with conventionally raised mice (Fetissov et al., 2008). In addition, previous research found a significant positive correlation between circulating leptin concentration and the quantity of *Bifidobacterium* and *Lactobacillus* and a negative correlation with the number of *Clostridium*, *Bacteroides*, and *Prevotella* and serum leptin levels (Queipo-Ortuño et al., 2013). However, leptin receptors become less sensitive in obese individuals, in which the hypothalamus loses the responsiveness to leptin, usually accompanied by hyperleptinemia (Andreoli et al., 2019). In a mouse model, a gut microbiota modulation by a prebiotic treatment improved leptin sensitivity and other metabolic parameters in diet-induced obesity (Everard et al., 2011). Another report mentioned that probiotic intervention also improved leptin sensitivity in an HFD mouse model (Cheng and Liu, 2020). The possible mechanism by which the gut microbiota is involved in is the reduction of leptin resistance-associated suppressor of cytokine signaling 3 expression in the hypothalamus and brainstem (Rosenbaum et al., 2015). In addition, Heiss et al. indicated that gut microbiota enhances leptin sensitivity by regulating GLP-1–dependent mechanism (Heiss et al., 2021).

Furthermore, ghrelin is a gastrointestinal peptide hormone secreted from the stomach and stimulates appetite by affecting the hypothalamic arcuate nucleus (Kojima and Kangawa, 2005). Serum ghrelin levels were proven to have a negative correlation with the ratio of Bacteroidetes and Firmicutes, as well as the number of *Faecalibacterium* and Prevotellaceae, and a positive correlation with the number of total bacteria, *Clostridium*, and *Ruminococcus*. For *Bacteroides*, *Bifidobacterium*, and *Lactobacillus*, both positive and negative correlations with ghrelin were observed (Leeuwendaal et al., 2021; Queipo-Ortuño et al., 2013). Numerous studies have indicated that microbial metabolites play a key role in ghrelin secretion. SCFAs are able to suppress ghrelin secretion and reduce ghrelin receptor (the growth hormone secretagogue receptor type 1a) stimulation; LPS has been proven to decrease circulating ghrelin levels. On the contrary, amino acids have the capacity to promote ghrelin release (Leeuwendaal et al., 2021).

## MODULATING FEED BEHAVIOR BY GUT–BRAIN AXIS

The gut microbiome modulates the gut–brain function and occupies an important modulator of the microbiota–gut–brain axis, which affects host energy homeostasis. By using the GF animal model, scientists showed the first evidence of the absence of microbiome implicated in brain regulation and altered animal behavior. Scientists have gained more understanding of the neuron alterations by specific strains on myelination, neurotransmitters, microglia, neurogenesis, dendritic growth, and the blood–brain barrier. Numerous studies have found that the administration of probiotics and prebiotics can reduce negative impacts and deterioration of brain function (Cryan et al., 2019). Moreover, recent research has indicated that the gut microbiome highly participates in with satiety, digestive function, and further cognitive and psychological effects. The gut conveys nutritional status signals with the central nervous system and engages energy modulation by using enteroendocrine cells (EECs), the vagus nerve, and the enteric nervous system (van Son et al., 2021). In addition, the metabolites produced by microbes can be involved in regulating signal transduction.

Interplay between the gut and brain is crucial for host energy homeostasis. In recent years, it has become clear that signals from the gut play a major role in appetite regulation, energy balance, glucose homeostasis, and satiety. One of the regulations might be the activation of neuroendocrine mechanisms. EECs, which are located in the GI tract from the stomach to rectum, secrete gut hormones and neurotransmitters such as somatostatin, serotonin, ghrelin, CCK, PYY, and GLP-1 that are stimulated by luminal nutrients and provide a wide range of human physiological modulations. After secretion, these gut hormones are transported to the target neuron or enteric nervous system and exert their effectiveness throughout the bloodstream. CCK, GLP-1, PYY, and oxyntomodulin are known as modulators of on postprandial satiety. During the fasting stage, the group of gut hormones that were highly increased was featured in promoting food intake and inhibiting gastric acid secretion, which included ghrelin, motilin, insulin-like peptide 5, and somatostatin. Conversely, hormones which secret postprandial such as gastrin, histamine, GLP-1, and CCK are characterized by enhancing digest efficiency, promoting satiety, and preparing for storage of nutrients (Gribble and Reimann, 2016; Symonds et al., 2015; van Son et al., 2021).

Beyond gut hormones, neuronal orchestration has been revealed as a key element in the gut–brain function. The vagus nerve is a mixed nerve that interfaces with the parasympathetic control of the heart, lungs, and digestive tract. Appetite, gastrointestinal motility, and anti-inflammatory modulation are all associated with the vagus nerve. In addition, gut hormones (ghrelin, PYY, CCK) can trigger the vagus nerve directly. According to previous studies, obesity and an HFD reduce the sensitivity of vagus nerve afferent fibers that respond to gut hormones. The gut microbiome influences the vagus nerve indirectly by driving EECs to stimulate neurotransmitters. In addition, dysbiosis has proven to be correlated with vagus nerve innervation and signaling by increasing LPS and inflammatory cytokines. (Sen et al., 2017) (Browning et al., 2017; van Son et al., 2021). Moreover, microbial metabolites converted by the gut microbiome, such as SCFAs, also play a crucial role in the gut–brain axis. SCFAs are derivatives from undigested fiber that modulate satiety and may increase energy expenditure. Additionally, a study revealed that SCFAs affect insulin signaling which leads to inhibition of fat accumulation in adipose tissue and promotes lipid and glucose metabolism in other tissues (Kimura et al., 2013). A portion of SCFAs can interact with EECs and stimulate PYY and GLP-1 secretion (Larraufie et al., 2018; Tolhurst et al., 2012; van Son et al., 2021).

## DIETARY MODULATING GUT MICROBIOTA COMPOSITION

### DIETARY STYLES IN RELATION TO GUT MICROBIAL COMPOSITION

Diet is a critical factor affecting the gut environment, gut transit time, pH, as well as changes in the composition of gut microbiota and diversity that influence host metabolism. An unhealthy style of diet may lead to microbiome dysbiosis and induce several sequelae, including obesity and type 2 diabetes. (Kim et al., 2019). Thus, a healthy diet could improve the composition of gut microbiota and reduce the risks of host metabolic disorders. Previous studies have revealed the differences in diet patterns such as Western diet, Mediterranean diet, vegetarian diet, and gluten-free diet have their own gut microbiome profiles that have different impacts on host metabolism (Lazar et al., 2019).

The Western diet, developed from the industrial evolution, is comprised of saturated fats, sugar, salt, protein, additional additives, and lower fiber and micronutrients. The Western diet has been proven to have a positive correlation with inflammation that leads to metabolic disorders and obesity. The major gut microbiota profile of the Western diet is the reduction in total bacterial volume and beneficial species including *Lactobacillus* spp., *Bifidobacterium* spp., and *Eubacterium* spp. Due to sufficient dietary fiber, some of the specific bacteria lack the sources to generate SCFAs. The observation of SCFAs in the lumen is significantly lower when consuming a Western diet that may enhance risks of inflammatory (Kim et al., 2019; Lazar et al., 2019; Statovci et al., 2017). Conversely, vegan and vegetarian diets contain abundant dietary fiber which is opposite to the Western diet. Dietary fiber provides a good energy source to beneficial bacteria that promote a stable gut microbiota profile and increase the number of lactic acid bacteria. A low quantity of *Bacteroides* spp. and *Bifidobacterium* spp. was observed in the group that consumed vegan or vegetarian diets. In addition, these diets usually consume rich polyphenols which is from coffee, artichokes, olive, asparagus, and berries, which can facilitate the growth of protective bacteria. *Bifidobacterium* and *Lactobacillus* which are known intestinal barrier protectors, and butyrate-producing bacteria, including *Faecalibacterium prausnitzii* and *Roseburia*, *Bacteroides vulgatus*, and *Akkermansia muciniphila*, are reported to have an increase in vegan and vegetarian diets. Additionally, a decline in LPS producers such as *Escherichia coli* and *Enterobacter cloacae* has also been observed in vegan and vegetarian diets that lead to alleviation of inflammation (Glick-Bauer and Yeh, 2014).

The gut microbiota profile of a gluten-free diet has a lower abundance of *Lactobacillus* spp., *Bifidobacterium* spp., *Ruminococcus bromii*, and *Roseburia faecis*, whereas the *Victivallaceae* and *Clostridiaceae*, *E. coli*, and total *Enterobacteriaceae* demonstrate the opposite trend due to decreasing of polysaccharide and fiber intake (De Palma et al., 2009). The gluten-free diet, which is characterized by a reduction or exclusion of alimentary fiber from specific foods (i.e., grain), now has been considered as a therapeutic method for celiac disease (Reddel et al., 2019). The Mediterranean diet consists of abundant vegetables, olive oil, legumes, fish, and a low amount of red meat and dairy products that contain monounsaturated and polyunsaturated fatty acids as well as antioxidants and fiber. The gut microbiota profile in the Mediterranean diet has a high amount of *Lactobacillus* spp., *Bifidobacterium* spp., and *Prevotella* spp., but a low amount of *Clostridium* spp. This profile of the gut microbiota can prevent obesity and improve lipid and cholesterol levels (Garcia-Mantrana et al., 2018). Additionally, numerous studies have demonstrated that difference in the ratio intake of macronutrients and micronutrients can change the composition of gut microbiota and diversity which can influence host metabolism.

## MACRONUTRIENTS

### Carbohydrates

Many research studies have highlighted the altered ability of carbohydrates. In general, carbohydrates are separated into two types, which are digestible and nondigestible carbohydrates, and the gut microbiota composition has different responses to different types of carbohydrates. Starch and sugars such as glucose, lactose, fructose, and sucrose constitute digestible carbohydrates. They release glucose into the circulation and induce insulin to further respond after digestion in the intestine. The level of glucose is positively correlated with *Bifidobacteria* and *Prevotella* but negatively correlated with *Bacteroides* (Holmes et al., 2012; Lazar et al., 2019). In addition, lactose is related to the reduction of *Clostridia* (Francavilla et al., 2012). Furthermore, unlike digestible carbohydrates, nondigestible carbohydrates are the main materials that offer commensal bacteria to produce SCFAs. Quantity and types of fiber intake have a huge effect on gut microbiota alternations. Negative association with Bacteroides and Actinobacteria and positive association with Proteobacteria and Firmicutes were discerned in fiber intervention, and Firmicutes and Actinobacteria were the main responders particularly (Holmes et al., 2012). According to previous reports, individuals who received a diet with resistant starch as a supplement had an enhanced abundance of *Bifidobacterium adolescentis, Ruminoccocus bromii, Eubacterium rectale*, and *Parabacteroides distasonis* (Makki et al., 2018). Conversely, galactooligosaccharides intervention can increase the volume of *Bifidobacterium* spp. (Davis et al., 2011). *Faecalibacterium prausnitzii*, a high SCFA producer, was not observed in the gut microflora profile of diabetic patients. These results illustrated that carbohydrates are attributed to the composition of gut microbiota (Machiels et al., 2014).

Artificial sweeteners such as sucralose, saccharin, and aspartame are designed as healthier food additives, are becoming a new trend, and are widely used to reduce energy intake for natural sugar. However, Suez et al. proved that artificial sweeteners have a relationship with microbiota dysbiosis and metabolic abnormalities. This gut microbiota compositional and functional alteration leads to metabolic disease and glucose intolerance in healthy human subjects. An increase of *Bacteroides* spp. and reduction of *Lactobacillus reuteri* are observed in the diet with artificial sweetener usage (Suez et al., 2014).

## FAT

Fats are generally divided into several types based on their structure. Consumption of saturated and trans fats has been proven to enhance the risks of cardiovascular disease. Conversely, monounsaturated and polyunsaturated fats are known as health-promoting fats that alleviate the risk of chronic diseases. In general, a positive correlation with Bacteroides and Actinobacteria and a negative correlation with Firmicutes and Proteobacteria were observed in the diet with rich fats. Fats from dairy products have been reported to promote *delta Proteobacteria* and induce inflammation (Holmes et al., 2012). Dietary with rich fat modifies the gut microbiota structure with abundant LPS-expressing bacteria that lead to enhanced circulating LPS levels in humans (Amar et al., 2008). LPS is related to weight gain, adiposity accumulation, and the induction of inflammatory markers in white adipose tissue that facilitate host physiology to a preinflammatory status. It is interesting that the adverse effect of saturated fat seems to be specific to mice fed a lard-rich diet, and meanwhile, enrichment of *Bacteroides, Turicibacter*, and *Bilophila* spp. were observed to be associated with the white adipose tissue inflammation, adiposity, and insulin intolerance. In contrast, mice fed a diet with unsaturated fat exhibited increased amounts of *Bifidobacterium, Akkermansia*, and *Lactobacillus* spp. with no metabolic disorders observed (Caesar et al., 2015). Nevertheless, there are inconsistent results in the human clinical trials and individuals who switch diet patterns from saturated fat to unsaturated fat as caloric sources did not influence the gut microbiota structure but reduced the total bacterial volume (Fava et al., 2013).

## PROTEIN

Contrarily, consumption protein presents a comprehensively different gut microbiota profile. Sources of protein are important characteristics to impact gut microbiota. Both the diet with vegetarian protein (whey and pea) and animal protein are contributed to overall microbiota diversity (Singh et al., 2017). Generally, plant protein intake has positively associated with commensal *Bifidobacterium* and *Lactobacillus*, whereas negatively associated with pathogenic including *Bacteroides* and *Clostridium perfringens*. *Bifidobacterium* and *Lactobacillus* are contributed to SCFA production that optimizes the host gut mucosa barrier and reduces inflammation. By contrast, the diet rich in animal protein enhances *Prevotella* and *Clostridia* levels as well as reduce the number of *Bifidobacterium*. Also, animal protein can enhance the abundance of bile-tolerant anaerobes such as *Alistipes* spp., *Bilophila* spp., and *Bacteroides* spp. that are related to trimethylamine N-oxide formation and promote the risk of atherosclerosis and IBD (David et al., 2014; De Filippis et al., 2016; Singh et al., 2017).

## MICRONUTRIENTS

Trace minerals and vitamins are known as micronutrients, and their intake is crucial for physiological maintenance. Various studies have demonstrated the interaction between micronutrients and gut microbiota and led to further metabolic regulation. Iron supplementation suppresses the levels of *Bifidobacterium* but enhances the counts of *Bacteroides* and *E. coli*. Another study revealed an increase in the fecal *Enterobacteriaceae* family and a reduction in *Lactobacillus*. These results are totally consistent with the argument that bacteria and some pathogens are efficient iron scavengers. Thus, iron supplementation may give rise to microbiota dysbiosis and pathogen invasion (Yilmaz and Li, 2018). Manganese supplementation in mice increased the colonization of the heart and lethality of *Staphylococcus aureus* infection, likely because the bacterium utilizes manganese to protect itself from reactive oxygen species and neutrophil killing (Juttukonda et al., 2017). *Bacteroides vulgatus* is a prominent responder to vitamin A, and it increases in number in the absence of vitamin A. *Bacteroides dorei* decreases when vitamin A is deficient (Hibberd et al., 2017). Vitamin D plays a vital role in immune homeostasis maintenance due to its interaction with the gut microbiota. It has been reported that vitamin D has a negative correlation with gram-negative genera, such as *Haemophilus* and *Veillonella*. This variation may be promoted by low intake or levels of vitamin D (Luthold et al., 2017).

## APPLICATIONS

Cumulative evidence elucidates that gut microbiota composition and diversity influence host metabolism and has close relationships with obesity and metabolic disorders. Currently, scientists gain more knowledge on the mechanism between resident bacteria and host metabolism, which leads to the development of different ways to manipulate gut microbiota, such as fecal microbiota transplantation, probiotics, and prebiotic intervention. In addition, lifestyle and dietary patterns are well understood to alter and optimize the gut microbiota profile, especially by enriching commensal bacteria. In this section, we will review studies with different applications to gain more comprehension on enhancing human wellness by fostering a healthy gut microbiota and environment.

## CLINICAL THERAPEUTICS

Fecal microbiota transplantation (FMT) is a novel method to alleviate dysbiosis and complications. Patients receive healthy donor feces and transfer the donor's gut microbiota into the intestinal tract to restore the dysbiosis. In clinical, FMT has become a robust method to treat recurrent or refractory *Clostridium difficile* infection (Smits et al., 2013). Additionally, various clinical experiments have proven that FMT can relieve ulcerative colitis and reduce the relative pathogenic gastrointestinal symptoms (Gupta et al., 2016). Recently, persuasive evidence has shown that FMT has become a treatment for obesity, metabolic syndrome, and diabetes mellitus. The possible mechanisms of FMT are the alternation of gut microbiota, enhancement of gut barrier integrity and immunomodulation, and inhibition of pathogen growth. Furthermore, the level of SCFA-producing bacteria is increased in the patients with metabolic syndrome after receiving microbiota from lean donors and significantly improves insulin sensitivity and fasting glycemia (Vrieze et al., 2012). Supporting this notion, Ng et al. revealed that FMT can increase butyrate-producing bacteria in the group of obese patients with type 2 diabetes mellitus. In particular, the abundances of *Bifidobacterium* and *Lactobacillus* were increased after FMT with lifestyle intervention. The improvement of total and low-density lipoprotein cholesterol and liver stiffness is observed in recipients with lifestyle intervention (Ng et al., 2021). Thus, manipulating the human gut microbiome may provide an effective treatment for obesity.

## PROBIOTICS AND PREBIOTICS INTERVENTION

Probiotics are commensal bacteria that have a beneficial influence on host health. *Bifidobacterium* and lactic acid bacteria such as *Lactobacillus* are the most well-known and widely used probiotics that exist in functional food, fermented food, and dietary supplements. Moreover, heat-killed probiotics have been proven to have the advantage of physiological modulation (Plaza-Diaz et al., 2019). Probiotics have been reported to interact with the host through four main mechanisms, including promoting intestinal barrier function, competition with pathogens, immunomodulation, and physiological influences (Sánchez et al., 2017). Previous studies prove the mitigation of severe digestive disorders, allergic disorders, Clostridium difficile–associated diarrhea, and inflammatory bowel disorders after administration of probiotics (Plaza-Diaz et al., 2019).

Additionally, probiotics have also declared a resolution of metabolic disorders and obesity due to their modulation capability. Supporting this notion, various studies have enumerated evidence that probiotics have the antimetabolic disorders and anti-obesity ability. In animal models, *Lactobacillus* (e.g., *L. casei* strain *Shirota* (LAB13), *L. gasseri*, *L. rhamnosus*, *L. plantarum*) and *Bifidobacterium* (e.g., *B. infantis*, *B. longum*, and *B. breve* B3) have been revealed to have anti-obesity ability and reduce fat accumulation in well-established animal models of obesity (Abenavoli et al., 2019). Clinically, *Lactobacillus gasseri* SBT2055 and *Lactobacillus plantarum* have been proven to reduce the BMI in obese adults, and *L. gasseri* SBT2055 decreases visceral fat area, while *L. plantarum* can especially alleviate hypertension (Kadooka et al., 2010; Sharafedtinov et al., 2013). *Bifidobacterium animalis* subsp. *lactis* CECT 8145 led to a decrease in BMI, body weight, as well as fat mass and waist circumference (Pedret et al., 2019). The combination of probiotics with multiple strains is widely applied in clinical trials. A commercial probiotic mixture, VSL#3®, combined with multiple bacterial strains, including *Lactobacillus* spp., *Bifidobacterium* spp., and *Streptococcus*, provides evidence of anti-obesity ability and inhibits adipose accumulation in young adults (Cheng et al., 2020; Osterberg et al., 2015). Obese individuals who supplemented *Lactobacillus acidophilus* La5 and *Bifidobacterium animalis* subsp *lactis* Bb12 can improve glycemic control (Ivey et al., 2014). Selected probiotics have been demonstrated to improve fasting blood glucose levels, insulin sensitivity, and carbohydrate metabolism and reduce the metabolic stress in type 2 diabetes mellitus. In addition, recent research shows that particular selected probiotics and symbiotics improve the liver biochemical and metabolic parameters in nonalcoholic fatty liver disease patients (Sáez-Lara et al., 2016).

Prebiotics are also critical for alleviating dysbiosis and improving obesity. In 2008, Food and Agriculture Organization defined prebiotics as a "nonviable food component that confers a health benefit on the host associated with modulation of the microbiota" (Pineiro et al., 2008). Prebiotics are common in fruits and vegetables, and their presence has numerous health benefits. The major characteristics of prebiotics is non-digested or partially digested and cannot be absorbed in the upper segments of the alimentary tract, while prebiotics can be well fermented by probiotics which are usually located in the colon. Carbohydrates and their derivates are the most common molecular structures of prebiotics and are normally found in animal and human diets including disaccharides, oligosaccharides, and polysaccharides (Markowiak and Śliżewska, 2017). Prebiotics may mediate microbiota composition and microbial metabolic products such as SCFAs, suppression of pathogenic bacteria, trace elements absorption, and the immune system. *Lactobacilli* and *Bifidobacteria* are the populations that have the most significant blooms induced by prebiotics (Bindels et al., 2015). In addition, accumulating evidence suggests the beneficial effects of prebiotics on host metabolism. In a human study, overweight and obese adults consumed oligofructose as supplementation and found a decrease in body weight, body fat, and plasma glucose. In particular, oligofructose supplementation also resulted in a lower energy intake due to the regulation of satiety hormones, including ghrelin and PYY (Parnell and Reimer, 2009). Supplementation with prebiotics increased plasma gut peptide production (GLP-1 and PYY), which contributes to altered appetite sensations and glucose responses following meals (Cani et al., 2009). Another study also found a similar result in overweight and obese children. A reduction in energy intake and improvement in appetite control was observed with prebiotics intervention (Hume et al., 2017). Moreover, prebiotics are helpful in the reduction of blood lipids, including total cholesterol, low-density lipoprotein-cholesterol, and triacylglycerol levels (Delzenne and Williams, 2002). Thus, scientists suppose that prebiotics play a pivotal role in satiety control, glucose, and lipid catabolism (Markowiak and Śliżewska, 2017).

In addition to administrating probiotics and prebiotics supplementation, consuming fermented food is also a good way to intake sufficient probiotics. Fermented foods contain stable microorganisms, usually including diverse lactic acid bacteria and their metabolites. The well-known fermented foods are yogurt, cheese, kefir, cocoa, pickles, kimchi, sauerkraut, and red wine. The variety of bacteria that fermented food contains may have health-promoting properties and modulated functions on the gut microbiota. Probiotics in fermented food can interact with the host gut microbiota and mediate the composition into a "healthy gut microbiota." It has been reported that dysbiosis can be prevented after consuming fermented food periodically (Stiemsma et al., 2020). Yogurt, fermented by cultured probiotics, ameliorates human metabolic disorders, including insulin intolerance and hepatic fat fraction. Additionally, a reduction in serum LPS levels and modulation of gut microbiota composition were observed in obese adults with metabolic syndrome and nonfatty liver disease (Chen et al., 2019). The investigations of kefir were discrepancies about the metabolism modulation. However, some studies have mentioned the improvement of lipid metabolic parameters, fasting blood glucose, and HbA1c levels; in contrast, body weight was not significantly different (Bourrie et al., 2020). Han et al. found an increase in *Bifidobacterium* after kimchi consumption for 8 weeks, and the gene correlated with metabolism, immunity, and digestion was upregulated in obese individuals (Han et al., 2015). For red wine, previous studies have revealed that the intake of red wine increases *Bifidobacterium*, *Prevotella*, *Bacteroides*, *Eggerthellalenta*, *Enterococcus*, *Bacteroidesuniformis*, and *Blautiacoccoides/Eubacterium rectale* abundance in the gut microbiota. Meanwhile, a reduction in BMI and body weight and amelioration of blood pressure, total cholesterol, high-density lipoprotein -cholesterol levels are observed due to the rich polyphenols (Moreno-Indias et al., 2016; Queipo-Ortuño et al., 2012).

Individuals with high-protein and low-carbohydrate diets have fewer levels of *Roseburia* and *Eubacterium rectale* and lower levels of butyrate in their feces, which may have detrimental effects (Russell et al., 2011). In addition, the abundance of *Prevotella* and *Bacteroides* is increased after intake of red meat. Furthermore, red meat contains L-carnitine, which induces the production of the proatherogenic microbial metabolite trimethylamine N-oxide production and may induce the risk of metabolic syndrome (Lazar et al., 2019). HFDs have been positively correlated with metabolic syndrome and type 2 diabetes and have also been known as obesogenic diets. In addition, saturated fats and trans fats are especially linked with cardiovascular disease. Consumption of monosaturated and polyunsaturated fats can decrease the risk of chronic disease. For gut microbiota modification, HFDs can enrich the numbers of Bacteroides and total anaerobic microorganisms. In contrast, blooms of *Bifidobacterium* are observed after intake of a low-fat diet and improve fasting glucose and total cholesterol (Fava et al., 2013). As mentioned above, fruits and vegetables are full of dietary fiber, flavones, and polyphenols. They are recommended for intake and bring multiple benefits to optimize gut microbiota and GI tract health. A recent study used a multiomics approach to demonstrate the intestinal microbiome response in vegetable-rich diets. An increase in catalytic activities for carbohydrates and food proteins, an increase of cell motility to access nutrients, and the release or synthesis of bioactive metabolites and proteins that are beneficial to human health have been observed (De Angelis et al., 2020).

## CONCLUSION

In this chapter, we elucidated the importance and characteristics of gut microbiota and the interaction between bacteria and the host. In particular, we mentioned how gut microbiota signals and contributes to host metabolism by microbial metabolites, altering richness, and elevating or suppressing specific bacteria. The gut microbiota plays a critical role in the host metabolism by modulating the gut environment, immune system, metabolism, and appetite. The knowledge drives the development of therapies that enhance human well-being by improving the gut microbiome composition and diversity. Thus, therapeutic applications of microbiota, including diet, probiotics, and prebiotics treatment, have become a novel approach to tackle the problem of obesity and metabolic disorders.

## REFERENCES

Abenavoli, L., Scarpellini, E., Colica, C., Boccuto, L., Salehi, B., Sharifi-Rad, J., Aiello, V., Romano, B., De Lorenzo, A., Izzo, A.A., Capasso, R., 2019. Gut microbiota and obesity: a role for probiotics. *Nutrients* 11, 2690.

Alcock, J., Maley, C.C., Aktipis, C.A., 2014. Is eating behavior manipulated by the gastrointestinal microbiota? Evolutionary pressures and potential mechanisms. *Bioessays* 36, 940–949.

Amar, J., Burcelin, R., Ruidavets, J.B., Cani, P.D., Fauvel, J., Alessi, M.C., Chamontin, B., Ferriéres, J., 2008. Energy intake is associated with endotoxemia in apparently healthy men. *The American Journal of Clinical Nutrition* 87, 1219–1223.

Andreoli, M.F., Donato, J., Cakir, I., Perello, M., 2019. Leptin resensitisation: a reversion of leptin-resistant states. *Journal of Endocrinology* 241, R81–R96.

Aron-Wisnewsky, J., Prifti, E., Belda, E., Ichou, F., Kayser, B.D., Dao, M.C., Verger, E.O., Hedjazi, L., Bouillot, J.-L., Chevallier, J.-M., 2019. Major microbiota dysbiosis in severe obesity: fate after bariatric surgery. *Gut* 68, 70–82.

Arumugam, M., Raes, J., Pelletier, E., Le Paslier, D., Yamada, T., Mende, D.R., Fernandes, G.R., Tap, J., Bruls, T., Batto, J.-M., 2011. Enterotypes of the human gut microbiome. *Nature* 473, 174–180.

Bäckhed, F., Ding, H., Wang, T., Hooper, L.V., Koh, G.Y., Nagy, A., Semenkovich, C.F., Gordon, J.I., 2004. The gut microbiota as an environmental factor that regulates fat storage. *Proceedings of the National Academy of Sciences* 101, 15718–15723.

Bäckhed, F., Manchester, J.K., Semenkovich, C.F., Gordon, J.I., 2007. Mechanisms underlying the resistance to diet-induced obesity in germ-free mice. *Proceedings of the National Academy of Sciences* 104, 979–984.

Bernard, A., Ancel, D., Neyrinck, A.M., Dastugue, A., Bindels, L.B., Delzenne, N.M., Besnard, P., 2019. A preventive prebiotic supplementation improves the sweet taste perception in diet-induced obese mice. *Nutrients* 11, 549.

Bervoets, L., Van Hoorenbeeck, K., Kortleven, I., Van Noten, C., Hens, N., Vael, C., Goossens, H., Desager, K.N., Vankerckhoven, V., 2013. Differences in gut microbiota composition between obese and lean children: a cross-sectional study. *Gut Pathogens* 5, 1–10.

Bindels, L.B., Delzenne, N.M., Cani, P.D., Walter, J., 2015. Towards a more comprehensive concept for prebiotics. *Nature Reviews Gastroenterology & Hepatology* 12, 303–310.

Bischoff, S.C., 2016. Microbiota and aging. *Current Opinion in Clinical Nutrition & Metabolic Care* 19, 26–30.

Blaak, E., Canfora, E., Theis, S., Frost, G., Groen, A., Mithieux, G., Nauta, A., Scott, K., Stahl, B., van Harsselaar, J., 2020. Short chain fatty acids in human gut and metabolic health. *Beneficial Microbes* 11, 411–455.

Blaut, M., 2015. Gut microbiota and energy balance: role in obesity. *Proceedings of the Nutrition Society* 74, 227–234.

Bourrie, B.C., Richard, C., Willing, B.P., 2020. Kefir in the prevention and treatment of obesity and metabolic disorders. *Current Nutrition Reports* 9, 184–192.

Browning, K.N., Verheijden, S., Boeckxstaens, G.E., 2017. The vagus nerve in appetite regulation, mood, and intestinal inflammation. *Gastroenterology* 152, 730–744.

Byrne, C., Chambers, E., Morrison, D., Frost, G., 2015. The role of short chain fatty acids in appetite regulation and energy homeostasis. *International Journal of Obesity* 39, 1331–1338.

Caesar, R., Tremaroli, V., Kovatcheva-Datchary, P., Cani, P.D., Bäckhed, F., 2015. Crosstalk between gut microbiota and dietary lipids aggravates WAT inflammation through TLR signaling. *Cell Metabolism* 22, 658–668.

Calle, E.E., Kaaks, R., 2004. Overweight, obesity and cancer: epidemiological evidence and proposed mechanisms. *Nature Reviews Cancer* 4, 579–591.

Campos, A.C., Rocha, N.P., Nicoli, J.R., Vieira, L.Q., Teixeira, M.M., Teixeira, A.L., 2016. Absence of gut microbiota influences lipopolysaccharide-induced behavioral changes in mice. *Behavioural Brain Research* 312, 186–194.

Cani, P.D., Bibiloni, R., Knauf, C., Waget, A., Neyrinck, A.M., Delzenne, N.M., Burcelin, R., 2008. Changes in gut microbiota control metabolic endotoxemia-induced inflammation in high-fat diet–induced obesity and diabetes in mice. *Diabetes* 57, 1470–1481.

Cani, P.D., Lecourt, E., Dewulf, E.M., Sohet, F.M., Pachikian, B.D., Naslain, D., De Backer, F., Neyrinck, A.M., Delzenne, N.M., 2009. Gut microbiota fermentation of prebiotics increases satietogenic and incretin gut peptide production with consequences for appetite sensation and glucose response after a meal. *The American Journal of Clinical Nutrition* 90, 1236–1243.

Caussy, C., Wallet, F., Laville, M., Disse, E., 2020. Obesity is associated with severe forms of COVID-19. *Obesity (Silver Spring, Md.)*, 28, 1175.

Chen, Y., Feng, R., Yang, X., Dai, J., Huang, M., Ji, X., Li, Y., Okekunle, A.P., Gao, G., Onwuka, J.U., 2019. Yogurt improves insulin resistance and liver fat in obese women with nonalcoholic fatty liver disease and metabolic syndrome: a randomized controlled trial. *The American Journal of Clinical Nutrition* 109, 1611–1619.

Cheng, F.-S., Pan, D., Chang, B., Jiang, M., Sang, L.-X., 2020. Probiotic mixture VSL# 3: an overview of basic and clinical studies in chronic diseases. *World Journal of Clinical Cases* 8, 1361.

Cheng, Y.-C., Liu, J.-R., 2020. Effect of Lactobacillus rhamnosus GG on energy metabolism, leptin resistance, and gut microbiota in mice with diet-induced obesity. *Nutrients* 12, 2557.

Chooi, Y.C., Ding, C., Magkos, F., 2019. The epidemiology of obesity. *Metabolism* 92, 6–10.

Consortium, H.M.P., 2012. Structure, function and diversity of the healthy human microbiome. *Nature* 486, 207.

Coyte, K.Z., Rakoff-Nahoum, S., 2019. Understanding competition and cooperation within the mammalian gut microbiome. *Current Biology* 29, R538–R544.

Cryan, J.F., O'Riordan, K.J., Cowan, C.S., Sandhu, K.V., Bastiaanssen, T.F., Boehme, M., Codagnone, M.G., Cussotto, S., Fulling, C., Golubeva, A.V., 2019. The microbiota-gut-brain axis. *Physiological Reviews*. 99, 1877–2013.

David, L.A., Maurice, C.F., Carmody, R.N., Gootenberg, D.B., Button, J.E., Wolfe, B.E., Ling, A.V., Devlin, A.S., Varma, Y., Fischbach, M.A., 2014. Diet rapidly and reproducibly alters the human gut microbiome. *Nature* 505, 559–563.

Davis, L.M., Martínez, I., Walter, J., Goin, C., Hutkins, R.W., 2011. Barcoded pyrosequencing reveals that consumption of galactooligosaccharides results in a highly specific bifidogenic response in humans. *PLoS One* 6, e25200.

De Angelis, M., Ferrocino, I., Calabrese, F.M., De Filippis, F., Cavallo, N., Siragusa, S., Rampelli, S., Di Cagno, R., Rantsiou, K., Vannini, L., 2020. Diet influences the functions of the human intestinal microbiome. *Scientific Reports* 10, 1–15.

De Filippis, F., Pellegrini, N., Vannini, L., Jeffery, I.B., La Storia, A., Laghi, L., Serrazanetti, D.I., Di Cagno, R., Ferrocino, I., Lazzi, C., 2016. High-level adherence to a Mediterranean diet beneficially impacts the gut microbiota and associated metabolome. *Gut* 65, 1812–1821.

De Palma, G., Nadal, I., Collado, M.C., Sanz, Y., 2009. Effects of a gluten-free diet on gut microbiota and immune function in healthy adult human subjects. *British Journal of Nutrition* 102, 1154–1160.

De Vadder, F., Kovatcheva-Datchary, P., Zitoun, C., Duchampt, A., Bäckhed, F., Mithieux, G., 2016. Microbiota-produced succinate improves glucose homeostasis via intestinal gluconeogenesis. *Cell Metabolism* 24, 151–157.

Delzenne, N.M., Williams, C.M., 2002. Prebiotics and lipid metabolism. *Current Opinion in Lipidology* 13, 61–67.

Dietz, W., Santos-Burgoa, C., 2020. Obesity and its implications for COVID-19 mortality. *Obesity (Silver Spring)* 28, 1005.

Everard, A., Lazarevic, V., Derrien, M., Girard, M., Muccioli, G.G., Neyrinck, A.M., Possemiers, S., Van Holle, A., François, P., de Vos, W.M., 2011. Responses of gut microbiota and glucose and lipid metabolism to prebiotics in genetic obese and diet-induced leptin-resistant mice. *Diabetes* 60, 2775–2786.

Fan, Y., Pedersen, O., 2021. Gut microbiota in human metabolic health and disease. *Nature Reviews Microbiology* 19, 55–71.

Fava, F., Gitau, R., Griffin, B.A., Gibson, G., Tuohy, K., Lovegrove, J., 2013. The type and quantity of dietary fat and carbohydrate alter faecal microbiome and short-chain fatty acid excretion in a metabolic syndrome 'at-risk'population. *International Journal of Obesity* 37, 216–223.

Ferretti, P., Pasolli, E., Tett, A., Asnicar, F., Gorfer, V., Fedi, S., Armanini, F., Truong, D.T., Manara, S., Zolfo, M., 2018. Mother-to-infant microbial transmission from different body sites shapes the developing infant gut microbiome. *Cell Host & Microbe* 24, 133–145.

Fetissov, S.O., Sinno, M.H., Coëffier, M., Bole-Feysot, C., Ducrotté, P., Hökfelt, T., Déchelotte, P., 2008. Autoantibodies against appetite-regulating peptide hormones and neuropeptides: putative modulation by gut microflora. *Nutrition* 24, 348–359.

Flint, H.J., Duncan, S.H., Scott, K.P., Louis, P., 2015. Links between diet, gut microbiota composition and gut metabolism. *Proceedings of the Nutrition Society* 74, 13–22.

Foster, J.A., Neufeld, K.-A.M., 2013. Gut–brain axis: how the microbiome influences anxiety and depression. *Trends in Neurosciences* 36, 305–312.

Francavilla, R., Calasso, M., Calace, L., Siragusa, S., Ndagijimana, M., Vernocchi, P., Brunetti, L., Mancino, G., Tedeschi, G., Guerzoni, E., 2012. Effect of lactose on gut microbiota and metabolome of infants with cow's milk allergy. *Pediatric Allergy and Immunology* 23, 420–427.

Gao, Z., Yin, J., Zhang, J., Ward, R.E., Martin, R.J., Lefevre, M., Cefalu, W.T., Ye, J., 2009. Butyrate improves insulin sensitivity and increases energy expenditure in mice. *Diabetes* 58, 1509–1517.

Garcia-Mantrana, I., Selma-Royo, M., Alcantara, C., Collado, M.C., 2018. Shifts on gut microbiota associated to mediterranean diet adherence and specific dietary intakes on general adult population. *Frontiers in Microbiology* 9, 890.

Glick-Bauer, M., Yeh, M.-C., 2014. The health advantage of a vegan diet: exploring the gut microbiota connection. *Nutrients* 6, 4822–4838.

Gonze, D., Coyte, K.Z., Lahti, L., Faust, K., 2018. Microbial communities as dynamical systems. *Current Opinion in Microbiology* 44, 41–49.

Gribble, F.M., Reimann, F., 2016. Enteroendocrine cells: chemosensors in the intestinal epithelium. *Annual review of physiology* 78, 277–299.

Gupta, S., Allen-Vercoe, E., Petrof, E.O., 2016. Fecal microbiota transplantation: in perspective. *Therapeutic Advances in Gastroenterology* 9, 229–239.

Han, K., Bose, S., Wang, J., Kim, B.S., Kim, M.J., Kim, E.J., Kim, H., 2015. Contrasting effects of fresh and fermented kimchi consumption on gut microbiota composition and gene expression related to metabolic syndrome in obese Korean women. *Molecular Nutrition & Food Research* 59, 1004–1008.

Heiss, C.N., Mannerås-Holm, L., Lee, Y.S., Serrano-Lobo, J., Gladh, A.H., Seeley, R.J., Drucker, D.J., Bäckhed, F., Olofsson, L.E., 2021. The gut microbiota regulates hypothalamic inflammation and leptin sensitivity in Western diet-fed mice via a GLP-1R-dependent mechanism. *Cell Reports* 35, 109163.

Heiss, C.N., Olofsson, L.E., 2018. Gut microbiota-dependent modulation of energy metabolism. *Journal of Innate Immunity* 10, 163–171.

Hibberd, M.C., Wu, M., Rodionov, D.A., Li, X., Cheng, J., Griffin, N.W., Barratt, M.J., Giannone, R.J., Hettich, R.L., Osterman, A.L., 2017. The effects of micronutrient deficiencies on bacterial species from the human gut microbiota. *Science Translational Medicine* 9, eaal4069.

Holmes, E., Li, J.V., Marchesi, J.R., Nicholson, J.K., 2012. Gut microbiota composition and activity in relation to host metabolic phenotype and disease risk. *Cell Metabolism* 16, 559–564.

Hume, M.P., Nicolucci, A.C., Reimer, R.A., 2017. Prebiotic supplementation improves appetite control in children with overweight and obesity: a randomized controlled trial. *The American Journal of Clinical Nutrition* 105, 790–799.

Hussain, M.M., Pan, X., 2009. Clock genes, intestinal transport and plasma lipid homeostasis. *Trends in Endocrinology & Metabolism* 20, 177–185.

Ivey, K.L., Hodgson, J.M., Kerr, D.A., Lewis, J.R., Thompson, P.L., Prince, R.L., 2014. The effects of probiotic bacteria on glycaemic control in overweight men and women: a randomised controlled trial. *European Journal of Clinical Nutrition* 68, 447–452.

Jumpertz, R., Le, D.S., Turnbaugh, P.J., Trinidad, C., Bogardus, C., Gordon, J.I., Krakoff, J., 2011. Energy-balance studies reveal associations between gut microbes, caloric load, and nutrient absorption in humans. *The American Journal of Clinical Nutrition* 94, 58–65.

Juttukonda, L.J., Berends, E.T., Zackular, J.P., Moore, J.L., Stier, M.T., Zhang, Y., Schmitz, J.E., Beavers, W.N., Wijers, C.D., Gilston, B.A., 2017. Dietary manganese promotes staphylococcal infection of the heart. *Cell Host & Microbe* 22, 531–542.

Kaakoush, N.O., Day, A.S., Huinao, K.D., Leach, S.T., Lemberg, D.A., Dowd, S.E., Mitchell, H.M., 2012. Microbial dysbiosis in pediatric patients with Crohn's disease. *Journal of Clinical Microbiology* 50, 3258–3266.

Kadooka, Y., Sato, M., Imaizumi, K., Ogawa, A., Ikuyama, K., Akai, Y., Okano, M., Kagoshima, M., Tsuchida, T., 2010. Regulation of abdominal adiposity by probiotics (Lactobacillus gasseri SBT2055) in adults with obese tendencies in a randomized controlled trial. *European Journal of Clinical Nutrition* 64, 636–643.

Kamada, N., Seo, S.-U., Chen, G.Y., Núñez, G., 2013. Role of the gut microbiota in immunity and inflammatory disease. *Nature Reviews Immunology* 13, 321–335.

Kim, B., Choi, H.-N., Yim, J.-E., 2019. Effect of diet on the gut microbiota associated with obesity. *Journal of Obesity & Metabolic Syndrome* 28, 216.

Kimura, I., Ozawa, K., Inoue, D., Imamura, T., Kimura, K., Maeda, T., Terasawa, K., Kashihara, D., Hirano, K., Tani, T., 2013. The gut microbiota suppresses insulin-mediated fat accumulation via the short-chain fatty acid receptor GPR43. *Nature Communications* 4, 1–12.

Kocełak, P., Zak-Gołąb, A., Zahorska-Markiewicz, B., Aptekorz, M., Zientara, M., Martirosian, G., Chudek, J., Olszanecka-Glinianowicz, M., 2013. Resting energy expenditure and gut microbiota in obese and normal weight subjects. *European Review for Medical and Pharmacological Sciences* 17, 2816–2821.

Kojima, M., Kangawa, K., 2005. Ghrelin: structure and function. *Physiological Reviews* 85, 495–522.

la Cuesta-Zuluaga, D., Mueller, N.T., Álvarez-Quintero, R., Velásquez-Mejía, E.P., Sierra, J.A., Corrales-Agudelo, V., Carmona, J.A., Abad, J.M., Escobar, J.S., 2019. Higher fecal short-chain fatty acid levels are associated with gut microbiome dysbiosis, obesity, hypertension and cardiometabolic disease risk factors. *Nutrients* 11, 51.

Larraufie, P., Martin-Gallausiaux, C., Lapaque, N., Dore, J., Gribble, F., Reimann, F., Blottiere, H., 2018. SCFAs strongly stimulate PYY production in human enteroendocrine cells. *Scientific Reports* 8, 1–9.

Lazar, V., Ditu, L.-M., Pircalabioru, G.G., Picu, A., Petcu, L., Cucu, N., Chifiriuc, M.C., 2019. Gut microbiota, host organism, and diet trialogue in diabetes and obesity. *Frontiers in Nutrition* 6, 21.

Le Chatelier, E., Nielsen, T., Qin, J., Prifti, E., Hildebrand, F., Falony, G., Almeida, M., Arumugam, M., Batto, J.-M., Kennedy, S., 2013. Richness of human gut microbiome correlates with metabolic markers. *Nature* 500, 541–546.

Leeuwendaal, N.K., Cryan, J.F., Schellekens, H., 2021. Gut peptides and the microbiome: focus on ghrelin. *Current Opinion in Endocrinology, Diabetes, and Obesity* 28, 243.

Ley, R.E., Turnbaugh, P.J., Klein, S., Gordon, J.I., 2006. Human gut microbes associated with obesity. *Nature* 444, 1022–1023.

Liang, X., Bushman, F.D., FitzGerald, G.A., 2015. Rhythmicity of the intestinal microbiota is regulated by gender and the host circadian clock. *Proceedings of the National Academy of Sciences* 112, 10479–10484.

Liang, X., FitzGerald, G.A., 2017. Timing the microbes: the circadian rhythm of the gut microbiome. *Journal of Biological Rhythms* 32, 505–515.

Liu, C.M., Kanoski, S.E., 2018. Homeostatic and non-homeostatic controls of feeding behavior: distinct vs. common neural systems. *Physiology & Behavior* 193, 223–231.

Luczynski, P., McVey Neufeld, K.-A., Oriach, C.S., Clarke, G., Dinan, T.G., Cryan, J.F., 2016. Growing up in a bubble: using germ-free animals to assess the influence of the gut microbiota on brain and behavior. *International Journal of Neuropsychopharmacology* 19, 1–17.

Luthold, R.V., Fernandes, G.R., Franco-de-Moraes, A.C., Folchetti, L.G., Ferreira, S.R.G., 2017. Gut microbiota interactions with the immunomodulatory role of vitamin D in normal individuals. *Metabolism* 69, 76–86.

Machiels, K., Joossens, M., Sabino, J., De Preter, V., Arijs, I., Eeckhaut, V., Ballet, V., Claes, K., Van Immerseel, F., Verbeke, K., 2014. A decrease of the butyrate-producing species Roseburia hominis and Faecalibacterium prausnitzii defines dysbiosis in patients with ulcerative colitis. *Gut* 63, 1275–1283.

Makki, K., Deehan, E.C., Walter, J., Bäckhed, F., 2018. The impact of dietary fiber on gut microbiota in host health and disease. *Cell Host & Microbe* 23, 705–715.

Manco, M., Putignani, L., Bottazzo, G.F., 2010. Gut microbiota, lipopolysaccharides, and innate immunity in the pathogenesis of obesity and cardiovascular risk. *Endocrine Reviews* 31, 817–844.

Mariat, D., Firmesse, O., Levenez, F., Guimarães, V., Sokol, H., Doré, J., Corthier, G., Furet, J., 2009. The Firmicutes/Bacteroidctes ratio of the human microbiota changes with age. *BMC Microbiology* 9, 1–6.

Markowiak, P., Śliżewska, K., 2017. Effects of probiotics, prebiotics, and synbiotics on human health. *Nutrients* 9, 1021.

Martin, F.P.J., Dumas, M.E., Wang, Y., Legido-Quigley, C., Yap, I.K., Tang, H., Zirah, S., Murphy, G.M., Cloarec, O., Lindon, J.C., 2007. A top-down systems biology view of microbiome-mammalian metabolic interactions in a mouse model. *Molecular Systems Biology* 3, 112.

McCarville, J.L., Chen, G.Y., Cuevas, V.D., Troha, K., Ayres, J.S., 2020. Microbiota metabolites in health and disease. *Annual Review of Immunology* 38, 147–170.

Méndez-Díaz, M., Rueda-Orozco, P.E., Ruiz-Contreras, A.E., Prospéro-García, O., 2012. The endocannabinoid system modulates the valence of the emotion associated to food ingestion. *Addiction Biology* 17, 725–735.

Milani, C., Duranti, S., Bottacini, F., Casey, E., Turroni, F., Mahony, J., Belzer, C., Delgado Palacio, S., Arboleya Montes, S., Mancabelli, L., 2017. The first microbial colonizers of the human gut: composition, activities, and health implications of the infant gut microbiota. *Microbiology and Molecular Biology Reviews* 81, e00036-00017.

Million, M., Maraninchi, M., Henry, M., Armougom, F., Richet, H., Carrieri, P., Valero, R., Raccah, D., Vialettes, B., Raoult, D., 2012. Obesity-associated gut microbiota is enriched in Lactobacillus reuteri and depleted in bifidobacterium animalis and Methanobrevibacter smithii. *International Journal of Obesity* 36, 817–825.

Minaya, D.M., Turlej, A., Joshi, A., Nagy, T., Weinstein, N., DiLorenzo, P., Hajnal, A., Czaja, K., 2020. Consumption of a high energy density diet triggers microbiota dysbiosis, hepatic lipidosis, and microglia activation in the nucleus of the solitary tract in rats. *Nutrition & Diabetes* 10, 1–12.

Moreno-Indias, I., Sánchez-Alcoholado, L., Pérez-Martínez, P., Andrés-Lacueva, C., Cardona, F., Tinahones, F., Queipo-Ortuño, M.I., 2016. Red wine polyphenols modulate fecal microbiota and reduce markers of the metabolic syndrome in obese patients. *Food & function* 7, 1775–1787.

Morrison, C.D., Morton, G.J., Niswender, K.D., Gelling, R.W., Schwartz, M.W., 2005. Leptin inhibits hypothalamic Npy and Agrp gene expression via a mechanism that requires phosphatidylinositol 3-OH-kinase signaling. *American Journal of Physiology-Endocrinology and Metabolism* 289, E1051–E1057.

Morton, G., Schwartz, M., 2001. The NPY/AgRP neuron and energy homeostasis. *International Journal of Obesity* 25, S56–S62.

Mu, C., Yang, Y., Zhu, W., 2016. Gut microbiota: the brain peacekeeper. *Frontiers in Microbiology* 7, 345.

Nejrup, R.G., Licht, T.R., Hellgren, L.I., 2017. Fatty acid composition and phospholipid types used in infant formulas modifies the establishment of human gut bacteria in germ-free mice. *Scientific Reports* 7, 1–11.

Ng, S.C., Xu, Z., Mak, J.W.Y., Yang, K., Liu, Q., Zuo, T., Tang, W., Lan, I., Lui, R.N., Wong, S.H., 2021. Microbiota engraftment after faecal microbiota transplantation in obese subjects with type 2 diabetes: a 24-week, double-blind, randomised controlled trial. *Gut* 71, 716–723.

O'Toole, P.W., Jeffery, I.B., 2015. Gut microbiota and aging. *Science* 350, 1214–1215.

Osterberg, K.L., Boutagy, N.E., McMillan, R.P., Stevens, J.R., Frisard, M.I., Kavanaugh, J.W., Davy, B.M., Davy, K.P., Hulver, M.W., 2015. Probiotic supplementation attenuates increases in body mass and fat mass during high-fat diet in healthy young adults. *Obesity* 23, 2364–2370.

Parnell, J.A., Reimer, R.A., 2009. Weight loss during oligofructose supplementation is associated with decreased ghrelin and increased peptide YY in overweight and obese adults. *The American Journal of Clinical Nutrition* 89, 1751–1759.

Pedret, A., Valls, R.M., Calderón-Pérez, L., Llauradó, E., Companys, J., Pla-Pagà, L., Moragas, A., Martín-Luján, F., Ortega, Y., Giralt, M., 2019. Effects of daily consumption of the probiotic Bifidobacterium animalis subsp. lactis CECT 8145 on anthropometric adiposity biomarkers in abdominally obese subjects: a randomized controlled trial. *International Journal of Obesity* 43, 1863–1868.

Perry, R.J., Peng, L., Barry, N.A., Cline, G.W., Zhang, D., Cardone, R.L., Petersen, K.F., Kibbey, R.G., Goodman, A.L., Shulman, G.I., 2016. Acetate mediates a microbiome–brain–β-cell axis to promote metabolic syndrome. *Nature* 534, 213–217.

Pineiro, M., Asp, N.-G., Reid, G., Macfarlane, S., Morelli, L., Brunser, O., Tuohy, K., 2008. FAO Technical meeting on prebiotics. *Journal of Clinical Gastroenterology* 42, S156–S159.

Plaza-Diaz, J., Ruiz-Ojeda, F.J., Gil-Campos, M., Gil, A., 2019. Mechanisms of action of probiotics. *Advances in Nutrition* 10, S49–S66.

Popkin, B.M., Du, S., Green, W.D., Beck, M.A., Algaith, T., Herbst, C.H., Alsukait, R.F., Alluhidan, M., Alazemi, N., Shekar, M., 2020. Individuals with obesity and COVID-19: a global perspective on the epidemiology and biological relationships. *Obesity Reviews* 21, e13128.

Queipo-Ortuño, M.I., Boto-Ordóñez, M., Murri, M., Gomez-Zumaquero, J.M., Clemente-Postigo, M., Estruch, R., Cardona Diaz, F., Andres-Lacueva, C., Tinahones, F.J., 2012. Influence of red wine polyphenols and ethanol on the gut microbiota ecology and biochemical biomarkers. *The American Journal of Clinical Nutrition* 95, 1323–1334.

Queipo-Ortuño, M.I., Seoane, L.M., Murri, M., Pardo, M., Gomez-Zumaquero, J.M., Cardona, F., Casanueva, F., Tinahones, F.J., 2013. Gut microbiota composition in male rat models under different nutritional status and physical activity and its association with serum leptin and ghrelin levels. *PLoS One* 8, e65465.

Rao, C., Coyte, K.Z., Bainter, W., Geha, R.S., Martin, C.R., Rakoff-Nahoum, S., 2021. Multi-kingdom ecological drivers of microbiota assembly in preterm infants. *Nature* 591, 633–638.

Rau, A.R., Hentges, S.T., 2019. GABAergic inputs to POMC neurons originating from the dorsomedial hypothalamus are regulated by energy state. *The Journal of Neuroscience* 39, 6449–6459.

Reddel, S., Putignani, L., Del Chierico, F., 2019. The impact of low-FODMAPs, gluten-free, and ketogenic diets on gut microbiota modulation in pathological conditions. *Nutrients* 11, 373.

Renz, H., Skevaki, C., 2021. Early life microbial exposures and allergy risks: opportunities for prevention. *Nature Reviews Immunology* 21, 177–191.

Rinninella, E., Raoul, P., Cintoni, M., Franceschi, F., Miggiano, G.A.D., Gasbarrini, A., Mele, M.C., 2019. What is the healthy gut microbiota composition? A changing eco-system across age, environment, diet, and diseases. *Microorganisms* 7, 14.

Rooks, M.G., Garrett, W.S., 2016. Gut microbiota, metabolites and host immunity. *Nature Reviews Immunology* 16, 341–352.

Rosenbaum, M., Knight, R., Leibel, R.L., 2015. The gut microbiota in human energy homeostasis and obesity. *Trends in Endocrinology & Metabolism* 26, 493–501.

Russell, W.R., Gratz, S.W., Duncan, S.H., Holtrop, G., Ince, J., Scobbie, L., Duncan, G., Johnstone, A.M., Lobley, G.E., Wallace, R.J., 2011. High-protein, reduced-carbohydrate weight-loss diets promote metabolite profiles likely to be detrimental to colonic health. *The American Journal of Clinical Nutrition* 93, 1062–1072.

Sáez-Lara, M.J., Robles-Sanchez, C., Ruiz-Ojeda, F.J., Plaza-Diaz, J., Gil, A., 2016. Effects of probiotics and synbiotics on obesity, insulin resistance syndrome, type 2 diabetes and non-alcoholic fatty liver disease: a review of human clinical trials. *International Journal of Molecular Sciences* 17, 928.

Sánchez, B., Delgado, S., Blanco-Míguez, A., Lourenço, A., Gueimonde, M., Margolles, A., 2017. Probiotics, gut microbiota, and their influence on host health and disease. *Molecular Nutrition & Food Research* 61, 1600240.

Scheiman, J., Luber, J.M., Chavkin, T.A., MacDonald, T., Tung, A., Pham, L.D., Wibowo, M.C., Wurth, R.C., Punthambaker, S., Tierney, B.T., Yang, Z., Hattab, M.W., Avila-Pacheco, J., Clish, C.B., Lessard, S., Church, G.M., Kostic, A.D., 2019. Meta-omics analysis of elite athletes identifies a performance-enhancing microbe that functions via lactate metabolism. *Nature Medicine* 25, 1104–1109.

Schéle, E., Grahnemo, L., Anesten, F., Hallén, A., Bäckhed, F., Jansson, J.-O., 2013. The gut microbiota reduces leptin sensitivity and the expression of the obesity-suppressing neuropeptides proglucagon (Gcg) and brain-derived neurotrophic factor (Bdnf) in the central nervous system. *Endocrinology* 154, 3643–3651.

Sen, T., Cawthon, C.R., Ihde, B.T., Hajnal, A., DiLorenzo, P.M., Claire, B., Czaja, K., 2017. Diet-driven microbiota dysbiosis is associated with vagal remodeling and obesity. *Physiology & Behavior* 173, 305–317.

Sharafedtinov, K.K., Plotnikova, O.A., Alexeeva, R.I., Sentsova, T.B., Songisepp, E., Stsepetova, J., Smidt, I., Mikelsaar, M., 2013. Hypocaloric diet supplemented with probiotic cheese improves body mass index and blood pressure indices of obese hypertensive patients-a randomized double-blind placebo-controlled pilot study. *Nutrition Journal* 12, 1–11.

Singh, R.K., Chang, H.-W., Yan, D., Lee, K.M., Ucmak, D., Wong, K., Abrouk, M., Farahnik, B., Nakamura, M., Zhu, T.H., 2017. Influence of diet on the gut microbiome and implications for human health. *Journal of Translational Medicine* 15, 1–17.

Smits, L.P., Bouter, K.E., de Vos, W.M., Borody, T.J., Nieuwdorp, M., 2013. Therapeutic potential of fecal microbiota transplantation. *Gastroenterology* 145, 946–953.

Sobhani, I., Tap, J., Roudot-Thoraval, F., Roperch, J.P., Letulle, S., Langella, P., Corthier, G., Van Nhieu, J.T., Furet, J.P., 2011. Microbial dysbiosis in colorectal cancer (CRC) patients. *PLoS One* 6, e16393.

Sonnenburg, E.D., Smits, S.A., Tikhonov, M., Higginbottom, S.K., Wingreen, N.S., Sonnenburg, J.L., 2016. Diet-induced extinctions in the gut microbiota compound over generations. *Nature* 529, 212–215.

Statovci, D., Aguilera, M., MacSharry, J., Melgar, S., 2017. The impact of western diet and nutrients on the microbiota and immune response at mucosal interfaces. *Frontiers in Immunology* 8, 838.

Stiemsma, L.T., Nakamura, R.E., Nguyen, J.G., Michels, K.B., 2020. Does consumption of fermented foods modify the human gut microbiota? *The Journal of nutrition* 150, 1680–1692.

Suárez-Zamorano, N., Fabbiano, S., Chevalier, C., Stojanović, O., Colin, D.J., Stevanović, A., Veyrat-Durebex, C., Tarallo, V., Rigo, D., Germain, S., 2015. Microbiota depletion promotes browning of white adipose tissue and reduces obesity. *Nature Medicine* 21, 1497–1501.

Suez, J., Korem, T., Zeevi, D., Zilberman-Schapira, G., Thaiss, C.A., Maza, O., Israeli, D., Zmora, N., Gilad, S., Weinberger, A., 2014. Artificial sweeteners induce glucose intolerance by altering the gut microbiota. *Nature* 514, 181–186.

Sun, L., Ma, L., Ma, Y., Zhang, F., Zhao, C., Nie, Y., 2018. Insights into the role of gut microbiota in obesity: pathogenesis, mechanisms, and therapeutic perspectives. *Protein & Cell* 9, 397–403.

Symonds, E.L., Peiris, M., Page, A.J., Chia, B., Dogra, H., Masding, A., Galanakis, V., Atiba, M., Bulmer, D., Young, R.L., 2015. Mechanisms of activation of mouse and human enteroendocrine cells by nutrients. *Gut* 64, 618–626.

Thaiss, C.A., Zeevi, D., Levy, M., Zilberman-Schapira, G., Suez, J., Tengeler, A.C., Abramson, L., Katz, M.N., Korem, T., Zmora, N., 2014. Transkingdom control of microbiota diurnal oscillations promotes metabolic homeostasis. *Cell* 159, 514–529.

Thursby, E., Juge, N., 2017. Introduction to the human gut microbiota. *Biochemical Journal* 474, 1823–1836.

Tirosh, A., Calay, E.S., Tuncman, G., Claiborn, K.C., Inouye, K.E., Eguchi, K., Alcala, M., Rathaus, M., Hollander, K.S., Ron, I., 2019. The short-chain fatty acid propionate increases glucagon and FABP4 production, impairing insulin action in mice and humans. *Science Translational Medicine* 11, eaav0120.

Tolhurst, G., Heffron, H., Lam, Y.S., Parker, H.E., Habib, A.M., Diakogiannaki, E., Cameron, J., Grosse, J., Reimann, F., Gribble, F.M., 2012. Short-chain fatty acids stimulate glucagon-like peptide-1 secretion via the G-protein–coupled receptor FFAR2. *Diabetes* 61, 364–371.

Topping, D.L., Clifton, P.M., 2001. Short-chain fatty acids and human colonic function: roles of resistant starch and nonstarch polysaccharides. *Physiological Reviews*. 81, 1031–1064.

Torres-Fuentes, C., Schellekens, H., Dinan, T.G., Cryan, J.F., 2017. The microbiota–gut–brain axis in obesity. *The Lancet Gastroenterology & Hepatology* 2, 747–756.

Turnbaugh, P.J., Hamady, M., Yatsunenko, T., Cantarel, B.L., Duncan, A., Ley, R.E., Sogin, M.L., Jones, W.J., Roe, B.A., Affourtit, J.P., 2009. A core gut microbiome in obese and lean twins. *Nature* 457, 480–484.

Turnbaugh, P.J., Ley, R.E., Mahowald, M.A., Magrini, V., Mardis, E.R., Gordon, J.I., 2006. An obesity-associated gut microbiome with increased capacity for energy harvest. *Nature* 444, 1027–1031.

Uzbay, T., 2019. Germ-free animal experiments in the gut microbiota studies. *Current Opinion in Pharmacology* 49, 6–10.

Vaiserman, A.M., Koliada, A.K., Marotta, F., 2017. Gut microbiota: a player in aging and a target for anti-aging intervention. *Ageing Research Reviews* 35, 36–45.

van Son, J., Koekkoek, L.L., La Fleur, S.E., Serlie, M.J., Nieuwdorp, M., 2021. The role of the gut microbiota in the gut–brain axis in obesity: mechanisms and Future Implications. *International Journal of Molecular Sciences* 22, 2993.

Vaughn, A.C., Cooper, E.M., DiLorenzo, P.M., O'Loughlin, L.J., Konkel, M.E., Peters, J.H., Hajnal, A., Sen, T., Lee, S.H., de La Serre, C.B., 2017. Energy-dense diet triggers changes in gut microbiota, reorganization of gut-brain vagal communication and increases body fat accumulation. *Acta Neurobiologiae Experimentalis* 77, 18.

Voigt, R., Forsyth, C., Green, S., Engen, P., Keshavarzian, A., 2016. Circadian rhythm and the gut microbiome. *International Review of Neurobiology* 131, 193–205.

Vrieze, A., Van Nood, E., Holleman, F., Salojärvi, J., Kootte, R.S., Bartelsman, J.F., Dallinga–Thie, G.M., Ackermans, M.T., Serlie, M.J., Oozeer, R., 2012. Transfer of intestinal microbiota from lean donors increases insulin sensitivity in individuals with metabolic syndrome. *Gastroenterology* 143, 913–916.

Willemsen, L., Koetsier, M., Van Deventer, S., Van Tol, E., 2003. Short chain fatty acids stimulate epithelial mucin 2 expression through differential effects on prostaglandin E1 and E2 production by intestinal myofibroblasts. *Gut* 52, 1442–1447.

World Health Organization, 2020. *"Overweight and obesity", in Health at a Glance: Asia/Pacific 2020: Measuring Progress Towards Universal Health Coverage*, OECD Publishing, Paris, https://doi.org/10.1787/a47d0cd2-en.

Wright, H., Li, X., Fallon, N.B., Crookall, R., Giesbrecht, T., Thomas, A., Halford, J.C., Harrold, J., Stancak, A., 2016. Differential effects of hunger and satiety on insular cortex and hypothalamic functional connectivity. *European Journal of Neuroscience* 43, 1181–1189.

Xuan, C., Shamonki, J.M., Chung, A., DiNome, M.L., Chung, M., Sieling, P.A., Lee, D.J., 2014. Microbial dysbiosis is associated with human breast cancer. *PLoS One* 9, e83744.

Yilmaz, B., Li, H., 2018. Gut microbiota and iron: the crucial actors in health and disease. *Pharmaceuticals* 11, 98.

Yu, K.B., Hsiao, E.Y., 2021. Roles for the gut microbiota in regulating neuronal feeding circuits. *Journal of Clinical Investigation* 131, e143772.

Zhao, L., 2013. The gut microbiota and obesity: from correlation to causality. *Nature Reviews Microbiology* 11, 639–647.

Zhao, L., Zhang, F., Ding, X., Wu, G., Lam, Y.Y., Wang, X., Fu, H., Xue, X., Lu, C., Ma, J., 2018. Gut bacteria selectively promoted by dietary fibers alleviate type 2 diabetes. *Science* 359, 1151–1156.

Zhou, Y., Rui, L., 2013. Leptin signaling and leptin resistance. *Frontiers of Medicine* 7, 207–222.

Zmora, N., Suez, J., Elinav, E., 2019. You are what you eat: diet, health and the gut microbiota. *Nature Reviews Gastroenterology Hepatology* 16, 35–56.

# 9 Challenge, Future Research, and Influence in Food Science and Product Development

*Marta Vernero*
University of Pavia

*Claudia Caglioti and Gianluca Ianiro*
Catholic University of Rome

## CONTENTS

## FOOD AND GUT MICROBIOME

Being more than $10^{14}$, bacteria are the most represented inhabitants of human microbiota, together with viruses and fungi. Human gut host approximately 1,000 species of bacteria, most of which are anaerobes, mainly belonging to Bacteroidetes and Firmicutes phyla, that all together represent the 90% of gut bacterial microbiome. The remaining 10% is represented by Actinobacteria, Fusobacteria, Proteobacteria, and Verrucomicrobia as well as by some other minor phyla. The individual composition of gut microbiota is widely different in each human depending on a variety of genetic and environmental factors, including age, lifestyle, food intake, drug administration, and illnesses of the patient. As drugs are concerned, of course the most relevant influence on gut microbiota composition is due to antibiotics administration (Ianiro, Tilg, and Gasbarrini 2016; Jernberg et al. 2010; Slimings and Riley 2014; Jakobsson et al. 2010; Zhang et al. 2013; Fouhy et al. 2012).

Another major factor influencing gut microbiome is diet; in fact, both short and mostly long-term diet changes can influence permanently influence gut microorganisms (Bibbò et al. 2016). For instance, an animal-based diet (high in meat and animal

DOI: 10.1201/b22970-12

fat), especially if associated with high sugar and low fiber intake, increases bile-tolerant microorganisms including *Bacteroides*, *Bilophila*, *Alistipes*, and *Ruminococcus*, decreasing those polysaccharides digesting species such as *Firmicutes* (Mukhopadhya et al. 2012; David et al. 2014). Children living in Burkina Faso have a prevalence of Bacteroidetes in their microbiome, while Italian children, with opposite dietary habit, have a majority of Enterobacteriaceae.

This finding suggests that carbohydrate and fiber intake is the key to richness in gut microbiota composition (Yatsunenko et al. 2012). Fibers divide into complex carbohydrates and oligosaccharides with different impacts on the gut. Complex carbohydrates usually contain a huge part of indigestible material that is eliminated through stools, called starch. These indigestible fibers can be divided into four subgroups, depending on the resistance features: type 1 is characterized by plant cell wall polymers, type 2 is characterized by a granular structure, type 3 is derived from retro gradiation by means of heating and coiling, and type 4 is represented by chemical cross-linking (Flint et al. n.d.). Particularly, resistant starch type 2 increases *Ruminococcus* spp. and *Eubacterium rectale*, whereas type 3 promotes *Roseburia* spp. and *Ruminococcus bromii* (Leitch et al. 2007). Type 4 starch increases *Parabacteroides distasonis* but reduces *Euacterium rectale* and *Ruminococcus bromii*. This last one also leads to a reduction of *Firmicutes* while increasing *Bacteroides* and Actinobacteria (Martínez et al. 2010). In addition, a diet high in soluble fibers is usually associated with an increase in butyrate producing bacteria such as *Clostridium leptum* and *Eubacterium rectale* and of other beneficial bacteria such as *Bifidobacterium longum*. Particularly, in vegetarian individuals, the most represented bacteria is *Prevotella* spp. (Dewulf et al. 2013). On the contrary, a low-fiber diet significantly decreases all of the aforementioned bacteria (Bibbò et al. 2016). Oligosaccharides, including fructooligosaccharides, galactooligosaccharides, and arabinoxylan-oligosaccharides, can influence microbiota composition. For instance, inulin and fructooligosaccharides increase *Bifidobacterium* spp. and *Lactobacillus* spp. and butyrate producing bacteria such as *Faecalibacterium prausnitzii* (Ramirez-Farias et al. 2009). On the other hand, galactooligosaccharides usually increases *Bifidobacteria* spp. (adolescentis and catenulatum) and *Faecalibacterium prausnitzii*, although its effect can be different in each subject (Ramirez-Farias et al. 2009; Davis et al. 2011).

Additionally, the role of fatty acids in gut microbiota modulation has been extensively studied: A high intake in monounsaturated fatty acids decreases *Bifidobacteria* spp. and slightly improves *Bacteroides* spp. (Simões et al. 2013). In addition to that a high-fat diet can lead to dysbiosis through reduction of *Roseburia* species (Neyrinck et al. 2011).

## MICROBIOTA INVESTIGATION TOOLS: PRESENT AND FUTURE

Analyzing gut microbiota ecosystem had become a major goal for scientists and researchers due to its pivotal role in human health.

Culture-dependent methods, such as plating and Gram-staining techniques, represent the first attempt to study the complexity of human gut microbial community. Unfortunately, this approach limited the range of detectable organisms to the aerobic ones. This bacterial genus accounts for approximately only 0.1% of the microbes inhabiting the average human intestine, whereas the majority of microbial species could never have been cultured, studied, or quantified in a laboratory. Great progress has been made by the advent of molecular biology, a DNA-based culture-independent method. By doing this, researchers received a key tool to investigate several aspects of microbial communities (e.g., taxonomic composition and functional metagenomics) and (theoretically) to deduce potential biological tasks carried out by a community as a whole.

Starting from the earliest DNA-based methods by using fluorescent in-situ hybridization (FISH), passing through polymerase chain reaction (PCR), we arrived to the revolutionary technology of high-throughput sequencing, known as next-generation sequencing (NGS). NGS exhibits substantial advances over the Sanger method in terms of ease and cost of sequencing, as complete bacterial genome sequences could be assayed and dissected in hours or days rather than months or years (Hiergeist et al. 2015).

With the development of these methods, two different approaches became available: the 16S gene analysis and metagenomics. 16S DNA sequencing needs the DNA extraction from the sample of choice and the use of a specific primer to allow the PCR to begin. It usually looks for a fundamental part of the set of prokaryotic functional genes; therefore, only bacteria can be detected. These hypervariable gene regions could define the genetic fingerprint of a single microorganism. In fact, such regions have been numbered from V1 to V9 and every one of them encodes specific primers. To notice, some authors pointed out that there is no hypervariable region that alone allows the diagnosis of all the bacterial genera examined, so it would be advisable to investigate different regions (Martellacci et al. 2019).

On the other hand, metagenomics is the study of genetic material recovered directly from environmental samples, such as fecal samples, in an untargeted (shotgun) way without the need to first cultivate these organisms or specific primers. It relies on a labor-intensive cloning process and on NGS technologies such as the 454/Roche, Illumina/Solexa, and Ion Torrent/Ion Proton platforms (Garza and Dutilh 2015).

In particular, Shotgun metagenomics, which "fragments" and then "reads" the entire DNA in the sample, is able to detect viruses, bacteria, and parasites.

Comparing these two methods is quite clear that metagenomics approach presents several advantages: (i) it needs less amount of PCR amplification than 16S DNA sequence analysis; (ii) it is able to quantify individual bacterial species in samples; and (iii) only with metagenomic approach is possible to identify genetic segments potentially associated with health or disease. However, it has to be considered that 16S DNA sequencing has lower costs and less computational requirements than metagenomics, and for these reasons, it is often preferred by researchers (Martellacci et al. 2019).

Overall, metagenomics revolutionized the understanding of the relations among the human microbiome, health, and diseases and supplanted the long and laborious culture-dependent methods of classic microbiology (Lagier et al. 2016). With metagenomic approaches, we can discover the identity, evolution, gene composition, distribution, and ecological patterns of uncultured microbes and viruses (Garza and Dutilh 2015). However, it generates a countless number of sequences that have not been assigned to a known microorganism, raising the awareness that a complementarity use of both culture-dependent and culture-independent methods was needed. Therefore, in 2012, a new strategy named "culturomics" was proposed for the study of the human gut microbiota.

## CULTUROMICS: A NEW APPROACH TO INVESTIGATE HUMAN GUT MICROBIOTA

Culturomics is a high-throughput culture method that utilizes culture conditions, matrix-assisted laser desorption ionization–time of flight mass spectrometry (MALDI–TOF MS) and 16S rRNA sequencing for the identification of a wider number of bacterial species. It allows the culture of organisms corresponding to sequences previously not assigned (Lagier et al. 2012).

The first step of culturomics method is to divide the sample into different culture conditions designed to suppress the culture of majority populations and to promote the growth of fastidious microorganisms at lower concentrations. This technique is the co-culture, which allows to culture bacteria from different environments at the same time. In fact, according to environmental microbiology, some bacterial species naturally grow in the same environment, as they provide each other growth promoting factors. An important feature of culturomics is the rapid (less than 1 hour) identification by MALDI–TOF mass spectrometry which relies on the comparison of the protein mass spectra of the isolate with an upgradable database. If identification fails, the isolate is subjected to 16S rRNA sequencing. If there is less than 98.65% similarity to the closest official strain, the isolate could be a new species. Then, the discovery of new taxa is confirmed by genome sequencing and taxonogenomics is used to formally describe the bacterium. Finally, all identification results are compared with a database that contains bacterial species recovered from humans (Lagier et al. 2018).

Through culturomics, we can identify much more bacterial species, isolated at least once in the human gut. Moreover, culturomics allows to cultivate even that species "noncultivable" with standard approach. In the first reported culturomics study by Lagier and his group, 212 different culture conditions generated more than 30,000 colonies. Among all the bacterial species isolated, 31 were new or belonged to rare phyla (Lagier et al. 2012). To date, thanks to culturomics, 73 additional species from the human gut, 13 new species from the urinary tract, 15 species from the vaginal tract, nine species from the respiratory tract, two species from human skin, one from human colostrum, and one from the foot of an individual with osteomyelitis have been isolated (Lagier et al. 2018).

Moreover, the culturomic method, despite the long analytical times, has a greater analytical depth allowing the detection of bacterial populations up to concentrations of $10^2$ cells per gram, while for metagenomics bacteria population, under $10^5$ cells per gram are undetectable (Dubourg et al. 2014). However, an important limitation of culturomics is that the result can only be qualitative, as this approach is based on the induction to the growth of the greatest number of bacterial species present on the sample. No quantitative information can be drawn. Nonetheless, this negative aspect can be avoided by combining culturomics with the real-time PCR that, unfortunately, causes an increase in costs (Martellacci et al. 2019).

In conclusion, to investigate microbial communities efficiently and completely (i.e., to detect all members including the least abundant), deep sampling and high-throughput DNA sequencing are the approaches of choice at present, probably in combination with other genome-wide analyses such as transcriptomics, proteomics, or metabolomics (Hiergeist et al. 2015). In fact, metaproteomics enables functional activity information to be gained from the microbiome samples, while metabolomics provides insight into the overall metabolic states affecting/representing the host–microbiome interactions. Combining these functional-omic platforms together with microbiome composition profiling allows for a holistic overview on the functional and metabolic state of the microbiome and its influence on human health (Peters et al. 2019).

## ROLE OF FUNCTIONAL FOOD IN MICROBIOTA MODULATION

The gut microbiota is a complex ecosystem continuously shaped by many factors, such as dietary habits, seasonality, lifestyle, stress, antibiotics use, or diseases. Changes in habitual or available diet have a significant impact on the structure-function activity of the gut microbiota, potentially impacting intestinal barrier functions and the immune system. In fact, there is the growing perception that diet may play a major role than host genetics in selective pressure on gut microbiota.

As diet has a major influence on microbiome dynamics, the study of how a specific nutrient affects the gut microbiota composition represents a powerful tool, known as nutritional ecology, even though it still needs to be fully understood (Murtaza, Ó Cuív, and Morrison 2017; Rinninella et al. 2019). Both current dietary habits, resulting from a specific mixture of micro- and macronutrients, and food appearing to exert positive effect on gut microbiome (functional foods) have been investigated.

In a review of Rinninella and colleagues, the effects of different types of modern diet on commensal bacterial species, mucus layer, and lamina propria hosting immune cells have been discussed.

What emerges is that Western diet rich in total fat, animal proteins, refined sugars, and additives may reduce gut microbial diversity in terms of phyla and genus leading to dysbiosis, alteration of barrier function and permeability, abnormal activation of immune cells, and a higher incidence of chronic diseases.

On the other hand, elimination diets such as low-FODMAP (fermentable oligo-, di-, monosaccharides, and polyols) diet and gluten-free diet (GFD) seem to improve the symptoms of some diseases like irritable bowel syndrome (IBS) and celiac disease (CD) in selected patients, but the long-term effects on gut microbiota require elucidations. FODMAPs are a large class of small nondigestible carbohydrates which are poorly absorbed in the small bowel. They can be found in a wide range of foods such as fruits, vegetables, legumes, cereals, honey, sweeteners, milk, and dairy products. Low-FODMAP diet strongly limits consumption of FODMAP foods that are potential triggers of abdominal symptoms in the IBS patient (Bellini et al. 2020). Unfortunately, such long-term limitation decreases the amount of potential prebiotics (fructooligosaccharides and galactooligosaccharides) leading to a reduction in beneficial bacteria, for example, *Bifidobacteria*, and fermentative effects that may require an integration with probiotics to counteract gut microbiota imbalances (Rinninella et al. 2019). Gluten-free diet is characterized by the complete elimination of gluten. It was recognized as a potential cure, restoring the normal intestinal mucosa in coeliac patients. However, it has been demonstrated that long-term GFD leads to a decrease of healthy bacteria such as *Bifidobacterium* and *Lactobacillus*, to a diminution of SCFAs production and their beneficial meta-bolic and host immunity effects, and to an increase of detrimental species such as *Enterococcus*, *Staphylococcus*, *Salmonella*, *Shigella*, and *Klebsiella*.

To date, the Mediterranean diet (MD) seems to remain the evergreen solution to optimally modulating microbiota diversity and stability as well as the regular perme-ability and activity of immune functions of the human host (Rinninella et al. 2019). The MD is based on the consumption of monounsaturated and polyunsaturated fatty acids (MUFAs and PUFAs), polyphenols, and other antioxidants, a high intake of prebiotic fiber and low-glycemic carbohydrates, and greater consumption of plant proteins than animal proteins. It seems that this combination of nutrients linked to many health benefits and to an increase of healthy bacteria and SCFAs, thus improv-ing the diversity and richness of gut microbiota.

"Functional food" is a new term that indicates a food that is known to beneficially affect one or more target functions in the body in addition to adequate nutritional effects in a way to either the state of well-being and health or to a reduction in disease incidence (Jones 2010).

To this extent, fermented foods (yogurt, kombucha, sauerkraut, tempeh, natto, miso, kimchi, and sourdough bread) need a special mention due to the putative impact they have.

They are defined as foods or beverages produced through controlled microbial growth, contain potentially probiotic microorganisms, fermentation-derived metabo-lites, prebiotics, and vitamins that may exert health benefit. For instance, lactic acid bacteria (both dairy and nondairy fermented foods) generate bioactive peptides and polyamines potentially influencing cardiovascular, immune, and metabolic health. Moreover, fermentation can reduce toxins and antinutrients such as the reduction of phytic acid concentrations and content of fermentable carbohydrates (e.g., ferment-able oligosaccharides, disaccharides, monosaccharides and polyols, FODMAPs), which may increase the tolerance in patients with functional disorders such as irri-table bowel syndrome.

The most widely investigated fermented food is kefir, with evidence from at least one randomized controlled trial, suggesting beneficial effects in both lac-tose malabsorption and *Helicobacter pylori* eradication (Bekar, Yilmaz, and Gulten 2011). Kefir is a fermented milk drink with a creamy texture, sour taste, and subtle effervescence. It is produced by adding a starter culture named "kefir grains" to milk. These grains contain symbiotic lactose-fermenting yeasts (e.g., *Kluyveromyces marxianus*), nonlactose fermenting yeasts (e.g., *Saccharomyces cerevisiae*, *Saccharomyces unisporus*), and lactic and acetic acid producing bac-teria, housed within a polysaccharide and protein matrix called kefiran. Kefir's antimicrobial activity has been investigated through several in vitro studies. Its antimicrobial activity is attributed to competition with pathogens for available nutrients, as well as the production of organic acids, bacteriocins, carbon dioxide, hydrogen peroxide, ethanol, and diacetyl (Leite et al. 2013). These studies have also shown that kefir exhibits antimicrobial activity against *Candida albicans*,

*Salmonella typhi, Salmonella enterica, Shigella sonnei, Escherichia coli, Bacillus subtilis, Enterococcus faecalis,* and *Staphylococcus aureus* (Chifiriuc, Cioaca, and Lazar 2011). Fermentation-derived bioactive peptides produced from casein have been shown to stimulate the immune system in animal models. It has also been suggested a potential anti-oxidative, anti-hypertensive, anti-carcinogenic, cholesterol, and glucose-lowering effects of kefir (Kwon et al. 2008; Liu, Chen, and Lin 2005; Khoury et al. 2014; Liu et al. 2006). Kefir and its constituent strains seem to have a considerable impact on gut microbiota composition, increasing *Lactobacillus, Lactococcus,* and *Bifidobacterium* and reducing in *Proteobacteria* and *Enterobacteriaceae* concentrations, being demonstrated in numerous animal studies (Dimidi et al. 2019).

Overall, the use of combinations of pre- and probiotics has the potential to induce more substantial effects on the gut microbiota and host health than isolated intake of one of them, as the prebiotic component stimulates probiotic bacteria survival and growth in the gastrointestinal tract. However, scientists are moving toward examining the capacity of dietary patterns and personalized nutrition to modulate the intestinal microbiota in pathological conditions. Their main struggle is to find a balance between the effects of specific foods, nutrients, bioactive compounds, and macronutrients since first ones are isolated nutrients rarely consumed, and Western diet, the most common dietary pattern, is high in fat and simple carbohydrates while low in important fibers.

A recent study in patients with type 2 diabetes demonstrates that a dietary intervention with functional foods significantly modifies gut microbiota by increasing alpha diversity and modifying the abundance of specific bacteria, independently of antidiabetic drugs. In this study, patients had an increase in two anti-inflammatory bacterial species (*Faecalibacterium prausnitzii* and *Akkermansia muciniphila*) together with a decrease in *P. copri*. Long-term adherence to a high-fiber polyphenol-enriched and vegetable-protein-based diet provides benefits for the composition of gut microbiota and may offer potential therapies for improvement of glycemic control, dyslipidemia, and inflammation. After 2.5 months of dietary intervention, patients with type 2 diabetes also exhibit significant reductions in areas under the curve for glucose, total and LDL cholesterol, FFAs, HbA1c, triglycerides, and C-reactive protein.

In conclusion, the observation that diet can modulate host–microbe interactions is an indicator that future therapeutic approaches can be developed to modify the gut microbiota and reduce the dysbiosis induced by diseases related with the nutrition (Sánchez-Tapia, Tovar, and Torres 2019).

## THE JOURNEY OF MICROBIOME THROUGH HUMAN EVOLUTION

Humans can be considered as ecosystems containing millions of microorganisms. Our current gut microbiome derives from years of microorganisms selection due to dietary, environmental, lifestyle cultural, and historical changes. How the composition of the microbiome has changed since humans diverged from other species, since human populations diverged from one another, is a key point in the comprehension of gut microbiome, but it is still difficult to investigate.

As previously discussed, gut microbiome plays a pivotal role in human body homeostasis, influencing key functions such as digestion, mood and behavior, development, immunity, and the susceptibility of a vast range of acute and chronic diseases (Marchesi and Ravel 2015). With the initiation of the Human Microbiome Project in 2007, as a direct consequence of the improvement of DNA sequencing, it has become increasingly clear that the study of human evolution could exclude the study of human gut microbiome (Peterson et al. 2009).

Gut microbiome and its co-resident microbes contain a huge quantity of different additional genes, functioning as a target for natural selection (Schnorr et al. 2016).

So, the study of gut microorganisms in human populations, non-human primates, and past human populations is a key point in understanding human evolution, even though this is a novel field still lacking strong evidences. In fact, up to date, the only archaeological materials containing stable components allowing ancient microbiome sequencing are coprolites (paleofeces) from mummified human rests and dental calculus (Zeng et al. 2015). The majority of these materials come from samples originated in Europe and Americas.

Interestingly, environmental and lifestyle changes that have occurred throughout human history and prehistory had a huge impact on microbiome composition and physiology.

In fact, unlike the nuclear and mitochondrial genomes of the host, the microbiome continuously responds to external and internal changes and signaling (Dewulf et al. 2013).

Particularly, gut microbiome can change through both vertical (parental transmission) and horizontal transmission (more typical of microorganisms, information derive from the environment) (Davenport et al. 2017).

Moeller et al. investigated the changes in the passage from apes microbiome to human microbiome and found out that among apes, *Prevotella* was negatively correlated with *Bacterioides*, but *Bacterioides* were positively correlated with *Ruminococcus* and *Parabacteroides*. Most of these changes in the composition of the human microbiome have functional implications for host nutrition. For instance, the abundance of *Bacteroides*, which has been positively associated with diets rich in animal fat and protein, has increased in humans. On the other hand, the archaeon *Methanobrevibacter*, which promotes the degradation of complex plant polysaccharides, has reduced within humans, as well as *Fibrobacter* (Moeller et al. 2014; Kobayashi, Shinkai, and Koike 2008).

Interestingly, among primates, Old World monkeys and apes have the most similar microbiome to actual human microbiome, rather than New World primates and lemurs. In fact, captive primates consume less diverse, lower-fiber diets compared to their wild counterparts mirroring the gradual transition to low-fiber diets of human evolution and the contrast of modern Western and non-Western diets (Davenport et al. 2017).

Basing on biogeographic analyses, it is clear that there are some specific microbial taxa depending host genotypes and environment. This is evident in a higher presence of *Prevotella*, *Catenibacterium*, *Succinivibrio*, and *Treponema* among both contemporary and ancient populations following the same lifestyle such as hunting and gathering or agriculture (Gomez et al. 2016; Yatsunenko et al. 2012; Raul Y. Tito et al. 2012; Raúl Y. Tito et al. 2008).

Recently, some samples recovered from Mexico provided DNA from numerous human gut microbial symbionts (Tito et al. 2008, 2012), with taxonomic profile similar to those observed in contemporary rural and traditional human communities (Yatsunenko et al. 2012; Obregon-Tito et al. 2015).

A further example of how environmental and dietary factors influence human microbiome is the huge difference between nowadays US humans and apes. In fact, this difference is more evident than what we would expect basing on the evolutionary time from African apes to hominid and to actual human being (Moeller et al. 2014). On average, there has been a reduction of ancestral diversity in the passage from apes microbiome to human microbiome; this finding is more evident among US population. A possible explanation could be due to the recent lifestyle changes that possibly have depleted the human microbiome of microbial diversity that was present in our wild-living ancestors (Blaser and Falkow 2009). Alongside with this hypothesis, we know that diet has a strong impact on gut microbiome. In fact, some authors sequenced oral microbiota from skeleton teeth deriving from different eras human beings and found out that the most significant changes had occurred during the passage from the hunter-gatherer Paleolithic era to the farming Neolithic era and the beginning of the industrialized period. In the first passage, the human diet shifted from meat based to fiber and carbohydrates based, while in the second one, diet shifted to a more processed sugar and flour (Bibbò et al. 2016; Chan, Estaki, and Gibson 2013; Adler et al. 2013). Last but not least, the most recent change in human gut microbiome was at the beginning of antibiotic revolution due to the well-known influence of antibiotics on gut microbiome (Ianiro, Tilg, and Gasbarrini 2016).

Not only host genes influence gut microbiome composition (together with diet and energy substance available), but also gut microbiome can influence some gene selection. For instance, human genetic variants that facilitate lactose tolerance and dairying in adulthood (that differentiate human being from the other mammalian and modern human being from ancient human being) were probably microbiome influenced. As we know, lactase production is intensive during childhood and progressively decreases during life and a continued milk consumption in the lack of this enzyme leads to an extensive microbial fermentation of lactose in colon. This mechanism produces some metabolites that can induce lactose intolerance symptoms, but at the same time facilitate the development of adaptive alleles allowing the persistence of lactase expression (Schnorr et al. 2016; He et al. 2008).

Another example of this interaction is the presence of gluten degrading microorganisms in oral (*Rothia mucilaginosa, Rothia aeria, Actinomyces odontolyticus, Streptococcus mitis, Streptococcus* sp., *Neisseria mucosa,* and *Capnocytophaga sputigena)* and gut (*Firmicutes* and *Actinobacteria,* mainly from the genera *Lactobacillus, Streptococcus, Staphylococcus, Clostridium,* and *Bifidobacterium)* microbiome of human species after the advent of agriculture (Fernandez-Feo et al. 2013; Caminero et al. 2014).

Moreover, as gut microbes produce more than 90% of the body's serotonin (Yano et al. 2015) and modulate synthesis of metabolites affecting gene expression for myelin production in the prefrontal cortex, host–microbe interactions have likely influenced human brain development (Stilling et al. 2014). Particularly, human behavior such as stress, anxiety, and novelty seeking is additionally reinforced by microbial production of neuroactive compounds (Schnorr et al. 2016).

So, the evolution of gut microbiome basically was dictated by the environmental changes (especially food related) that occurred during human evolution. The most important difference between present microbiome composition and apes is the decreased variability mainly due to fast lifestyle changes. In addition to that, nowadays, composition of microbiome is much more different between different individuals, depending on where they live and how they eat (Moeller et al. 2014; Bibbò et al. 2016; Ianiro, Tilg, and Gasbarrini 2016).

## REFERENCES

Adler, Christina J., Keith Dobney, Laura S. Weyrich, John Kaidonis, Alan W. Walker, Wolfgang Haak, Corey J.A. Bradshaw, et al. 2013. "Sequencing Ancient Calcified Dental Plaque Shows Changes in Oral Microbiota with Dietary Shifts of the Neolithic and Industrial Revolutions." *Nature Genetics* 45 (4): 450–55. https://doi.org/10.1038/ng.2536.

Bekar, Onder, Yusuf Yilmaz, and MacIt Gulten. 2011. "Kefir Improves the Efficacy and Tolerability of Triple Therapy in Eradicating Helicobacter Pylori." *Journal of Medicinal Food* 14 (4): 344–47. https://doi.org/10.1089/jmf.2010.0099.

Bellini, Massimo, Sara Tonarelli, Attila G. Nagy, Andrea Pancetti, Francesco Costa, Angelo Ricchiuti, Nicola de Bortoli, Marta Mosca, Santino Marchi, and Alessandra Rossi. 2020. "Low FODMAP Diet: Evidence, Doubts, and Hopes." *Nutrients*. MDPI AG. https://doi.org/10.3390/nu12010148.

Bibbò, S., G. Ianiro, V. Giorgio, F. Scaldaferri, L. Masucci, A. Gasbarrini, and G. Cammarota. 2016. "The Role of Diet on Gut Microbiota Composition." *European Review for Medical and Pharmacological Sciences* 20 (22): 4742–49.

Blaser, Martin J., and Stanley Falkow. 2009. "What Are the Consequences of the Disappearing Human Microbiota?" *Nature Reviews Microbiology* 7 (12): 887–94. https://doi.org/10.1038/nrmicro2245.

Caminero, Alberto, Alexandra R. Herrán, Esther Nistal, Jenifer Pérez-Andrés, Luis Vaquero, Santiago Vivas, José María G. Ruiz de Morales, Silvia M. Albillos, and Javier Casqueiro. 2014. "Diversity of the Cultivable Human Gut Microbiome Involved in Gluten Metabolism: Isolation of Microorganisms with Potential Interest for Coeliac Disease." *FEMS Microbiology Ecology* 88 (2): 309–19. https://doi.org/10.1111/1574-6941.12295.

Chan, Yee Kwan, Mehrbod Estaki, and Deanna L. Gibson. 2013. "Clinical Consequences of Diet-Induced Dysbiosis." *Annals of Nutrition & Metabolism* 63 (Suppl 2): 28–40. https://doi.org/10.1159/000354902.

Chifiriuc, Mariana Carmen, Alina Badea Cioaca, and Veronica Lazar. 2011. "In Vitro Assay of the Antimicrobial Activity of Kephir against Bacterial and Fungal Strains." *Anaerobe* 17 (6): 433–35. https://doi.org/10.1016/j.anaerobe.2011.04.020.

Davenport, Emily R., Jon G. Sanders, Se Jin Song, Katherine R. Amato, Andrew G. Clark, and Rob Knight. 2017. "The Human Microbiome in Evolution." *BMC Biology*. BioMed Central Ltd. https://doi.org/10.1186/s12915-017-0454-7.

David, Lawrence A., Corinne F. Maurice, Rachel N. Carmody, David B. Gootenberg, Julie E. Button, Benjamin E. Wolfe, Alisha V. Ling, et al. 2014. "Diet Rapidly and Reproducibly Alters the Human Gut Microbiome." *Nature* 505 (7484): 559–63. https://doi.org/10.1038/nature12820.

Davis, Lauren M.G., Inés Martínez, Jens Walter, Caitlin Goin, and Robert W. Hutkins. 2011. "Barcoded Pyrosequencing Reveals That Consumption of Galactooligosaccharides Results in a Highly Specific Bifidogenic Response in Humans." *PLoS One* 6 (9). https://doi.org/10.1371/journal.pone.0025200.

Dewulf, Evelyne M., Patrice D. Cani, Sandrine P. Claus, Susana Fuentes, Philippe G.B. Puylaert, Audrey M. Neyrinck, Laure B. Bindels, et al. 2013. "Insight into the Prebiotic Concept: Lessons from an Exploratory, Double Blind Intervention Study with Inulin-Type Fructans in Obese Women." *Gut* 62 (8): 1112–21. https://doi.org/10.1136/gutjnl-2012-303304.

Dimidi, Eirini, Selina Rose Cox, Megan Rossi, and Kevin Whelan. 2019. "Fermented Foods: Definitions and Characteristics, Impact on the Gut Microbiota and Effects on Gastrointestinal Health and Disease." *Nutrients*. MDPI AG. https://doi.org/10.3390/nu11081806.

Dubourg, Grégory, Jean Christophe Lagier, Catherine Robert, Fabrice Armougom, Perrine Hugon, Sarah Metidji, Niokhor Dione, et al. 2014. "Culturomics and Pyrosequencing Evidence of the Reduction in Gut Microbiota Diversity in Patients with Broad-Spectrum Antibiotics." *International Journal of Antimicrobial Agents* 44 (2): 117–24. https://doi.org/10.1016/j.ijantimicag.2014.04.020.

Fernandez-Feo, M., G. Wei, G. Blumenkranz, F.E. Dewhirst, D. Schuppan, F.G. Oppenheim, and E.J. Helmerhorst. 2013. "The Cultivable Human Oral Gluten-Degrading Microbiome and Its Potential Implications in Coeliac Disease and Gluten Sensitivity." *Clinical Microbiology and Infection* 19 (9). https://doi.org/10.1111/1469-0691.12249.

Flint, Harry J., Karen P. Scott, Sylvia H. Duncan, Petra Louis, and Evelyne Forano. n.d. "Microbial Degradation of Complex Carbohydrates in the Gut." *Gut Microbes* 3 (4): 289–306. Accessed January 24, 2020. https://doi.org/10.4161/gmic.19897.

Fouhy, Fiona, Caitriona M. Guinane, Seamus Hussey, Rebecca Wall, C. Anthony Ryan, Eugene M. Dempsey, Brendan Murphy, et al. 2012. "High-Throughput Sequencing Reveals the Incomplete, Short-Term Recovery of Infant Gut Microbiota Following Parenteral Antibiotic Treatment with Ampicillin and Gentamicin." *Antimicrobial Agents and Chemotherapy* 56 (11): 5811–20. https://doi.org/10.1128/AAC.00789-12.

Garza, Daniel R., and Bas E. Dutilh. 2015. "From Cultured to Uncultured Genome Sequences: Metagenomics and Modeling Microbial Ecosystems." *Cellular and Molecular Life Sciences* 72 (22): 4287–308. https://doi.org/10.1007/s00018-015-2004-1.

Gomez, Andres, Klara J. Petrzelkova, Michael B. Burns, Carl J. Yeoman, Katherine R. Amato, Klara Vlckova, David Modry, et al. 2016. "Gut Microbiome of Coexisting BaAka Pygmies and Bantu Reflects Gradients of Traditional Subsistence Patterns." *Cell Reports* 14 (9): 2142–53. https://doi.org/10.1016/j.celrep.2016.02.013.

He, T., K. Venema, M. G. Priebe, G. W. Welling, R. J.M. Brummer, and R. J. Vonk. 2008. "The Role of Colonic Metabolism in Lactose Intolerance." *European Journal of Clinical Investigation. European Journal of Clinical Investigation*. https://doi.org/10.1111/j.1365-2362.2008.01966.x.

Hiergeist, Andreas, Joachim Gläsner, Udo Reischl, and André Gessner. 2015. "Analyses of Intestinal Microbiota: Culture versus Sequencing." *ILAR Journal* 56 (2): 228–40. https://doi.org/10.1093/ilar/ilv017.

Ianiro, Gianluca, Herbert Tilg, and Antonio Gasbarrini. 2016. "Antibiotics as Deep Modulators of Gut Microbiota: Between Good and Evil." *Gut* 65 (11): 1906–15. https://doi.org/10.1136/gutjnl-2016-312297.

Jakobsson, Hedvig E., Cecilia Jernberg, Anders F. Andersson, Maria Sjölund-Karlsson, Janet K. Jansson, and Lars Engstrand. 2010. "Short-Term Antibiotic Treatment Has Differing Long-Term Impacts on the Human Throat and Gut Microbiome." *PLoS One* 5 (3): e9836. https://doi.org/10.1371/journal.pone.0009836.

Jernberg, Cecilia, Sonja Löfmark, Charlotta Edlund, and Janet K. Jansson. 2010. "Long-Term Impacts of Antibiotic Exposure on the Human Intestinal Microbiota." *Microbiology* 156: 3216–3223. https://doi.org/10.1099/mic.0.040618-0.

Khoury, Nathalie, Stephany El-Hayek, Omayr Tarras, Marwan El-Sabban, Mirvat El-Sibai, and Sandra Rizk. 2014. "Kefir Exhibits Anti-Proliferative and pro-Apoptotic Effects on Colon Adenocarcinoma Cells with No Significant Effects on Cell Migration and Invasion." *International Journal of Oncology* 45 (5): 2117–27. https://doi.org/10.3892/ijo.2014.2635.

Kobayashi, Y., T. Shinkai, and S. Koike. 2008. "Ecological and Physiological Characterization Shows That Fibrobacter Succinogenes Is Important in Rumen Fiber Digestion - Review." *Folia Microbiologica* 53 (3): 195–200. https://doi.org/10.1007/s12223-008-0024z.

Kwon, Ok Kyoung, Kyung Seop Ahn, Mee Young Lee, So Young Kim, Bo Young Park, Mi Kyoung Kim, In Young Lee, Sei Ryang Oh, and Hyeong Kyu Lee. 2008. "Inhibitory Effect of Kefiran on Ovalbumin-Induced Lung Inflammation in a Murine Model of Asthma." *Archives of Pharmacal Research* 31 (12): 1590–96. https://doi.org/10.1007/s12272-001-2156-4.

Lagier, Jean-Christophe, F. Armougom, M. Million, P. Hugon, I. Pagnier, C. Robert, F. Bittar, G. Fournous, G. Gimenez, M. Maraninchi, J.-F. Trape, E. V. Koonin, B. la Scola, D. Raoult. 2012. "Microbial Culturomics: Paradigm Shift in the Human Gut Microbiome Study." *Clinical Microbiology and Infection : The Official Publication of the European Society of Clinical Microbiology and Infectious Diseases* 18 (12): 1185–93. https://doi.org/10.1111/1469-0691.12023.

Lagier, Jean Christophe, Grégory Dubourg, Matthieu Million, Frédéric Cadoret, Melhem Bilen, Florence Fenollar, Anthony Levasseur, Jean Marc Rolain, Pierre Edouard Fournier, and Didier Raoult. 2018. "Culturing the Human Microbiota and Culturomics." *Nature Reviews Microbiology*. Nature Publishing Group. https://doi.org/10.1038/s41579-018-0041-0.

Lagier, Jean-Christophe, Saber Khelaifia, Maryam Tidjani Alou, Sokhna Ndongo, Niokhor Dione, Perrine Hugon, Aurelia Caputo, et al. 2016. "Culture of Previously Uncultured Members of the Human Gut Microbiota by Culturomics." *Nature Microbiology* 1 (November): 16203. https://doi.org/10.1038/nmicrobiol.2016.203.

Leitch, E. Carol McWilliam, Alan W. Walker, Sylvia H. Duncan, Grietje Holtrop, and Harry J. Flint. 2007. "Selective Colonization of Insoluble Substrates by Human Faecal Bacteria." *Environmental Microbiology* 9 (3): 667–79. https://doi.org/10.1111/j.1462-2920.2006.01186.x.

Leite, Analy Machado de Oliveira, Marco Antônio Lemos Miguel, Raquel Silva Peixoto, Alexandre Soares Rosado, Joab Trajano Silva, and Vania Margaret Flosi Paschoalin. 2013. "Microbiological, Technological and Therapeutic Properties of Kefir: A Natural Probiotic Beverage." *Brazilian Journal of Microbiology*. Sociedade Brasileira de Microbiologia. https://doi.org/10.1590/S1517-83822013000200001.

Liu, Je-Ruei, Ming Ju Chen, and Chin Wen Lin. 2005. "Antimutagenic and Antioxidant Properties of Milk-Kefir and Soymilk-Kefir." *Journal of Agricultural and Food Chemistry* 53 (7): 2467–74. https://doi.org/10.1021/jf048934k.

Liu, Je-Ruei, Sheng-Yao Wang, Ming-Ju Chen, Hsiao-Ling Chen, Pei-Ying Yueh, and Chin-Wen Lin. 2006. "Hypocholesterolaemic Effects of Milk-Kefir and Soymilk-Kefir in Cholesterol-Fed Hamsters." *British Journal of Nutrition* 95 (5): 939–46. https://doi.org/10.1079/bjn20061752.

Marchesi, Julian R., and Jacques Ravel. 2015. "The Vocabulary of Microbiome Research: A Proposal." *Microbiome* 3 (1). https://doi.org/10.1186/s40168-015-0094-5.

Martellacci, Leonardo, Gianluca Quaranta, Romeo Patini, Gaetano Isola, Patrizia Gallenzi, and Luca Masucci. 2019. "A Literature Review of Metagenomics and Culturomics of the Peri-Implant Microbiome: Current Evidence and Future Perspectives." *Materials (Basel, Switzerland)* 12 (18). https://doi.org/10.3390/ma12183010.

Martínez, Inés, Jaehyoung Kim, Patrick R. Duffy, Vicki L. Schlegel, and Jens Walter. 2010. "Resistant Starches Types 2 and 4 Have Differential Effects on the Composition of the Fecal Microbiota in Human Subjects." *PLoS One* 5 (11). https://doi.org/10.1371/journal. pone.0015046.

Moeller, Andrew H., Yingying Li, Eitel Mpoudi Ngole, Steve Ahuka-Mundeke, Elizabeth V. Lonsdorf, Anne E. Pusey, Martine Peeters, Beatrice H. Hahn, and Howard Ochman. 2014. "Rapid Changes in the Gut Microbiome during Human Evolution." *Proceedings of the National Academy of Sciences of the United States of America* 111 (46): 16431–35. https://doi.org/10.1073/pnas.1419136111.

Mukhopadhya, Indrani, Richard Hansen, Emad M. El-Omar, and Georgina L. Hold. 2012. "IBD-What Role Do Proteobacteria Play?" *Nature Reviews. Gastroenterology & Hepatology* 9 (4): 219–30. https://doi.org/10.1038/nrgastro.2012.14.

Murtaza, Nida, Páraic Ó. Cuív, and Mark Morrison. 2017. "Diet and the Microbiome." *Gastroenterology Clinics of North America* 46 (1): 49–60. https://doi.org/10.1016/j. gtc.2016.09.005.

Neyrinck, Audrey M., Sam Possemiers, Céline Druart, Tom Van de Wiele, Fabienne De Backer, Patrice D. Cani, Yvan Larondelle, and Nathalie M. Delzenne. 2011. "Prebiotic Effects of Wheat Arabinoxylan Related to the Increase in Bifidobacteria, Roseburia and Bacteroides/Prevotella in Diet-Induced Obese Mice." *PLoS One* 6 (6): e20944. https:// doi.org/10.1371/journal.pone.0020944.

Obregon-Tito, Alexandra J., Raul Y. Tito, Jessica Metcalf, Krithivasan Sankaranarayanan, Jose C. Clemente, Luke K. Ursell, Zhenjiang Zech Xu, et al. 2015. "Subsistence Strategies in Traditional Societies Distinguish Gut Microbiomes." *Nature Communications* 6. https://doi.org/10.1038/ncomms7505.

Peters, Danielle L., Wenju Wang, Xu Zhang, Zhibin Ning, Janice Mayne, and Daniel Figeys. 2019. "Metaproteomic and Metabolomic Approaches for Characterizing the Gut Microbiome." *Proteomics* 19 (16): e1800363. https://doi.org/10.1002/pmic.201800363.

Peterson, Jane, Susan Garges, Maria Giovanni, Pamela McInnes, Lu Wang, Jeffery A. Schloss, Vivien Bonazzi, et al. 2009. "The NIH Human Microbiome Project." *Genome Research* 19 (12): 2317–23. https://doi.org/10.1101/gr.096651.109.

Ramirez-Farias, Carlett, Kathleen Slezak, Zoë Fuller, Alan Duncan, Grietje Holtrop, and Petra Louis. 2009. "Effect of Inulin on the Human Gut Microbiota: Stimulation of Bifidobacterium Adolescentis and Faecalibacterium Prausnitzii." *The British Journal of Nutrition* 101 (4): 541–50. https://doi.org/10.1017/S0007114508019880.

Rinninella, Emanuele, Marco Cintoni, Pauline Raoul, Loris Riccardo Lopetuso, Franco Scaldaferri, Gabriele Pulcini, Giacinto Abele Donato Miggiano, Antonio Gasbarrini, and Maria Cristina Mele. 2019. "Food Components and Dietary Habits: Keys for a Healthy Gut Microbiota Composition." *Nutrients.* MDPI AG. https://doi.org/10.3390/nu11102393.

Sánchez-Tapia, Mónica, Armando R. Tovar, and Nimbe Torres. 2019. "Diet as Regulator of Gut Microbiota and Its Role in Health and Disease." *Archives of Medical Research* 50 (5): 259–68. https://doi.org/10.1016/j.arcmed.2019.09.004.

Schnorr, Stephanie L., Krithivasan Sankaranarayanan, Cecil M. Lewis, and Christina Warinner. 2016. "Insights into Human Evolution from Ancient and Contemporary Microbiome Studies." *Current Opinion in Genetics and Development.* Elsevier Ltd. https://doi.org/10.1016/j.gde.2016.07.003.

Simões, Catarina D., Johanna Maukonen, Jaakko Kaprio, Aila Rissanen, Kirsi H. Pietiläinen, and Maria Saarela. 2013. "Habitual Dietary Intake Is Associated with Stool Microbiota Composition in Monozygotic Twins." *The Journal of Nutrition* 143 (4): 417–23. https:// doi.org/10.3945/jn.112.166322.

Slimings, Claudia, and Thomas V. Riley. 2014. "Antibiotics and Hospital-Acquired Clostridium Difficile Infection: Update of Systematic Review and Meta-Analysis." *The Journal of Antimicrobial Chemotherapy* 69 (4): 881–91. https://doi.org/10.1093/jac/dkt477.

Stilling, Roman M., Seth R. Bordenstein, Timothy G. Dinan, and John F. Cryan. 2014. "Friends with Social Benefits: Host-Microbe Interactions as a Driver of Brain Evolution and Development?" *Frontiers in Cellular and Infection Microbiology* 4 (Oct). https://doi.org/10.3389/fcimb.2014.00147.

Tito, Raúl Y., Dan Knights, Jessica Metcalf, Alexandra J. Obregon-Tito, Lauren Cleeland, Fares Najar, Bruce Roe, et al. 2012. "Insights from Characterizing Extinct Human Gut Microbiomes." *PLoS One* 7 (12). https://doi.org/10.1371/journal.pone.0051146.

Tito, Raúl Y., Simone Macmil, Graham Wiley, Fares Najar, Lauren Cleeland, Chunmei Qu, Ping Wang, et al. 2008. "Phylotyping and Functional Analysis of Two Ancient Human Microbiomes." *PLoS One* 3 (11): e3703–e3703. https://doi.org/10.1371/journal.pone.0003703.

Vasquez, Alex, Sidney MacDonald Baker, Peter Bennett, Jeffrey S. Bland, Leo Galland, Robert J. Hedaya, Mark Houston, Mark Hyman, Jay Lombard, and Robert Rountree. 2010. *Textbook of Functional Medicine.* Example Product Manufacturer.

Yano, Jessica M., Kristie Yu, Gregory P. Donaldson, Gauri G. Shastri, Phoebe Ann, Liang Ma, Cathryn R. Nagler, Rustem F. Ismagilov, Sarkis K. Mazmanian, and Elaine Y. Hsiao. 2015. "Indigenous Bacteria from the Gut Microbiota Regulate Host Serotonin Biosynthesis." *Cell* 161 (2): 264–76. https://doi.org/10.1016/j.cell.2015.02.047.

Yatsunenko, Tanya, Federico E. Rey, Mark J. Manary, Indi Trehan, Maria Gloria Dominguez-Bello, Monica Contreras, Magda Magris, et al. 2012. "Human Gut Microbiome Viewed across Age and Geography." *Nature.* https://doi.org/10.1038/nature11053.

Zeng, Qinglong, Jeet Sukumaran, Steven Wu, and Allen Rodrigo. 2015. "Neutral Models of Microbiome Evolution." *PLoS Computational Biology* 11 (7). https://doi.org/10.1371/journal.pcbi.1004365.

Zhang, Lu, Ying Huang, Yang Zhou, Timothy Buckley, and Hua H. Wang. 2013. "Antibiotic Administration Routes Significantly Influence the Levels of Antibiotic Resistance in Gut Microbiota." *Antimicrobial Agents and Chemotherapy* 57 (8): 3659–66. https://doi.org/10.1128/AAC.00670-13.

# Index

Note: Bold page numbers refer to tables; italic page numbers refer to figures.